Michael T Winstanley SDB

GW00601690

Walking with Luke

Thematic Studies in the Lukan Narrative With Reflections

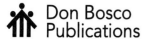
Don Bosco
Publications

Don Bosco Publications
Thornleigh House, Sharples Park, Bolton BL1 6PQ
United Kingdom

ISBN 978-1-909080-35-5
©Don Bosco Publications, 2017
©Michael T Winstanley SDB, 2017

Front cover photograph by Michael T Winstanley SDB

Printed in Great Britain by Jump Design and Print

For the many friends who over the years
have encouraged, supported and loved me,
and whose lives as disciples of Jesus
have been an inspiration.

Foreword

Even a first reading of the Gospel of Luke indicates that its author generated unique images in an attempt to catch the reader's imagination. This impression is strengthened by more careful readings, especially in light of Luke's synoptic roommates: the Gospels of Mark and Matthew. For example, only Luke portrays the image of Mary, the Mother of Jesus, in the fashion that we have come to uncritically accept as the way it was. Our Christmas pageantry and our Joyful Mysteries of the Rosary tell of the Annunciation, the Visitation and Birth of our Lord, the Presentation and the Finding of the Child Jesus in the Temple. If we were to develop Mysteries of the Rosary on the infancy of Jesus from the Gospel of Matthew, we would hardly have the Mysteries of Light: a genealogy; the suspicion of an illegitimate birth; Herod the Great's slaying of the innocent children in Bethlehem; the flight into Egypt; the return from Egypt to Israel leading to a further flight to Nazareth because of another wicked king, Archelaus. Powerful images are found in both birth stories, but the Lukan version is the one that has captured popular imagination.

Then there are the many other imaginative narratives and parables that one finds only in Luke: the restoration of the only son to a widow at Nain (Luke 7:11–17); John the Baptist, still wondering if Jesus is the one who is to come (7:18–23); the shock generated by Jesus' attention to, and forgiveness of, a sinful woman who enters the house of a Pharisee to perform an erotic ritual (7:36–50); the scandal of the women who journey with this itinerant preacher (8:1–3); the Good Samaritan (10:25–37); Martha and Mary (10:38–42); the parable of the great banquet (14:15–25); the parable of the lost sheep (15:3–7); the parable of the lost coin (15:8–10); the parable of the father with two lost sons (15:11–32); the parable of the cunning steward (16:1–9); the rich man and Lazarus (16:19–31); the one cured leper, a Samaritan, who returns to thank Jesus (17:11–19); the parable of the Pharisee and the tax collector (18:9–14); Jesus and Zachaeus (19:1–10); and Jesus' weeping over Jerusalem (19:41–44). These evocative Gospel stories, at the top of the list among the images that have been captured by Christian iconography over the centuries, are found only in Luke.

There is more. The Gospel of Luke tells the story of the Passion of Jesus, but it has been transformed. Jesus' final words of despair, as they are found in Matthew and Luke ("My God, my God, why have you forsaken me?" [Mark 15:34; Matt 27:46]), become: "Father, forgive them; for they do not know what they are doing" (23:34); "Truly, I tell you, today you will be with me in Paradise" (23:43); "Father, into your hands I commend my spirit" (23:46). The Roman centurion does not say: "Truly this man was the Son of God." (Mark 15:39; Matt 27:54), but he praises God, exclaiming, "Certainly this man was innocent" (Luke 23:47). Finally, Luke has his own way of telling of the resurrection, featuring the story of the journey to Emmaus (24:13–35), and his solemn commission as risen Lord:

> Thus it is written, that the Messiah is to suffer and rise from the dead on the third day, and that repentance and forgiveness of sins is to be proclaimed in his name to all nations, beginning from Jerusalem. You are witnesses of these things. And see, I am sending upon you what my Father promised; so stay here in the city, until you have been clothed with power from on high. (24:46–49)

This rapid sketch indicates that there is 'something special' about the Gospel of Luke. Of course, there is something special about all four Gospels, but nothing matches Luke's imaginative storytelling. Michael Winstanley's 'Walking with Luke: Studies in the Lukan Narrative' provides a remarkable uncovering of the 'specialness' of the Gospel of Luke. Not only are all the singularly Lukan features of the Gospel stories just mentioned dealt with, but there is more as this book is marked by several unusual features of its own that single it out as 'different' from the many books on Luke currently available. In the first place, its text is determined by Luke's story. The subtitle of the book betrays that concern: 'Studies in the Lukan Narrative'. Michael is keenly aware that Luke wants to tell a story to show his readers (personified in Theophilus) the trustworthiness of their faith in Jesus Christ (see Luke 1:4). Although not slavishly following the narrative sequence of the Gospel, as this is a series of studies and not a commentary, Michael's readers will find that as they proceed through the book, they will become familiar with Luke's overall literary and theological design. There may be difficult turns in the narrative, especially the narrative sequence of the so-called 'journey narrative' of 9:51–19:44, but a singleness of purpose can be traced from Luke 1:1–24:52 (not to mention the Acts of the Apostles). Readers will find that singleness of purpose as they move from one brief chapter to another in this fine book.

A second feature of this book is Michael's domination of classical and contemporary discussion of the Third Gospel. There may be times when the everyday reader might wonder about the long endnotes and the discussion of various points of view found there, or even discussions that are sometimes found in Michael's text. Nevertheless, once the reader is aware of what is provided, this aspect of the book becomes a treasure house. It has been said of the Fourth Gospel that it is like a magic pool in which an elephant can swim and a child can paddle. Michael shows that this is also the case for the Gospel of Luke. His familiarity with classical and contemporary writings on Luke is outstanding, as is his respectful presentation of a variety of differing views. Many of us will be grateful to have it on our desk to guide us through our own teaching, study and writing on Luke's Gospel.

Finally, as always with the writings of Michael, there is a carefully expressed and profound application of the Lukan message to the challenges of Christian life in the third millennium. While some will enjoy the analysis of the text, and others will join them but rejoice further at the scholarly information provided in each study, everyone who ponders Michael's wise and profound appreciation of the perennial value of the Lukan account of Jesus' birth, life, teaching, death, resurrection and ascension will come away from reading this book greatly enriched.

One cannot say everything in a foreword. I would thus like to focus upon one further feature of this book that struck me forcibly as I read it: Michael's focus upon the 'radical' nature of Luke's message. Whether it be the infancy stories, the challenge of the parables, the message of compassion, the interest in the marginalised of society, an honest reading of Luke's Gospel leaves us somewhat shaken. This comes as something of a surprise as, picking and choosing episodes from this Gospel can generate a pastiche of a Jesus full of 'loving mercy and compassion'. This is a false impression. Luke provides our most demanding Gospel portrait of Jesus. As Michael repeatedly points out, Luke can be singled out as the one who recalls, from the authentic memories of Jesus, the radical demands he makes upon all who claim to be his followers. Allow me to briefly address this theme and its contemporary relevance.

More than anywhere else in the New Testament, Jesus is presented as the perfection of God's prophetic presence among God's people. Jesus is the most questioning and the most relentless of prophets. The meaning generally attributed to the words 'prophet' and 'prophetic' in contemporary language is associated with the ability of the person in question to speak of oncoming situations with accuracy. Such a meaning, however common it may be today, has little to do with the biblical notion of a prophet or Luke's presentation of Jesus. As long as Israel was a pilgrim people in the desert, or a charismatic people under the early leadership of the Judges, she could claim to be a 'people' only because of the unity that was created by their commitment to a common Covenant. They believed that who they were was the result of Y*hwh*'s extraordinary intervention into their history at Sinai. In other words, central to the People of God's very existence as a people was the lived consciousness of the Covenant. Even after the settlement of Canaan under the Judges, they had no sense of being a political nation. There was only a charismatic unity under the Covenant that was defended by charismatic leaders when the need arose. Once it passed, each tribe drifted back to its former independence. With the gradual settling down of this people in Canaan, the political power structures of the people around them caused Israel to sense its uncomfortable strangeness and to seek to be like all the other nations. The covenanted people eventually came to seek the ways of the other nations. The all-pervading consciousness of the Covenant that held them together as God's people was threatened (see 1 Sam 8:4–7).

Israel became a powerful nation especially under David—but with strength came a kingly court, the international glitter of a royal capital in Jerusalem, a royal army using conscripted soldiers and foreign mercenaries, and this led to the tragedy of Solomon and the division of the nation. It is within the historical context of the divided kingdoms, each led by kings who were prepared to settle for the Baals, that the prophets emerge in Israel. The function of the prophetic movement in Israel was not primarily to speak about future events. Above all, the prophets were men and women who were entirely engaged with their loyalty to the Covenant. They are best described as lovers, women and men who are so consumed with the overpowering presence of the lordship of Y*hwh* that they are deeply hurt when they see Y*hwh*'s people living in division, adoring false gods, behaving like 'all the nations', alienated from one another, and from their unique God, with whom they have been called to live in Covenant. Thus, they can do no other than cry out in the name of the Lord, criticising the situation which they see on every side.

While Matthew's Jesus blesses those who are poor "in spirit", those who hunger and thirst "for righteousness" (Matt 5:3, 6), in Luke, Jesus announces beatitudes:

> Blessed are you who are poor, for yours is the kingdom of God. Blessed are you who are hungry now, for you will be filled. Blessed are you who weep now, for you will laugh. (6:20–21)

These beatitudes are balanced by woes that are not found in Matthew:

> Woe to you who are rich, for you have received your consolation. Woe to you who are full now, for you will be hungry. Woe to you who are laughing now, for you will mourn and weep. (6:24–25)

The physically poor, hungry and suffering can recognise that nothing this world has to offer will resolve their anguish, and thus they are open to the action of God. How timely Jesus' fourth woe is for all who think that they have 'made it' in the Christian life: "Woe to you when all speak well of you, for that is what their ancestors did to the false prophets." The perfection of the prophetic presence of God will not be spoken well of. He will be insulted, reviled and crucified, and he indicates that his followers must take on a similar prophetic lifestyle:

> If anyone wants to become my followers, let them deny themselves and take up their cross daily and follow me. For those who want to save their life will lose it, and those who lose their life for my sake will save it. (9:23–24)

The same urgent demands are found across the travel narrative (9:51–19:44), especially 11:14–14:35. There is a fierceness about Jesus' attack on those who would oppose him in the way he addresses the crowds, who must recognise the urgency of the times, and the demands he makes upon his followers. To those who suggest that he casts out demons in the name of Beelzebub, he accuses: "Whoever is not with me is against me, and whoever does not gather with me scatters" (11:23). Pharisees are attacked in a series of "woes" across 11:37–44: "Woe to you! For you are like unmarked graves, and people walk over them without realising it" (v 44). The lawyers receive the same treatment across 11:45–52: "Woe to you lawyers! For you have taken away the key of knowledge; you did not enter yourselves, and you hindered those who were entering" (v 52). He attacks the rich fool who stores up goods for this life, but does not live to see the next day (12:13–21). In place of such anxieties, he offers a different model: the ravens that neither sow nor reap; the lilies, more glorious than Solomon in all his splendour. "Your father knows that you need them. Instead, strive for his kingdom, and these things will be given to you as well" (vv. 30–31).

He castigates those who turn to him superficially. To the woman who calls out from the crowd, praising the body of the mother who bore him, he replies: "Blessed rather are those who hear the word of God and obey it" (11:28). In these words, Jesus returns to the response of Mary that is the sign of her greatness, not her physical cooperation with the design of God, however much subsequent

Christianity has made of this, but her response to the angel of the Lord: "Let it be with me according to your word" (1:38). He rails against hypocrisy:

> Beware of the yeast of the Pharisees, that is, their hypocrisy. Nothing is covered up that will not be uncovered, and nothing secret that will not become known. Therefore, whatever you have said in the dark will be heard in the light, and what you have whispered behind closed doors will be proclaimed upon the housetops. (12:1b–3)

When Peter asks whether these threatening words were just for the disciples or for everyone, he is told of the fierceness of the approaching time of the Lord, and the need to respond generously and unconditionally (12:41–48). Jesus came to cast fire on the earth, and has not come to bring peace, but division where houses and families will be divided (vv. 49–53). Only in the Gospel of Luke does Jesus speak so unconditionally about the cost of discipleship (14:25–33):

> Whoever comes to me and does not hate father and mother, wife and children, brothers and sisters, yes, and even life itself, cannot be my disciple. (v. 26)

> Whoever does not carry the cross and follow me, cannot be my disciple. (v. 27)

> None of you can become my disciple if you do not give up all your possessions. (v. 33)

Across the journey to Jerusalem, these themes emerge with solemn authority. No meek or mild Jesus speaks here, but rather the prophet called to a difficult destiny, summoning people to join him in his task of restoring God's established order. One of the measures we must use for an understanding of Jesus, as he is presented in the Gospel of Luke, is his divinely given task to act out the prophetic imagination in his life, teaching, death and resurrection. He relentlessly attacks a consciousness committed to achievable satiation. In its place, he proposes an alternative prophetic consciousness devoted to the pathos and passion of covenanting, cost what it may. For the Lukan Jesus, it will cost no less than everything. This must never be lost from view in our understanding of the Gospel of Luke. Jesus explains to the Pharisees during the journey to Jerusalem: "I must go on my way today and tomorrow and the day following; for it cannot be that a prophet should perish away from Jerusalem." (13:33)

As Michael and I talked about the book that follows, he shared his discomfort: how difficult it is to write an interpretation of Luke's Gospel, and its relevance to contemporary Christian life, in the comfort of a private study, with a well-stocked wine cellar waiting for consumption at a reliably provided evening meal.

So true! Why does Luke do this? There are many responses to that question, but the one that I find most relevant is closely associated to Luke's theme of a 'journey' that has been outlined in the subsequent pages. Luke makes use of this theme because he was addressing early Gentile communities who thought that the Gospel message had at last made it into their world. It was time to stop. There was a tendency among the audiences (some would have been able to read, while others would have heard it read or even seen it performed) to settle for all that had been achieved. The Gospel of Luke and the Acts of the Apostles shake them up. Luke insists that the journey is not yet over. Any tendency to settle into an inculturated 'bourgeois' Christianity had to be challenged, as the prophets had challenged a comfortable Israel. All the baggage and cultural accoutrements had to be laid to one side so that the journey could go on.

It is not only the original disciples that Jesus instructs:

> Thus it is written, that the Messiah is to suffer and to rise from the dead on the third day, and that repentance and forgiveness of sins is to be proclaimed in his name to all nations, beginning from Jerusalem. You are witnesses of these things. (24:46–48)

Quite early, this instruction is forgotten. Those same disciples gazed into heaven as Jesus ascended. Thus, the angels told them:

> Men of Galilee, why do you stand looking up toward heaven? This Jesus, who has been taken up from you into heaven, will come in the same way as you saw him go into heaven. (Acts 1:11)

Yes, Luke's story is full of care for the marginalised and compassion for sinners, but above all, it asks for unconditional Christianity. Indeed, as Michael suggests, this is perhaps the major overall Lukan message to disciples of Jesus of all times. Our compromised secular world matches Israel's desire to be 'like the other nations', and the Lukan Christians' tendency to accept the mediocrity of a settled Greco-Roman Christianity. We would all like to settle for what we have achieved. The radical urgency of Luke's prophetic message should be ringing in the ears of all third millennium Christians. Readers of this book have a unique access to that message, and they will not be able to escape it.

Francis J Moloney SDB AM FAHA
Catholic Theological College, University of Divinity, Melbourne, Australia
Feast of Saints Peter and Paul, 2017.

Contents

Introduction

For the title of this book, I have chosen 'Walking with Luke'. This I have preferred to a possible 'Journeying with Luke' for three reasons. First, 'journey' constitutes a major theme of the Gospel itself; as the title of the book, this would be confusing. Secondly, my last book had 'journey' in the title, so an appropriate alternative is called for.[1] Thirdly, and this is very subjective, I tend to think of a journey as going from A to B in a systematic manner; this would be more suitable for a commentary on the whole Gospel, which this book is not. To my mind, going for a 'walk' implies a return to the same place. Most summers for the last forty years, I have taken a holiday with friends in the Lake District or North Wales. I have never been attracted to walking journeys like the Pennine Way, the West Highland Way or the Coast to Coast, or even the famous Compostella *camino*. Rather, I prefer several one-day excursions of a circular nature, which enable me to return, mission accomplished, to the point of departure, have a shower, a meal and a drink, assess the day's experience, pray and relax.

Walking with Luke, Gospel in hand, offers a wide and rich area for exploration. I have chosen fourteen themes (or walks) that appeal to me both for their exegetical interest and their spirituality. Some themes are fairly compact, paths easily defined; others thread their way through the Gospel pages. Rather than follow each walk in the order of the contents, it is possible for the reader to choose a theme at will. Over the years, I have repeated many Lakeland walks several times, often finding new views and fresh points of interest that I missed before. Sometimes, this has depended on my frame of mind, the quality of light, my energy levels or simply the weather! The same is true in my experience of Gospel stories; one can return to them time and time again, and always find something new. Like fellwalking, some Lukan themes are demanding, others exhilarating, others challenging, but all can surprise and leave much to ponder. Like Lakeland hills, there are connections, continuities, obvious and subtle differences.

The choice of themes is mine; some topics I have used in other contexts and revised and developed here, some are exciting new adventures, others I have found particularly significant in my own life's 'journey'. Other authors would probably have chosen differently, I'm sure. But by the end of these Lukan walks, we should have a good idea of the evangelist's style and agenda, his concerns, theological mindset and spirituality. We will become more aware of Luke's idea of God, his appreciation of the prophetic character and role of Jesus, his understanding of the joys and challenges of discipleship.

The written Gospels were the outcome of a complex process of development beginning with the initial impact that Jesus made on his followers during his ministry, which became the core of the apostolic testimony and preaching. This Jesus tradition, the remembering of what Jesus said and did, was handed on orally in a world that was largely illiterate. In such community oral transmission, there is inevitably variation, but since its purpose is primarily to recall and preserve what is valued from the past, the nucleus or core content tends to remain stable and fixed.[2] In the light of the resurrection and the subsequent outpouring of the Holy Spirit, deeper dimensions of the historical ministry and death of Jesus came to be appreciated, and this new understanding was reflected in the telling of the story of Jesus. Development occurred over a period of some forty to seventy years, as the early Christian communities grew and spread and reacted to their own changing environment and to the various challenges that faced them, from within and without. Liturgy, worship and catechetical instruction exerted a significant influence. Eventually, from a variety of traditions about the teaching and life of Jesus, which were circulating in many communities of faith, Mark composed the first written Gospel, creating with originality, technical skill and theological acumen a connected narrative.[3] For their story of Jesus, Matthew and Luke drew on Mark, their own special sources and oral traditions and a further written source, no longer extant, known as 'Q', containing many of Jesus' sayings.[4] John's Gospel was written independently of the others and has its own very distinctive style, symbolism and theology. Occasionally, there are clear points of contact with similar early traditions.[5] "The Gospels are a wonderful weaving together of history and theology, as they report the events of Christ's life intertwined with later understandings of Christ from the communities of the first century."[6]

Whatever the sources of Luke's Gospel and the amount of editing that has gone into its composition, it is the present text that is the main object of my interest.[7] For each chosen theme I have used the same approach and format that I have adopted elsewhere.[8] First, I try to locate the passage in its wider Gospel context, since I am not following the sequence of the narrative verse by verse, as in a commentary. Then, I make relevant exegetical comments in order to explore and clarify the content and meaning of the episode as it stands. My main preoccupation is to highlight the theological message of each passage, the word from God, and the enlightenment and challenge it offers to our understanding and our living. But God's word is conveyed through human language, and I sometimes refer to significant literary features of the narrative text, for Luke is an author and storyteller of great skill.[9] Occasionally, historical issues arise and must be addressed.[10] Secondly, I offer some brief personal reflections arising from the text, which I hope will be helpful to the reader as a stimulus for prayer and pondering. The English version of the Bible that I use is the NRSV, which I believe renders the original Greek most faithfully.[11]

Luke's name has been attached to the third Gospel since the late second century; he was thought to be a physician, a fellow worker and travelling companion of Paul (Phlm 24; Col 4:14; 2 Tim 4:11; the 'we' sections in Acts). In recent decades both aspects of this assertion have been seriously questioned by scholars, and agreement is elusive.[12] Consensus suggests that he wrote his Gospel during the years between 80–90 CE, for a mainly gentile audience, be that his own urban community or other Church communities in areas of Greece with direct or indirect links to the earlier Pauline mission.[13] These communities were heterogeneous in religious heritage, social status, financial situation, ethnicity and nationality.[14] Luke is also responsible for the book of Acts, composed as a complementary volume and devoted to the growth of the early Church. Clearly well-educated, he is recognised as a skilled and creative writer and storyteller and a talented theologian. His good knowledge of the Greek Old Testament suggests that he could have been a convert from (Hellenistic) Judaism, or, more probably, that he was a gentile, converted or attracted to Judaism prior to becoming Christian. A second or third generation Christian (1:1–3), he was not an eyewitness to the life of Jesus, but depends on Mark, 'Q' and other oral and written traditions, which scholars refer to as 'L'. He is conversant with Hellenistic literature and philosophy, with biographical and historical narratives, and he uses the Jewish scriptures extensively.[15] In telling the story of Jesus, Luke is clearly sensitive to the context of the gentile world of the Roman Empire within which his audience is situated, while seeking to maintain strong links with the story of Israel. He wishes to confirm the faith of his readers and hearers, deepen their understanding and commitment, and challenge any incipient complacency arising among them.

My aim in writing this book is to make available to a wide audience the inspirational learning and instructive insights of many New Testament scholars,

4

whose works I have had the opportunity to read, and whom I have sought faithfully to acknowledge in the endnotes. To them I owe an enormous debt. My major personal contribution is found in the thematic approach to Luke and in the reflections within or at the end of each chapter, where I share some thoughts about the implications of these Gospel passages for our lives in today's world, a world very different from that of the evangelists and their audience. I have tried to write in a nontechnical style, hoping that this book will be accessible to a wide readership, lay, religious and clergy of all denominations, female and male, who wish to deepen their understanding of Jesus and his message and to explore the implications of discipleship for today. And so, it can be used for personal study, prayer and reflection and also for Christian groups of various kinds: prayer groups, bible study groups, and also for retreatants, teachers, catechists and students at different levels.

I wish to thank in a special way Fr Frank Moloney SDB, a friend for over fifty years since student days, who has read the text and made helpful comments. His scholarship and encouragement have been invaluable, and he has kindly provided the foreword. I am grateful to Fr Kieran Anderson SDB, who generously proofread the text and made many perceptive and useful suggestions, and to Professor John Lydon and Doctor Eamonn Mulcahy CSSp, who, having pondered the manuscript, have kindly submitted comments for the back sleeve. Finally, I wish to express my appreciation to Fr Bob Gardner SDB and the staff of Don Bosco Publications, Sarah Seddon and Bernadette Gaskell, for their patience, care and expertise in preparing the manuscript for publication.

Finally, I thank my Salesian confrères and many other friends, contemporary disciples of Jesus, for their encouragement, inspiration and support over many years. I have dedicated this book to them in appreciation and gratitude. It is my wish that this book may help many readers to come to know more deeply the merciful love of God, revealed and made present in the ministry, death and resurrection of Jesus, to respond to his challenge with generosity, courage and love, and to find in Jesus a friend and guide.

Michael T Winstanley SDB
Thornleigh House, Bolton
The Feast of St Mary Magdalene, July 22, 2017.

Notes

1   Michael T Winstanley, *An Advent Journey* (Bolton: Don Bosco Publications, 2014), follows the Gospel readings for the weekdays of Advent until Christmas, journey's end.

2   See the treatment of these issues in James D G Dunn, *A New Perspective: What the Quest for the Historical Jesus Missed* (London: SPCK, 2005), 46–56, and Robert K McIver, *Memory, Jesus and the Synoptic Gospels* (Resources for Biblical Study 59; Atlanta: SBL, 2011); his conclusions are found on pp 183–187.

3   Brendan Byrne, *A Costly Freedom: A Theological Reading of Mark's Gospel* (Collegeville, MN: Liturgical Press, 2008), xvi, xx. This is not to deny that before Mark the oral tradition had already developed narrative or kerygmatic blocks or sequences; see Dunn, *A New Perspective*, 124. Mark probably wrote soon after 70 CE, the year of the destruction of Jerusalem by the Romans. A long tradition maintains that he wrote in Rome, and a majority of scholars still accept this view. Others suggest a place closer to Palestine, like southern Syria. Most commentaries on Mark deal with these issues in some detail.

4   This is the commonly accepted scholarly opinion. 'Q' comes from the German *Quelle* meaning a source. It is possible that there were different versions of 'Q'. Matthew and Luke probably wrote in the mid-eighties CE.

5   There is much discussion about the authorship of the Fourth Gospel. The long tradition which identifies three figures: John the son of Zebedee, the Beloved Disciple and the Gospel's author, is no longer generally held to be accurate. Today some scholars believe that a minor disciple during Jesus' ministry (later known as the Beloved Disciple) had an important role in the founding of the Johannine community and was the source of its tradition about Jesus. This tradition developed through decades of reflection, liturgical celebration, struggles and lived experience, and was eventually fashioned into our Gospel, probably at Ephesus, between 90–100 CE by an unknown but very gifted member of the community, himself a disciple of the Beloved Disciple. Another member of the community (usually referred to as 'the redactor') revised the text shortly afterwards, making a few additions. See Raymond E Brown, *An Introduction to the New Testament* (New York: Doubleday, 1997), 368–371; R Alan Culpepper, *The Gospel and Letters of John* (Nashville, TN: Abingdon Press, 1998), 29–41.

6   The Catholic Bishops' Conference of England and Wales, and of Scotland *The Gift of Scripture* (London: CTS, 2005), 35. See also Craig R Koester, *The Word of Life: A Theology of John's Gospel* (Grand Rapids: Eerdmans, 2008), 7; James D G Dunn, *Jesus Remembered* (Cambridge: Eerdmans, 2003); Richard Bauckham, *Jesus and the Eyewitnesses: The Gospels as Eyewitness Testimony* (Grand Rapids: Eerdmans, 2006).

7   The study of sources and editing (known as source and redaction criticism) is fascinating, but it is not a major concern in this book. See John R Donahue and Daniel Harrington, *The Gospel of Mark* (Collegeville MN: The Liturgical Press, 2002), 1–22.

8   See Michael T Winstanley, *Lenten Sundays* (Bolton: Don Bosco Publications, 2011).

9   A development of the last 25 years or so is the study of the Gospels as story; it is called narrative criticism. See David Rhoads and Donald Michie, *Mark as Story: An Introduction to the Narrative of a Gospel* (Philadelphia: Fortress, 1982); Mark A Powell, *What is Narrative Criticism?* (Minneapolis: Fortress, 1990); James L Resseguie, *Narrative Criticism of the New Testament. An Introduction* (Grand Rapids: Baker Academic, 2005).

10   Luke's literary profile of Jesus may not totally coincide with the historical figure, though there are, I believe, major points of agreement. See John T Carroll, *Luke*, (Louisville: Westminster John Knox Press, 2012), 12; Robert C Tannehill, *Luke* (Nashville, TN: Abingdon Press, 1996), 19. This applies also to other characters in Luke's story.

11   The NRSV (Oxford: Oxford University Press, 1999) is based on *The Greek New Testament* (United Bible Societies, 1983). Throughout this book I will follow the traditional expressions 'Old Testament' and 'New Testament'; this is not a value judgement but simply an indication that one is older than the other. I shall use the abbreviation LXX to indicate the Septuagint, the Greek version of the Old Testament.

12   For a much more complete treatment, see Mark A Powell, *Fortress Introduction to the Gospels* (Minneapolis: Fortress, 1998), 96–98; Brown, *Introduction*, 225–26, 267–274. Carroll, *Luke*, 2, maintains the old position cannot be definitively disproved nor established.

13   Some widen this to the eastern Mediterranean: Antioch, Caesarea, Ephesus, Corinth and Rome have been suggested. Luke dedicates his Gospel to Theophilus (1:4), a literary patron, who is also representative of the wider audience that Luke wishes to reach.

14   Tannehill, *Luke*, 24–27.

15   About half of Mark's Gospel is found in Luke; there are some 230 verses common to Matthew and Luke, but absent from Mark; it is believed that these come from 'Q'. About half of Luke's Gospel is not found elsewhere, and comprises the Infancy Narrative, 14 parables, some healing stories and aspects of the passion and resurrection narratives. For more details see Carroll, *Luke*, 2–3.

Chapter One
Advent

In any literary work, beginnings are important.[1] The opening paragraphs of a book or article can grab our attention and stimulate our interest immediately, encouraging us to read on. They can also influence the whole reading process. Usually, we are furnished with important information, a privileged perspective, which will enable us, as readers, to better understand and interpret the whole story and the action as it unfolds. This applies to the two opening chapters of Luke's Gospel, frequently referred to as his Infancy Narrative.[2]

After a brief introduction addressed to 'Theophilus', the storyline of the Infancy Narrative commences. This unfolds in the following sequence: the annunciation of the Baptist's birth; the annunciation of the birth of Jesus; the visit of Mary to Elizabeth; the *Magnificat* canticle; the birth, circumcision and naming of the Baptist; the *Benedictus* canticle; the birth, circumcision and naming of Jesus; the two temple visits. The evangelist uses this block of material to share his understanding of the identity and mission of Jesus and also, overture-like, to give a first airing to themes and issues that are central to his Gospel message.[3] In this chapter I propose to follow the story as far as and including the *Benedictus*, which coincides with the first chapter of the Gospel, then devote Chapter Two to the other episodes, which coincides with Luke's second chapter. The second visit of Jesus to the temple is not, strictly speaking, an infancy event, since it takes place when Jesus is twelve years of age, but it is usually included in the period prior to Jesus' public ministry.

The Annunciation to Zechariah (1:5–25)

Omitting Luke's brief introduction to the Gospel, the storyline commences:

> In the days of King Herod of Judea, there was a priest named Zechariah, who belonged to the priestly order of Abijah. His wife was a descendant of Aaron, and her name was Elizabeth. Both of them were righteous before God, living blamelessly according to all the commandments and regulations of the Lord.

But they had no children, because Elizabeth was barren, and both were getting on in years.

Once when he was serving as priest before God and his section was on duty, he was chosen by lot, according to the custom of the priesthood, to enter the sanctuary of the Lord and offer incense. Now at the time of the incense-offering, the whole assembly of the people was praying outside. Then there appeared to him an angel of the Lord, standing at the right side of the altar of incense. When Zechariah saw him, he was terrified; and fear overwhelmed him. But the angel said to him, "Do not be afraid, Zechariah, for your prayer has been heard. Your wife Elizabeth will bear you a son, and you will name him John. You will have joy and gladness, and many will rejoice at his birth, for he will be great in the sight of the Lord. He must never drink wine or strong drink; even before his birth he will be filled with the Holy Spirit. He will turn many of the people of Israel to the Lord their God. With the spirit and power of Elijah he will go before him, to turn the hearts of parents to their children, and the disobedient to the wisdom of the righteous, to make ready a people prepared for the Lord." Zechariah said to the angel, "How will I know that this is so? For I am an old man, and my wife is getting on in years." The angel replied, "I am Gabriel. I stand in the presence of God, and I have been sent to speak to you and to bring you this good news. But now, because you did not believe my words, which will be fulfilled in their time, you will become mute, unable to speak, until the day these things occur."

Meanwhile, the people were waiting for Zechariah, and wondered at his delay in the sanctuary. When he did come out, he could not speak to them, and they realized that he had seen a vision in the sanctuary. He kept motioning to them and remained unable to speak. When his time of service was ended, he went to his home.

After those days his wife Elizabeth conceived, and for five months she remained in seclusion. She said, "This is what the Lord has done for me when he looked favourably on me and took away the disgrace I have endured among my people."

Luke begins his narrative by setting the scene, describing the geographical and political context and introducing the characters.[4] He informs us that the events he is to recount take place in Judea during the reign of King Herod the Great, a Roman appointee who ruled Palestine from about 40 or 37 to 4 BCE.[5] The territory that he governed stretched more widely than Judea itself and included Samaria and Galilee.[6] The leading human characters in the story are then brought on stage: Zechariah and his wife, Elizabeth. Zechariah, whose name means 'Yahweh remembers', is a priest. Elizabeth too, as a descendant of Aaron, comes from a priestly family.[7] They are presented as an upright and deeply religious couple, obediently observing the Law with meticulous care. God is clearly at the centre of their lives.[8] However, they have to bear the sorrow of having no children, which were popularly thought to be a sign of God's blessing, their absence a token of God's displeasure.[9] Elizabeth is said to be barren, which was a stigma, a painfully-felt reproach for a Jewish woman; the family has no future. Given that the couple are elderly, their situation is, humanly speaking, beyond hope.

The situation of Elizabeth and Zechariah contains echoes of situations found in a number of Old Testament narratives. There, we come across several stories of barren women who become capable of bearing children as a result of God's intervention: Sarah, Rebecca, Rachel, the unnamed mother of Samson, and Hannah. In the case of Abraham and Sarah, both were also very old. Luke's narrative recalls in a particular way the stories of Abraham and Sarah, and Elkanah and Hannah, the parents of Isaac and Samuel respectively.[10] Perhaps God will perform the impossible again.

The story moves forward with the information that Zechariah is on duty fulfilling his priestly responsibilities in the Jerusalem temple. The Gospel itself, as well as the Infancy Narrative, opens and closes in this temple setting.[11] This is a clear link with Israel's past. All the male descendants of Aaron were priests, entitled to officiate at temple worship. They numbered up to 18,000 and were divided into twenty-four groups or orders, named after the grandsons of Aaron; the Abijah section was eighth in the list. Only four of the original twenty-four had returned from the exile; they were re-divided into twenty-four new groups and given the old names. Each group served in rotation for one week every six months. Given such numbers, the morning and evening duties were assigned by lot.[12] This leaves space for the intervention of God; God is at work in the choice. The high point of a priest's life was to enter the sanctuary or Holy Place *(naos)*, situated next to the Holy of Holies, at the time of sacrifice and burn incense on the altar that stood in its centre.[13] After this, he would come outside and bless the people, who would be engaged in prayer. This was a once-in-a-lifetime experience, since a priest could not perform the task again until all the others of his division had done so. Consequently, this would be the greatest day in Zechariah's life. As he carries out this coveted task, probably in the early evening, the people in considerable numbers, a frequent Lukan feature, remain outside in prayer to their God.

It is in the setting of this Holy Place that the Good News of the inauguration of God's saving plan is announced.[14] For, suddenly an "angel of the Lord" appears to Zechariah on the right side, the place of honour and favour. God is taking the initiative and is actively present in his sanctuary through this heavenly messenger. The "angel of the Lord" is a figure commonly found in scriptural stories of this kind. Originally, the angel was not thought of as a personal being, but was simply a reverential way of describing God's presence. After the exile and contact with Persia, an angelology developed in which angels were conceived of as personal intermediaries.[15] Not unnaturally, Zechariah is disturbed by this visionary experience and fearful. The angel seeks to allay his fear by assuring him that his prayer has been heard by God, a motif which occurs frequently in this Gospel. Zechariah's formal prayer, in unison with the people outside, would have been for the salvation of Israel, but he was probably also praying for the gift of a son. Both storylines are brought together through God's intervention, as individual and national longings are set to be fulfilled.[16]

God's angel proceeds to announce to him the Good News that his wife will bear a son, and that he must be given the name "John". This was not an uncommon name; it was popularly taken to mean 'God has been gracious', though this etymology is not explicitly supplied.[17] His name is thus imposed by God and indicates something about his role in God's design. The boy will be a source of joy and delight for them, and his birth will be the occasion of widespread rejoicing beyond the family circle, for it has implications for the salvation of all the people.

The angel then speaks at some length in a rhythmic, poetic style about this child's future role and significance. He will be great in the sight of God, set apart and utterly dedicated to God's service, abstaining from wine and strong drink as did the Nazirites of old,[18] without being one himself in the full sense of the term. Even before birth, he will be filled with the Holy Spirit, a clear indication of God's special choice,[19] and thus empowered he will carry out a prophetic role, the mission of conversion, bringing a repentant people of Israel back to their God. Mention of "many" rather than "all" hints at resistance on the part of some of the people.[20] His role will be evocative of the great reformer prophet Elijah, as he prepares a people for the coming of God through repentance,[21] turning the hearts of fathers to the children,[22] and turning the disobedient to the wisdom of the upright.[23] He will thus take his place in a succession of prophetic figures through whom God visits his people.[24]

Zechariah then asks, not how this is to occur, given the factor of the couple's age, but how he is to know it, how he can be sure. In his unbelief, his lack of trust, he seeks a proof, a frequent Jewish failing, which is a way of usurping the initiative that belongs to God.[25] In reply, the angel now discloses his identity and credentials: he is Gabriel, who stands in God's presence as a special servant and who has been sent by God to deliver this Gladdening News. Since his message comes from God, it is utterly reliable and will inevitably come true; the prophecy will be duly fulfilled.[26] The giving of a sign is part of the literary form. Here,

Gabriel decrees that Zechariah will be struck dumb until the event occurs. This sign can be interpreted in different ways. It could be a punishment for unbelief, a means of preserving the content and wonder of the revelation from the people at large until later or a warning that something new is breaking in that demands great faith.[27] In fact, Zechariah is himself the sign for others that something quite mysterious has taken place in the temple.[28]

The scene now changes, reverting to the wider temple area. The people outside have become aware of the delay, and they are surprised and, no doubt, curious. When the priest eventually emerges from the sanctuary to give the customary blessing, he is unable to speak. "He kept motioning to them, but he remained speechless." The people realise that he has had a vision. After concluding his turn of office, Zechariah returns home to the country. Some time later, his wife becomes pregnant. She gratefully recognises that this is the result of God's gracious kindness towards her, a kindness that has also removed her public humiliation.[29] She withdraws from social life, remaining silently in the seclusion of her home. The reason for this is not evident. Some suggest that it is an indication of awe before the workings of God; others it is to avoid further reproach until the pregnancy is evident, or to remain in prayer. Most probably, it is a literary device to prepare for the revelation of the unknown pregnancy to Mary, who becomes the first to know.[30] Five months would be half the pregnancy according to the more common reckoning of ten lunar months.

Already in this opening section of the Infancy Narrative we have met some of the themes that will recur throughout Luke's Gospel: Jerusalem and the temple, the grouping of the whole people, the importance and efficacy of prayer, God's reversing human expectations and perceptions, the importance of women, the presence of the Spirit, joy, prophecy and fulfilment. But above all, it is clear that God is the central actor. Everything stems from God's free, faithful and compassionate love.

Reflections

Poverty can assume many forms. This Gospel excerpt and the stories that constitute its scriptural background highlight the poverty of childlessness. In the culture of the near east it was a source of shame for a woman not to bear children. We sense the disappointment and hopelessness of the elderly couple Elizabeth and Zechariah, and we can readily feel with them. However, the God of surprises intervenes dramatically, as in the past, announcing the reversal of this situation, the lifting of this heavy burden. The couple's prayer will be answered, Elizabeth will have a child, who will be their "joy and delight". And this child will have a significant role in the unfolding of God's saving plan, "preparing for the Lord a people fit for him." He is the answer to the elderly couple's prayers and the communal prayers of centuries.

We all experience our own forms of poverty; we have burdens to carry, dreams unfulfilled, longings unanswered, perhaps a sense of failure and hopelessness. This is not an indication of God's displeasure. It is an unavoidable aspect of human living, an aspect that we need to learn to cope with in a positive way. Our narrative invites us to trust in the God of surprises, who seems to delight in turning things upside-down. It assures us that God will listen to our prayers but will do so in God's own way and time, for there is always a bigger picture beyond our ken. Situations can be changed beyond our wildest dreams and imagining. From other situations, even if they remain unchanged, lasting and unexpected good can be drawn.

The God behind Luke's story is above all a God of joy, a God who remembers us graciously and with favour and whose love is generous and overflowing. It is important that we allow this God to touch our lives. This opening episode of the Infancy Narrative ends on a wonderfully symbolic and perhaps comical note: a pregnant old lady and a dumb old man who have become the makers of history.[31]

The Annunciation to Mary (1:26–38)

The annunciation of the angel Gabriel to Zechariah is followed immediately and in parallel by the annunciation to Mary. This is a scriptural passage with which we are all very familiar, a scene famously and imaginatively depicted in art and music. The narrative follows very closely the basic literary pattern for biblical annunciations of birth.[32]

> In the sixth month, the angel Gabriel was sent by God to a town in Galilee called Nazareth, to a virgin engaged to a man whose name was Joseph, of the house of David. The virgin's name was Mary. And he came to her and said, "Greetings, favoured one! The Lord is with you." But she was much perplexed by his words and pondered what sort of greeting this might be. The angel said to her, "Do not be afraid, Mary, for you have found favour with God. And now, you will conceive in your womb and bear a son, and you will name him Jesus. He will be great, and will be called the Son of the Most High, and the Lord God will give to him the throne of his ancestor David. He will reign over the house of Jacob for ever, and of his kingdom there will be no end." Mary said to the angel, "How can this be,

since I am a virgin?" The angel said to her, "The Holy Spirit will come upon you, and the power of the Most High will overshadow you; therefore the child to be born will be holy; he will be called Son of God. And now, your relative Elizabeth in her old age has also conceived a son; and this is the sixth month for her who was said to be barren. For nothing will be impossible with God." Then Mary said, "Here am I, the servant of the Lord; let it be with me according to your word." Then the angel departed from her.

Luke introduces the second episode of his Infancy Narrative with an indication of time, "the sixth month", which links the story with the preceding incident, Elizabeth's miraculous pregnancy, which is not known yet by any outsider because of her five months' confinement and Zechariah's dumbness. The location has switched northwards from the city of Jerusalem and its temple and priestly setting to provincial Galilee and an insignificant little hamlet, which Luke typically calls a "city" *(polis)*, named Nazareth. The two characters of the story are then brought on stage: the angel Gabriel once more, which means that God is the major protagonist, and a young virgin named Mary.[33] She is said to be betrothed to Joseph, a member of the house of David; the text probably does not imply that Mary too is of David's line.[34] The Jewish marriage process consisted in two stages: there was a betrothal ceremony in which consent was exchanged in the presence of witnesses, and then, after an interval of about a year, the two came to live together in the husband's family home. This betrothal ceremony was a legally binding contract, so technically Mary was Joseph's wife, though the couple had not yet begun to live together.[35]

The contrast between Zechariah and Mary is quite breathtaking. He is a priest functioning in the temple at the pulsating centre of national life. Mary holds no official position among the people. Whereas he is described as righteous and law-abiding, she is among the most powerless people in her society: she is young in a world that values age, female in a world ruled by men, poor in a stratified economy. Luke understands God's activity as surprising and often paradoxical, almost always reversing human expectations.[36]

The narrative proceeds according to the normal structural pattern of annunciation stories, and the parallels with the description of Gabriel's visiting of Zechariah are strikingly close. The two accounts are frequently referred to as a diptych.[37] The angel appears to Mary indoors in the home of her family, in the midst of her everyday life, and greets her with great respect. *Chaire*, "hail", is a customary formal manner of address; it can also mean 'rejoice".[38] He calls her "favoured one", or "you who enjoy God's favour". The two words have closely related stems in Greek, and alliteration is employed. In all that is happening, the initiative rests with God, with God's unconditional, gratuitous choice. She is assured that God is with her, an expression found frequently in the Old Testament;[39] it conveys the guarantee of God's help, support and empowerment for the one chosen to serve him.

Mary is "deeply disturbed" by what she hears, utterly confused, terrified even, and wonders about its meaning and implications.[40] The angel calms her fears, telling her not to be afraid, an injunction typical of annunciation stories. In words which have a poetic ring, he again assures her of God's gracious choice and initiative and spells out his message. She is to conceive and bear a son. She is to call the child Jesus, which was quite a common name at the time and means 'God helps' or, in popular etymology, 'God saves'. Surprisingly, such etymology is not given. It was normally the father who named the child, but there are precedents for women doing so.[41] Later, when Jesus is circumcised and named, the passive is used "he was called Jesus", with a reminder that this name was given by God's angel.

The identity and role of the child are then spelled out. He will be great, a greatness measured by his title "Son of the Most High".[42] By God's gift, he will accede to the Davidic throne as the royal Messiah and will rule forever. The phrasing of these verses echoes Nathan's promise to David, but the idea of a line of descendants ruling forever is changed to the idea that the Messiah himself will reign everlastingly.[43] The House of Jacob is an archaic synonym for Israel.[44] These are conventional Jewish messianic hopes and expectations.[45]

Following the usual pattern, Mary seeks information as to how such a conception is to take place given that she does not have a sexual relationship with Joseph or any man. Her question is different from that of Zechariah, who sought a way of knowing God's action. She is not doubting like him and sceptically demanding a proof. Her question highlights the action of God in all this and affords the opportunity for the angel to further clarify the true origin, identity and manner of conception of the child in a response which far exceeds the religious and cultural expectations of Israel.[46] The two phrases "the Holy Spirit will come upon you" and "the power of the Most High will cover you with its shadow" are in poetic parallel and lead into the third phrase: because of that coming and overshadowing, the child will be "holy" and will be recognised as "Son of God". What is to happen is the result of God's presence, activity and power. "Come upon" is used of the Spirit also in Luke's description of Pentecost; it is an empowering factor.[47] "Overshadow" recalls the creation scene, the Spirit's brooding presence over the waters. It is also used of God's glory and presence resting on the tabernacle and protecting God's people, and is used later in the Gospel in the transfiguration scene.[48] Thus the imagery and language, which in the baptism and transfiguration scenes of the Gospel are connected with Jesus' being proclaimed as God's Son, are combined here in the annunciation. Jesus' being holy and Son of God is linked with the action of the Spirit. "Something new is breaking in, surpassing anything that has happened before."[49] Luke's main idea seems to be that of creativity, total newness. Mary is not longing for a child, like Zechariah and Elizabeth, nor is there a prayerful request. Just as the Spirit's action brought life to earth's void, so the Spirit's action brings life to the void of Mary's womb. What is happening is entirely God's surprise, the result of God's initiative.

Mary, without having asked for a sign, is given information that functions as a sign, and this will confirm the trustworthiness of the angel's proclamation. Something deemed impossible has occurred in the life of her kinswoman Elizabeth, now six months pregnant in her old age.[50] This illustrates that for God, nothing is impossible. The phrasing echoes God's question to Abraham after Sarah's laughter: "Can anything said by God be impossible?"[51] This is the first hint of any family link between the two women; their stories and the stories of their children are interwoven.[52]

Mary then accepts the role graciously offered to her in the unfolding of God's plan; she receives God into her life in a new way. Open, humble and with great trust and courage, she expresses her willingness to cooperate and be of service unreservedly, cost what it may.[53] "You see before you the Lord's servant, let it happen to me as you have said." Mary joins the line of women who have served God's purposes throughout Israel's history. In the normal literary pattern, there is no vocalised reply; this is a Lukan innovation. Her response heralds the Lukan theme of discipleship. For later in the Gospel, in Luke's thorough adaptation of the Markan episode in which Jesus speaks about his true family, we read:

> His mother and his brothers came looking for him, but they could not get to him because of the crowd. He was told, "Your mother and brothers are standing outside and want to see you." But he said in answer, "My mother and my brothers are those who hear the word of God and put it into practice." (8:19–21)

Mary fulfils the criteria for family membership, for discipleship. In receiving the message of God in the annunciation and in her generous response, she shows that she is a woman of faith, as Elizabeth will shortly recognise. She is, in fact, the first disciple; her discipleship will continue during the ministry of her son and onwards after the resurrection.[54] She is also commissioned as a prophet to carry forward God's saving design.[55] After her accepting response, the angel departs.

The scenes of Luke's Infancy Narrative generally terminate with departures. "Mary becomes the literal embodiment of the promise of God."[56]

Reflections

We will never know what really happened on that Nazareth day.[57] We do not have access to Mary's religious experience.[58] In some mysterious way, God gratuitously calls and Mary freely responds. For Luke, she listens, she places her trust in God's faithfulness, she acts upon what she has heard; she is a model of discipleship. Her world-changing "yes", uttered with the whole of her being, resonates till the end of time.

"Yes" is one of the most powerful words in our language. It has the potential to transform faces, situations, lives. It can communicate a response of acceptance, a willingness to share, to collaborate, to become involved. It can convey an openness to change, to welcome what is new, to risk, to carry on and move forward. It can carry undertones of fear controlled, of hope entertained, of excitement aroused. It can indicate generosity, self-giving, the fullness of love. "Yes" is a word that crosses the lips of a small child, a young woman, an old man, a person in the prime of life, someone sick and struggling. It can be expressed in gesture as well as word. At times, it is the empathetic response to mystery, an embracing of the challenge of being alive. We are invited to make Mary's response a paradigm for our daily lives: "You see before you the Lord's servant; let it happen to me as you have said."[59]

In Luke's story, God, through the angel Gabriel, encounters Mary in her home in Nazareth village not in the Jerusalem temple. There is something ordinary about this extraordinary moment. It can be the same with us. Although angels don't just drop in from time to time, God is always calling and does so in myriad ways. It may be the song of a bird, a stunning sunset, a fascinating cloud formation, the drone of an aeroplane, the colour of a flower, the cry of a child or the look in someone's eyes. If we aren't sensitive and open, if we are inwardly deaf or blind, we'll miss the call and we won't even think of a possible response. But God will call again. God's call may come as a surprise, totally unexpected. It may be a note of affirmation and encouragement; it could be a challenge and demanding, even life-changing. If we do hear it, we inevitably respond, one way or another.

At this point, Gabriel's words to Mary can offer enlightenment. "Do not be afraid", she is told. I'm not a mathematician, but I suspect that this must rank as the most reiterated command or commandment in the Bible. These words are addressed frequently to individuals or groups or even the whole people in all kinds of critical situations in Israel's history. It's my belief that fear is at the core of the power of darkness. Fear holds us back from surrendering to God. Perhaps it is the fear of losing ourselves, being taken over, losing control over our lives; maybe it is the fear of being found wanting, being inadequate. Fear makes trust extremely difficult. Fear often prevents us from reaching out to others; it is an obstacle to friendship and intimacy, to community and collaboration, to service and self-giving. Fear can stifle compassion. Fear thwarts growth, deadens dreams, cramps initiative, crushes potential, saps life energy. Fear can hinder genuine discernment. So much of the violence and aggression within us and around us in our country and our wider world is born of fear and is sustained and fuelled by it. We can be afraid of people being different or holding different views. We can be afraid of failure, of what others may think or say. We can be afraid of challenge, of being sidelined, of becoming useless. We can be afraid of illness, diminishment, suffering and of death. It is important to be aware how fear finds expression in our lives now. As we do get in touch with our fears, let us hear the word of God brought by the angel: "Do not be afraid". [60]

The reason why we need not fear is made clear: "the Lord is with you." In so many of the scriptural narratives where a call is involved and a person is given a special role to fulfil in the unfolding of God's plan, God offers this kind of reassurance. In Mary's situation, God is present with her in a truly unique manner. But these reassuring words are addressed to us too. At every stage in our journey, in every situation in which we find ourselves, in all our ups and downs and twists and turns, the Lord is with us. We are always in the heart of God; God's love surrounds us. Maybe the problem here is not God's being with us, but our being aware of God's presence, our trusting that this is in fact the case. Awareness can grow as a result of frequent reflection on what is going on in our daily life; it often comes with hindsight. It can grow through silent, wordless prayer. Such awareness strengthens our trust in God's faithfulness for the future. But at the end of the day, the only way to learn how to trust is to trust. We have to take God at his word and surrender. Mary shows us the way.

Mary is chosen to "bear a son", to bring Jesus into the world, to give Jesus to the world. This is her role in life, her wonderful mission so crucial to the world's salvation and hope. In a different way, we too are called and missioned to be bearers of her son to others. For all our fragility and weakness and stumbling, we are sacraments, signs and instruments of the presence of Jesus in our world.

Jesus abides within us; he is always with us. We are called to reflect to others something of his compassionate love, his acceptance and care, his passion for justice, beginning with those nearest to us. We are invited by the Lord to 'be' Good News, to be bearers of healing and hope. It is an awesome responsibility. That is why God tells us not to fear and assures us that he is with us. If we are to mirror the true face of Jesus to one another and to all those whom we meet, then we need to come to know and love him ever more; and we, like Mary, need the creative and enlivening Spirit to work constantly within us, fashioning and transforming us.

The Visitation (1:39–45)

The next scene in Luke's Infancy Narrative brings together the two women who have featured in the annunciation diptych; their two parallel stories are now intertwined within the single story of God's redemption.[61] This episode consists of two parts: the visit of Mary to Elizabeth and then her *Magnificat* canticle, and her departure. The first part reads:

> In those days Mary set out and went with haste to a Judean town in the hill country, where she entered the house of Zechariah and greeted Elizabeth. When Elizabeth heard Mary's greeting, the child leapt in her womb. And Elizabeth was filled with the Holy Spirit and exclaimed with a loud cry, "Blessed are you among women, and blessed is the fruit of your womb. And why has this happened to me, that the mother of my Lord comes to me? For as soon as I heard the sound of your greeting, the child in my womb leapt for joy. And blessed is she who believed that there would be a fulfilment of what was spoken to her by the Lord."

The action is simply told. After God's saving plan has been revealed to her by the angel, Mary departs from Nazareth in great haste, a promptness which reflects her obedience to God's word.[62] The phrase "in those days" links the two stories. She heads for an unspecified town in the hills of Judah, a seventy to eighty miles' (112–128 km) journey of about three to four days.[63] Many of the priests who served in the temple lived away from Jerusalem. The parents of Samuel also lived in the hill country.[64] Luke's phrasing, "rose up and went", has a Semitic ring and recalls the departures of Lot and Abraham.[65] Mary arrives at Zechariah's house and greets Elizabeth, the older woman, thus bringing her seclusion to an end. The heart of the episode consists in the ensuing dialogue.[66]

The effect on Elizabeth of Mary's greeting is twofold. First, her child leaps in her womb. There is perhaps here an allusion to the jostling of Rebecca's twins that heralded their future destinies.[67] This is also an anticipation of the destiny of John, his being gifted with the Spirit from the womb as promised, enabling him to bear prophetic witness to the Coming One whom Mary is carrying. It is a leap of gladness which captures something of the eschatological joy foretold in Gabriel's announcement of his birth. Denis McBride speaks of "womb-shaking rejoicing, appropriate for the beginning of the messianic era, the onset of the messianic age of salvation."[68] The second effect is that Elizabeth is herself filled with the Holy Spirit, through whom she comes to realise what God has done for Mary.

Elizabeth is inspired to break into expressions of unrestrained joy and praise, and she proclaims in the form of a short poetic canticle the deep insight revealed to her about God's action in Mary, which far surpasses what God has done for her.[69] Mary, she acknowledges in a kind of prophetic blessing, is blessed by God among women, and the child she is carrying within her is also proclaimed to be blessed.[70] In fact, it is precisely because of the child that the mother is so blessed. These words of blessing echo words spoken concerning Judith and Jael, heroines through whom God intervened to save Israel from its enemies.[71] Recognising the superior position of her youthful relative, she is puzzled and readily acknowledges that she cannot possibly be worthy of a visit from the mother of "my Lord". Kyrios is used frequently of God in the Old Testament. In the New Testament, the designation is properly used as a title of the 'Risen One'. Luke frequently uses it of Jesus during the ministry both as a greeting and a title; this is the first instance of such usage, as Elizabeth recognises the child of Mary as Lord and Messiah. There may be an echo of David's words "How can the Ark come to me?"[72] and the words of Araunah addressed to David as he stands by the threshing floor, "What is this that my lord the king has come to his servant?" [73]

Elizabeth informs Mary of the movement of her own child within her at her greeting, about which the narrator has already informed the reader. She concludes her canticle as she began it with words of blessing: "Blessed is she who believed that the promise made her by the Lord would be fulfilled." The opening word here is makaria, the word common in the beatitudes, which is used to recognise a state of being resulting from God's graciousness. Later, during the ministry of Jesus, a woman from the crowd will pronounce blessed the womb and breasts of his mother. To this Jesus replies: "More blessed still are those who hear the word of God and keep it." (11:28)

Elizabeth's blessing is Luke's adaptation of these words. Elizabeth discerns that Mary has heard God's word and has believed that God could and would accomplish what was promised. She perceptively recognises the quality of Mary's listening and trust, a faith and obedience that contrasts with that of her own husband. For Luke, Mary is a model of faith, and already a disciple.[74] Mary responds by breaking into a hymn of praise herself, and this, along with the reference to her departure, is the topic for the second part of this episode.

Reflections

After her momentous meeting with Gabriel, her generous "yes", which changed the world forever, Mary doesn't hang around in wonder and amazement but hastily sets off to make the journey into the Judean hill country, a difficult trek over rough terrain. In self-forgetfulness, she desires to be of service to her elderly cousin, to assist her in the normal everyday tasks around the house, cleaning, washing, fetching water and just being there. She shares with her the ordinariness of existence, which is far from ordinary any more. To her journeying and her serving, she brings the child within her. There is a new dimension to every aspect of her being. When the two expectant mothers meet, Elizabeth recognises God's presence in what is happening to Mary, just as earlier she acknowledged God's compassionate faithfulness in her own life's adventure, and she expresses her wonder. This moment of encounter is more than simply a meeting of two pregnant mothers, one youthful, one worn and elderly. It is a deeply contemplative moment. This meeting, brimming over with promise and hope and future, is an encounter that occurs within the circle of God's faithful love, God's tender mercy. Both women are in touch with mystery, the transformative presence of God.[75]

All of us, as we go about our ordinary journeys and the humdrum tasks of every day, as we meet people in a wide variety of situations, are invited to perceive the extraordinary dimension of it all. For Jesus is always present in the core of our being, closer to us than we are to ourselves, even though we may fail to notice. And his presence makes such a difference. Like Mary, wherever we go and whatever we do, we carry Jesus with us into the space where we live our lives; and we carry him into the lives of others. Other people bring Jesus to us too—the members of our community, members of our family and the circle of our friends and acquaintances, the people we seek to serve, even those whom we meet casually. This is true particularly in the context of service; for wherever people seek to serve one another in self-forgetfulness, Jesus is especially present. Like Elizabeth, we need to develop the ability to recognise that deeper dimension, we need to be alert, we need to foster that gentle sensitivity to God's presence. We are called to recognise like Moses that the ground on which we tread is Holy Ground;[76] we are always in the heart of God. We are called to be everyday contemplatives.

The Magnificat (1:46–55)

Elizabeth has honoured Mary, praising her as mother of the Lord, and for her trust in God. Mary's response to Elizabeth's words of blessing is to redirect this praise to God, as she herself breaks into a hymn of praise, a hymn immortalised in the evening prayer of the Church. This creates a lull in the narrative movement, which enables Luke to highlight the significance of what has so far taken place.[77]

And Mary said,
"My soul magnifies the Lord,
    and my spirit rejoices in God my Saviour,
for he has looked with favour on the lowliness of his servant.
    Surely, from now on all generations will call me blessed;
for the Mighty One has done great things for me,
    and holy is his name.
His mercy is for those who fear him
    from generation to generation.
He has shown strength with his arm;
    he has scattered the proud in the thoughts of their hearts.
He has brought down the powerful from their thrones,
    and lifted up the lowly;
he has filled the hungry with good things,
    and sent the rich away empty.
He has helped his servant Israel,
    in remembrance of his mercy,
according to the promise he made to our ancestors,
    to Abraham and to his descendants for ever."
And Mary remained with her for about three months and then returned to her home.

The *Magnificat*, as this hymn or canticle is usually called,[78] bears a close resemblance to the psalms of the Hebrew Bible commonly referred to as hymns of praise; it exhibits the kind of parallelism that is a feature of Jewish poetry.[79] These hymns usually take the form of an introduction in which God is praised; a body, in which are listed the motives for praise (deeds that God has done for Israel and/or for the individual, and some of God's attributes); and a conclusion, which may recapitulate the motives for praise, take the form of a blessing or contain a request. The language of the *Magnificat* is heavily influenced by the Old Testament, especially the song of rejoicing uttered by Hannah after giving her son Samuel to the Lord at the Shiloh temple.[80] The hymn also introduces some key Lukan themes.[81]

By way of introduction, Mary celebrates with delight and rejoices in her Lord and God as "Saviour". The first two lines are in poetic parallelism: "my soul proclaims, my spirit rejoices"; the phrases mean simply "I". Mary sings with the whole of her being. This is the first mention of the theme of salvation, which is central to the Gospel of Luke. The angel later proclaims to the shepherds that "a saviour is born to you in the city of David". Simeon, as he holds the child Jesus in his arms, joyfully acknowledges that "my eyes have seen your salvation".[82] The apostles will later preach the coming of salvation through the death and resurrection of Jesus; Luke links it here with the child's birth.[83] In this opening verse it is God who is proclaimed as Saviour, and this is the thrust of the whole hymn; Mary manifests a profound sense of God's having freely gifted her. Mary's delight and rejoicing expresses the awareness that a new age is beginning.[84]

Following the usual pattern in this kind of hymn, she explains the reasons for her rejoicing. Initially, she focuses on what God has done for her personally. Her joy stems from God's looking with loving care upon her lowly, powerless condition, her humble state as a young woman from rural Galilee, her poverty of spirit. Mary is thus associated with those figures in Israel's past who were poor and needy, and also with oppressed Israel as a whole. She sees herself as God's servant, confirming her statement to Gabriel earlier. She is aware that as a result of God's graciousness, all future generations will follow Elizabeth in acknowledging her blessedness.[85] This is because of her central role in the coming of salvation through her son, though this is not explicitly mentioned. "The verse expresses a fundamental attitude of all Christians toward the believing Mother of the Lord."[86]

As the hymn evolves, Mary celebrates three of God's attributes: God is almighty, God is holy, God is merciful. First, God is the Mighty One. The kind of powerful intervention witnessed in military acts of salvation in the past, especially in the exodus, has been experienced by Mary, for the power of the Most High, for whom nothing is impossible, has overshadowed her.[87] God's name, secondly, is acclaimed as holy; later Jesus will be recognised as the embodiment of God's holiness.[88] Mary knows this already because she has been told that he will be conceived through the Holy Spirit, and will be called "holy". Mary, thirdly, acknowledges that God's doing great things for her stems from his mercy and compassion, his gracious faithfulness towards all those who are open to him. This has been true for countless generations right up to the time of her experience. What God has done in the past, God continues to do. In Jesus, God's compassion and mercy are present, and his loving faithfulness will establish a new covenant.

The motives for praising God now become less personally those of Mary, as the angle of focus widens. The thought is carried forward by a series of parallel antitheses.[89] The arrogant, conceited, haughty and self-confident are routed; this is probably in antithesis to the earlier "those who fear the Lord". Princes are dethroned, the lowly and oppressed are raised up high. The starving are filled, whereas the rich are dismissed with empty hands. Such arrogance, pride, power and wealth are forms that opposition to God constantly take and which God in his mercy combats. The adult Jesus will encounter them in his ministry.[90] This pattern of reversal, God's action in preferring the marginalised and the poor and needy, is a pattern or theme which will be evident during the ministry of Jesus in his preaching and his actions.[91]

The Greek *aorist* past tense is used in these verbs; this offers the possibility of several interpretations.[92] In the context it seems unlikely that this should simply refer to what God has done in the past as recorded in the Old Testament. Some scholars suggest that it could refer to the future: Mary is predicting what will come about in the future through the child who is to be born. Her experience is a paradigm of what will happen for others who are "poor". God has taken decisive action in the sending of his son, and Mary foresees as an accomplished fact the results that will follow in his mission.[93] Others believe that it refers to the present and describes God's normal way of proceeding. Alternatively, it is possible that the *Magnificat* is actually vocalising the sentiments of the Jewish Christians, proclaiming God's saving action achieved through the death and resurrection of Jesus.[94]

The hymn draws to a conclusion by explicitly recalling God's faithful love shown to Abraham, the father of Israel, and to his descendants throughout history, God's constant faithfulness to the covenant promise.[95] It is in this context of the covenant and God's faithful love that God has once more come to the help of Israel, God's servant or child, in the event that has begun in Mary.[96] The canticle ends as it began with this reference to God's saving/helping. This new, definitive helping/saving intervention has begun in the conception of Jesus; Mary can therefore proclaim its fulfilment.

After Mary's canticle response to Elizabeth's acknowledgement of her role, Luke picks up the storyline. Mary remains in Judah's hill country for three months, and then returns to her own home.[97] The implication seems to be that she leaves prior to the birth of Elizabeth's child. From the historical point of view this would seem unlikely and unhelpful, unless she needed to go to Joseph's home because of her own pregnancy. However, the ending of the episode is dictated by literary considerations, for Luke requires that Mary should leave the scene before he narrates the birth of John, so as to preserve the balance of the two coming birth scenes in which only the two parents will be present.[98] The two women and the two stories go their separate ways, as Mary departs for home.

On Lukan Hymns

The *Magnificat* is the first in a series of hymns, sometimes called canticles or psalms, found in Luke's Infancy Narrative.[99] The others are the *Benedictus* and the *Nunc Dimittis*, spoken by Zechariah and Simeon respectively, and the *Gloria in Excelsis* sung by the angelic choir at Jesus' birth; all of them form part of our current liturgical prayer. Most scholars would maintain that none of the speakers proclaiming the three more substantial hymns (Mary, Zechariah or Simeon) actually composed them historically. This was the pre-critical view based on the belief that the Infancy Narrative was derived from family circles. The hymns have a common style and a poetic polish, which would argue against on-the-spot composition by three quite separate individuals. There are also some lines that do not suit individual speakers.

Therefore, some critics have suggested that the hymns were composed by Luke himself. This view has not been widely accepted, mainly because in that case one would expect to find a more uniform style and a smoother transition between narrative text and hymn. It has been observed that the narrative would flow easily without them. The more widely held view is that Luke has taken over already existing compositions and inserted them into his narrative with some additions and adaptations. The differences between the hymns suggest different original authorship within the same environment.

The hymns are composed in a Jewish poetic style and with an outlook thought to be typical of the period between 200 BCE and 100 CE. They resemble a mosaic constructed from pieces taken from earlier poetry, from Old Testament and intertestamental passages. It is unclear whether they were originally composed in Hebrew or Greek. It has even been suggested that Luke took them from a collection that had nothing to do with Christianity at all, similar to material in 1 Maccabees and the Qumran literature, and applied their sentiments to the situation of the speakers in his narrative.[100] The mainstream view maintains that they are probably early Jewish Christian hymns (for there seems to be little openness to the gentile world), celebrating the saving action of God through Jesus the Messiah. There is a strong tone of salvation accomplished. Their Christology is phrased in Old Testament terms unlike the hymns in Paul. Luke saw that they could be introduced into the Infancy Narrative without much adaptation because the piety and concept of salvation expressed there corresponds to that of the people in the narrative. Motifs already in the narrative are continued.[101]

Raymond Brown thinks that it is not far-fetched to suggest that Luke got his canticles from a community of Jewish *anawim* who had been converted to Christianity, a group that, unlike the sectarians at Qumran, would have continued to reverence the temple and whose messianism was Davidic.[102] They may have found in Jesus the fulfilment of their expectations and used hymns to celebrate what God had accomplished in him. The *Magnificat* and *Benedictus* make sense in such a setting. Luke applied these general expressions of joy over the salvation brought in Jesus to the more specific setting of the infancy. The characters embodied the piety of the *anawim*.

> Thus, the canticles come to us in Luke with a background of two levels of Christian meaning: the original general jubilation of the Christian converts among the remnant of Israel, the 'Poor Ones' who recognised that in Jesus God had raised them up and saved them according to His promises; and the particular jubilation of a character in the infancy drama of salvation who is portrayed as a representative of the 'Poor Ones'.[103]

Perhaps they stem from the original Jewish Christian community in Jerusalem.

Reflections

The hymn that Luke places on Mary's lips in the Gospel narrative strongly echoes the hymn pronounced by Hannah after presenting her newly weaned child Samuel to Eli in the Shiloh temple. Mary praises God above all as saviour. She is aware of the wonders God has wrought in her and the ongoing impact this will have on the world. As we join her in praying this canticle, perhaps we too can sharpen our awareness of all that God has done for us personally and for our families, communities and our wider world. God's saving love continues to touch us in so many ways. And through us, God's love has impacted the lives of others. We join Mary in praising and thanking God with joy, for God does great and wonderful things for us.

Mary moves on to praise the qualities most strongly associated with Israel's God, especially God's faithful love and compassionate mercy. This has been characteristic of God's dealings with Israel since the beginning. It will continue to be God's characteristic style until the end of time. The God of Luke's infancy story is essentially a God who is compassionate and faithful. As the story of Jesus continues during his ministry, it is clear that the God he reveals in words and actions is the God of compassionate love. This is the God who continues to reach out to us; we need to allow him to touch our lives.

An aspect of the hymn that we can overlook is Mary's description of the way in which God turns the world upside-down, reversing situations of injustice and oppression. The salvation, which God in his compassion brings, entails social and political change and reformation. In the 1980s, the Guatemalan government forbade the public recitation of the *Magnificat* because of its revolutionary potential.[104] So, praying the *Magnificat* is demanding; it requires of us a heart that will be sensitive to the situations of the hungry, the lowly, the weak, the powerless, both locally and across the world, a heart which will enable us to be present and to stay alongside those in need and work courageously for the overturning of situations of oppression, untruth and injustice. It is a radical and challenging prayer that calls for liberating action because it celebrates the saving action of a compassionate God. Through us, that love must continue to transform our world into the Kingdom.

The Birth and Naming of The Baptist (1:57–66)

After the diptych of the two annunciation stories, Luke presents us with another diptych in the stories of the birth and naming of John and then of Jesus, as promise reaches fulfilment.[105] The *Benedictus* hymn proclaimed by Zechariah separates the two. First, then, the narrative:

> Now the time came for Elizabeth to give birth, and she bore a son. Her neighbours and relatives heard that the Lord had shown his great mercy to her, and they rejoiced with her.

> On the eighth day, they came to circumcise the child, and they were going to name him Zechariah after his father. But his mother said, "No; he is to be called John." They said to her, "None of your relatives has this name." Then they began motioning to his father to find out what name he wanted to give him. He asked for a writing-tablet and wrote, "His name is John." And all of them were amazed. Immediately his mouth was opened and his tongue freed, and he began to speak, praising God. Fear came over all their neighbours, and all these things were talked

about throughout the entire hill country of Judea. All who heard them pondered them and said, "What then will this child become?" For, indeed, the hand of the Lord was with him.

The storyline proceeds in two stages, with a week's gap in between. The angel's promise, which was first fulfilled in the conception of the child, now reaches further precise fulfilment in his birth.[106] Naturally, Elizabeth, the focus of our attention, is overjoyed by the birth of her child and by the restoration of her honour in the community. She is joined in her rejoicing on both counts by her neighbours and relatives, who recognise that "the Lord had lavished on her his faithful love". Such a joyful atmosphere fulfils the word of the angel to Zechariah concerning the impact of the birth of his future child. Luke reminds us that all that is taking place stems from God's free initiative, God's faithfulness and merciful love.

A week later, as was customary in accordance with the Law,[107] the time comes for the child to be circumcised and thus incorporated into membership of Israel and to receive his name. The neighbours and relatives gather for the occasion. The head of the household usually performed the ceremony in the presence of a number of witnesses, and there was a prayer of blessing. The naming of the child normally took place shortly after birth rather than a week later, which was a Greek custom. There are instances in the Old Testament of women naming their child, but by New Testament times it was generally the father who did so. It was traditional in priestly circles to name the child after his grandfather, but there are examples of the father's name being used, as in this case. The relatives have the intention of calling him Zechariah; perhaps they were already doing so.[108] Elizabeth, however, firmly insists that he be called John, which means 'God's gracious gift'. For the mother, he is indeed a gift from the gracious God; he is also a gift for his people. Without being aware of it, Elizabeth has chosen the name imposed by the angel.[109]

A woman's word in a patriarchal society counted for little, so those present persist in their intention, reminding Elizabeth that she is contravening the custom. Bypassing her, they appeal by means of signs to the child's deaf and dumb father.[110] Zechariah requests a writing tablet, a wooden board coated with wax. Without having heard what his wife has said, he writes unequivocally that his name is (already) John, and thus he obeys Gabriel's injunction. The neighbours react with astonishment, probably at the confirmation of this unexpected name for his son.[111] Some commentators feel that Luke wishes to imply that both parents acted without prior consultation or communication under the inspiration of God, though according to our logic it is hard to believe that Zechariah would not have already informed his wife of this by writing, unless Elizabeth was unable to read! Zechariah's speech suddenly returns, for he has shown that he no longer wishes to be in control, that he is content to follow the Lord's command. His immediate reaction is to praise God, who is so clearly at work in all that is happening.

As a result of all that has occurred, the neighbours are filled with awe and fear at the obvious presence of the supernatural in the twofold miracle, and the news spreads like wildfire throughout the area, providing the topic of conversation for some time. Those who hear what has happened "treasure it in their hearts", and they wonder what this child will turn out to be.[112] The reader already has some idea of the eventual denouement. The narrator adds a comment, which expresses the thought behind their questioning: "And indeed the hand of the Lord was with him". These words convey the wider significance of the occasion and communicate the assurance of God's accompanying power and guidance. The comment rounds off the scene on a note of hope and anticipation.[113]

Reflections

This reading, in its warm, realistic humanity, gives us much to ponder. The naming of a child can be an exciting or fraught event. There are personal preferences and family traditions to be accounted for. Whatever the reasons for a particular choice, the name we are given is ours for life. It both links us with our family history and defines our individual and unique identity. I was baptised Michael Thomas. Michael, I think, because mum and dad liked the name; Thomas because my paternal grandfather and my mother's favourite uncle had that name. I've never been fond of the Thomas bit, though it has proved useful as a way of distinguishing me from a fellow Salesian of my vintage called Michael Winstanley, without the Thomas, though most people adopted 'big' and 'little' to differentiate us! Most names get abbreviated; for many friends I'm Mike, and I like that. Mick has always been unacceptable! A number of my friends with two Christian names are known by the second rather than the first. Names provide a fascinating topic for discussion! For me the most important aspect is the uniqueness of my identity in relation to others and to God. The great medieval philosopher/theologian, Duns Scotus (1266–1308), used to speak about the 'this-ness' (*haecceitas*) of things. Each blade of grass, each pebble on a beach is utterly unique. Much more so is a human being.

The question of the elderly couple's neighbours and friends "what will this child become?" echoes across centuries and cultures. It encapsulates unspoken hopes and dreams. It also captures something of life's unpredictability, fragility and mystery. It acknowledges that we are not entirely in control of our destiny. For a Christian family, it is an invitation to make space for God in life's unfolding and to trust in God's providential love: "into your hands, O Lord, we commend our little son/daughter", your gracious gift to us. We humbly and gratefully believe that "the hand of the Lord" will be with our child, now and always.

For Luke, this story illustrates God's faithfulness to his promises, his trustworthiness, and this is important as the story of Jesus develops later. It also manifests God's remarkable ability to surprise, to operate outside the box, to turn experience and expectations upside-down. That, too, is a pattern which will recur later in the narrative.

The Benedictus (1:67–80)

On the eighth day after the birth of John, the naming and circumcision ceremony is held, as we have seen. As this draws to a conclusion, with the neighbours fearful and wondering about the child's future, Zechariah is filled with the Holy Spirit and bursts into a prophetic hymn of praise.[114] In some ways, Zechariah is also providing an answer to the people's pensive pondering, with which the previous scene concluded. The positioning of the canticle here rather than after verse sixty-four, where mention is made of his prayerful outburst, means that it has a place of emphasis. It also points forward to the story that follows as the Gospel unfolds, carrying the theological weight of the narrative.[115]

Then his father Zechariah was filled with the Holy Spirit and spoke this prophecy:

"Blessed be the Lord God of Israel,
    for he has looked favourably on his people and redeemed them.
He has raised up a mighty saviour for us
    in the house of his servant David,
as he spoke through the mouth of his holy prophets from of old,
    that we would be saved from our enemies and from the hand of all who hate us.
Thus, he has shown the mercy promised to our ancestors,
    and has remembered his holy covenant,
the oath that he swore to our ancestor Abraham,
    to grant us that we, being rescued from the hands of our enemies,
might serve him without fear, in holiness and righteousness
    before him all our days.

And you, child, will be called the prophet of the Most High;
    for you will go before the Lord to prepare his ways,
to give knowledge of salvation to his people
    by the forgiveness of their sins.
By the tender mercy of our God,
    the dawn from on high will break upon us,
to give light to those who sit in darkness and in the shadow of death,
    to guide our feet into the way of peace."

The canticle closely resembles traditional Old Testament psalms or hymns of praise, called *berakah*.[116] It commences by blessing or praising the God of Israel, and then in two balanced strophes provides the reasons for such praise. There is a lengthy insertion that is addressed directly to the child. This is followed by the original recapitulating conclusion.[117]

The opening blessing, "Blessed be the Lord God of Israel", is a stereotyped formula, frequently found in the psalms.[118] In this way, a link is made with Israel's past, especially the exodus event, in a hymn that will celebrate God's new redemptive intervention through Jesus. Reference to God as "the God of Israel" has an exclusive ring, discounting the gentiles. Two reasons for praising God are put forward in parallel: God visits his people; and God raises up a saviour. First, God is praised for having "visited" his people. The idea of God's visiting is used in the Old Testament with reference both to God's judging and, especially, to his saving interventions on behalf of his people;[119] it is an important idea for Luke.[120] The nature of God's visitation is clearly specified here as being redemptive, liberating, delivering. The verbs throughout this section are in the past tense, indicating an accomplished fact, but, building on what God has achieved in Israel's past, they refer to God's liberating work already begun with the birth of the child and the conception of the Messiah. Though not yet finally accomplished, God has set in motion the train of events that will achieve such deliverance.[121]

The means of such redemption consists in God's establishing for the people "a horn of salvation" or "mighty saviour" or a "saving power", who is the Davidic Messiah.[122] This is the second reason for Zechariah's praising God. The image is derived from the upright horns of a bull or ox, later transferred to the horns on a victorious warrior's helmet.[123] It is a symbol of power and strength. The image fits the idea of a triumphant messianic king.[124] In doing so, God is fulfilling what God promised in ancient times through the prophets, and in this way a long line of preparation is brought to completion.[125] The content of these promises was the saving of the people from their enemies or, again using poetic parallelism, "from the hands of those who hate us". In the psalms, such enemies can be personal or pagan foes.[126] In this way, God shows his mercy and faithful love, keeping the solemn covenant promise made to the fathers of old.

The second strophe highlights the covenant attributes of mercy or loving kindness in choosing Israel and faithfulness to the choice made, despite the inadequacies of human beings. These are two key characteristics of God that were highlighted also in the *Magnificat*. Here, the emphasis moves away from David and the promises made to him, for the covenant explicitly recalled is that made to Abraham, which in the eyes of the early Christians was wider and more fundamental than the Mosaic covenant.[127] "The salvation that is now coming from Yahweh, in raising his horn in David's house, is seen as an extension of his covenant promises to Israel's ancestors of long ago."[128] The purpose of this covenant oath is here described in terms of deliverance from the hands of enemies and freedom from the fear of persecution, so that they might forever serve God in holiness and upright living or justice, qualities which ought to characterise the covenanted people.[129] While the ideas of service and worship have a cultic and liturgical ring, they embrace a whole way of living.[130] "God keeps God's word, and it is a gracious word. God's people have their part to play as well, answering the divine gift of freedom with genuine worship of the holy God and an enduring commitment to justice."[131]

At this point, the style of the hymn alters, as Zechariah turns to his child, addressing him directly in a prophetic oracle. Such a switch is not uncommon in Jewish literature. It is thought that Luke is responsible for the addition of these verses to the original hymn. In words that echo the message of Gabriel earlier, Zechariah celebrates the role that his son will fulfil in the unfolding of God's saving intervention. John, too, will be a prophet of God the Most High, announcing God's new salvation.[132] He will exercise this role by going before the Lord in order to prepare his way, for God's visitation takes the form of the coming of Jesus.[133] This is, in fact, how the ministry of John the Baptiser is later described in the Gospel narrative.[134] The next sentence is in parallel: the Lord's way is prepared through John's providing the people with the knowledge of salvation, a salvation which consists in the forgiveness of sins. Knowledge of salvation here does not refer to something intellectual; it means that salvation is personally experienced deep within through the forgiveness of sins. In his later ministry, John proclaims a baptism "for the forgiveness of sins", and offers teaching on how different groups of people should live.[135] Forgiveness is central to the message and ministry of Jesus too; it is a key Lukan concept throughout the Gospel and Acts.[136]

As is usually the case, the final verses of the hymn summarise the ideas already expressed. The source of all that takes place is the faithful mercy of God, God's loving compassion.[137] Such compassion, such "tender mercy", brings about the visitation from above of a figure described as "the dawn from on high" or "a rising light". There is now a switch from second to third person and a different focus. The key word in Greek can mean a growing shoot or branch, or a rising star, which are both messianic images.[138] Perhaps this twofold significance is intended. The term was used among Greek-speaking Jews to describe the expected Davidic king. Some manuscripts have a future verb, "will come", others a past, "has come".[139] The Messiah comes from God as a source of light and liberation for those "sitting in darkness and the shadow of death",[140] "a light to guide our feet into the way of peace".[141] The theme of peace is taken up again later in the hymn of the angels at the birth of Jesus. This image balances the "horn of salvation" imagery found earlier in the canticle with its possible implications of force and political might.[142] In the Old Testament, salvation has to do mainly with the overthrowing of Israel's enemies, whereas for Luke, it concerns liberation from sin in its various dimensions.

According to this canticle, the main reason for blessing God is what God has done for his people in Jesus the Messiah. In the period of Old Testament preparation, promises were made to David and his descendants through the prophets and a covenant oath to Abraham and his. The hymn concludes with a eulogy of Jesus, and is therefore Christological. John the Baptiser is the bridge between old and new.[143]

After the hymn, which closes by pointing to the coming Messiah, the narrative is briefly resumed, and the section that deals with John is brought to a conclusion. John is removed from the scene before Luke moves on to concentrate his attention on the birth of Jesus. The boy John is said to grow physically and also to develop in spirit before the Lord. The phrasing is stereotyped, and echoes many of the parallels that have run through this opening chapter: Isaac, Samson, Samuel.[144] The child goes off into the Judean desert area (presumably some years later) and lives in the seclusion of the wilderness far from public gaze until the moment when he inaugurates his prophetic mission to Israel. We hear no more of Elizabeth and Zechariah; their role is fulfilled. As usual the scene thus ends on a note of departure. John's story is taken up again in 3:2 when "the word of God came to John the son of Zechariah, in the desert", and he embarks on his ministry for the renewal of his people, "preparing a way for the Lord".[145]

Reflections

Under the influence of the Holy Spirit, the second great hymn of Luke's Infancy Narrative is spoken by John's father, Zechariah. The Spirit has already touched Mary and Elizabeth, and will be active later in the story when Simeon and Anna meet the child in the temple. The traditional format of the canticle gives way to Zechariah's vision of his son's future role in God's saving visitation of our world. Parents often wonder what their children will become when grown up; Zechariah has a clear vision of his son's role, and in sharing it, he provides answers to the neighbours' pondering.

In the process of outlining John's mission, he also highlights salient aspects of the role of the one for whom he will prepare. Jesus will be a source of light for those who sit in darkness and in the shadow of death. These words which have an Isaian resonance recur in Matthew's Gospel as Jesus leaves Nazareth and makes his home in Capernaum at the start of his ministry. The occasions when Jesus heals blind people illustrate his light-bringing. His teaching scatters much shadow and darkness, for Jesus is the great revealer. Through his healing, teaching and his way of living and relating, he revealed to the people who encountered him the face of God, a God of forgiveness and compassion, a God who wanted to share their lives, a God of faithful love. He revealed to them a set of values and attitudes which mirror something of that God. He revealed to them the contours of a different world which he called God's Kingdom.

In the course of our life's journey, centuries later we have probably been drawn to acknowledge the areas of shadow and darkness in our minds and our lives and in our wider world. We have been exposed to Jesus' words and have had the opportunity to reflect on his message and healing ministry. In and through it all we have been able to encounter the God whom Jesus reveals. The core of Jesus' message is that God loves each of us very deeply, with a love that will always be there. God walks with us on our journey. God waits to welcome us into His embrace. Perhaps over the years we have become more aware of God's presence deep within our heart, and have been able to surrender to God's love a little more. It is that love which bursts into our world with gentle power in the next scene.

34

Notes

1 I have chosen to use 'Advent' as the title for this chapter for two reasons. Advent means 'coming', and this chapter is devoted to the coming of the Baptist and of Jesus. Advent is also the liturgical period of waiting and expectancy, and in this chapter the waiting of centuries comes to fulfilment, and two women begin a special time of waiting for their child to be born.

2 As well as the Gospel commentaries, for the first two chapters of this book I am particularly indebted to Raymond E Brown, *The Birth of the Messiah* (London: Geoffrey Chapman, 1993); *A Coming Christ in Advent* (Collegeville, MN: The Liturgical Press, 1988); *An Adult Christ at Christmas* (Collegeville, MN: The Liturgical Press, 1978); Marcus J. Borg and John Dominic Crossan, *The First Christmas: What the Gospels Really Teach About Jesus's Birth* (New York: HarperOne, 2007); Jeremy Corley, ed., *New Perspectives on the Nativity* (London: T&T Clark, 2009); Andrew T. Lincoln, *Born of a Virgin? Reconceiving Jesus in the Bible, Tradition, and Theology* (London: SPCK, 2013).

3 Lincoln, *Born of a Virgin?* 100, observes that in his structuring of Luke-Acts, Luke wishes to show that the history of salvation has a chain of continuity that runs through it from God's promises to Israel to their fulfilment in the mission of Jesus and on into the mission of Jesus' followers leading to the gentile church of his own day. Borg & Crossan, *First Christmas*, 25–53, maintain that the Infancy Narratives are neither fact nor fable; they are best understood as parable and overture, rich in theological significance, and a summary of what is to follow.

4 Brown, *Birth*, 264, offers this structure: 1:5–7: Introduction of the *dramatis personae*; 1:8–23: Annunciation by the angel; (8–10, Setting; 11–20, Core; 21–23 Conclusion); 1:24–25: Epilogue. Joel B. Green, *The Gospel of Luke*, NICNT (Cambridge: Eerdmans, 1997), 67, suggests a chiastic pattern to vv. 8–23. Scholars note the Semitic character and Septuagint language of the narrative. Carroll, *Luke*, 25, points out that this is the first of three contextualising markers, each more detailed than the preceding (1:5; 2:1–2; 3:1–2).

5 I. Howard Marshall, *The Gospel of Luke: A Commentary on the Greek Text* (Exeter: Paternoster Press, 1978), 51, suggests 40; Denis McBride, *The Gospel of Luke: A Reflective Commentary* (Dublin: Dominican Publications, 1991), 22; Green, *Luke*, 62; Joseph A. Fitzmyer, *The Gospel according to Luke*, 2 vols (New York: Doubleday, 1981, 1985), 1:321, n. 37, opt for 37.

6 Herod was noted for building programmes, tyranny, and attempts at Hellenisation. Carroll, *Luke*, 25, refers to a powerful political undercurrent in the story; the claims advanced for Jesus will challenge this kind of power.

7 The only Elizabeth mentioned in the Hebrew Bible was the wife of Aaron (Exod 6:23).

8 Luke T. Johnson, *The Gospel of Luke*, Sacra Pagina 3 (Collegeville, MN: The Liturgical Press, 1991), 32, observes that these characteristics reflect the simple piety associated with the "poor of Yahweh", the *anawim*, people who trust in God and are open to revelation.

9 Lev 20:20; Gen 16:4; 29:32; 30:1; 1 Sam 1:5–6; Ps 127:3–5; 128. Green, *Luke*,

63, notes the dissonance between blamelessness and lack of blessedness. Brown, *Birth*, 268, states that the couple combine priestly origins and the blameless observance of the Law, and are for Luke representatives of the best in the religion of Israel.

10   Zechariah's reply (1:18) is identical with that of Abraham (Gen 15:8); Elizabeth's joy is reminiscent of that of Sarah (Gen 21:6). The similarities with the story of Elkanah and Hannah in 1 Sam include: the opening of the story introducing the characters; the temple setting (Shiloh in their case) and sacrifice; Hannah's distress because of her barrenness; her prayer for a boy child, whom she would dedicate to God and who would be a Nazirite. Eli, the priest, assures her that her prayer will be granted. On their return home, she becomes pregnant. (See Brown, *Coming*, 43–44). Luke's language and style deliberately recall the Old Testament. These biblical episodes provide models for Luke's storytelling. Green, *Luke*, 69, describes the Old Testament as a "data bank" for Luke, who has constructed a complex network of echoes. Brown, *Coming*, 44, and *Birth*, 270, notes that Luke recalls the Law, the Prophets, and the Wisdom traditions, thus covering the timespan of Matthew's genealogy. Borg & Crossan, *First Christmas*, 212–213, observe that Luke does not use the prediction-fulfilment formula which we encounter in Matthew; he echoes phrases from the Old Testament in narrative and hymns. See also Lincoln, *Born of a Virgin?* 49–50.

11   24:53

12   Brown, *Birth*, 258–259; McBride, *Luke*, 23. For further details see Green, *Luke*, 68; Marshall, *Luke*, 54; G.B. Caird, *The Gospel of St. Luke* (Pelican Gospel Commentaries; Harmondsworth: Penguin, 1963), 50–51; Fitzmyer, *Luke*, 1:322.

13   Exod 30:7–8; 2 Chron 13:11. The only person who was allowed closer to the locus of God's presence was the High Priest who entered the Holy of Holies on the Day of Atonement. Carroll, *Luke*, 28, notes the linking of "Lord" and "people" (*laos*): "the sanctuary of the Lord" and "the assembly of the people"; John's role, in the words of the angel, will be to prepare a people for the Lord.

14   In the Old Testament. there are several episodes in which the birth of a child is announced. These follow a similar pattern, a pattern which is found here, and also in the annunciation to Mary later. See Brown, *Birth*, 156, Table VIII; he describes the template as follows: an appearance (or vision) of the Lord (or God's angel); a reaction of fear (or a prostration); the recipient is addressed, usually by name, and told not to fear; the message affirms that someone is or will be with child and will give birth; the name of the child is given (sometimes with an etymological explanation); the child's role and accomplishments are rehearsed; the visionary poses an objection or question, or asks for a sign. See Gen 17 and 18 regarding Isaac; 16:7–15 regarding Hagar and Ishmael; Judg 13:3–20 regarding Samson. Some vocation stories show similar features: the call of Gideon in Judg 6:12–23 and of Moses in Exod 3:2–12. Tannehill, *Luke*, 44, prefers to call these "promise and commission epiphanies". Carroll, *Luke*, 29, suggests: appearance, response of fear, divine message, question, giving of a sign, departure. The annunciation narrative is also influenced by Dan 8:16f; 9:21f; 10:8, 12, 15; here we find reference to Gabriel, a vision during evening liturgical prayer, fear, dumbness, the Holy of Holies. See also Chistopher F. Evans, *Saint Luke* (London: SCM, 1990), 144. Fitzmyer, *Luke*, 1:309, 316–317, takes the view that Luke is using a Baptist source for this episode, a view which

Brown resists (*Birth*, 244–245, 265–279).

15   Brown, *Birth*, 260. Evans, *Luke*, 151, refers to the speculative theology of angels which developed in Judaism in the 2nd century BCE in apocalyptic circles and popular piety. Some were given names. Unlike the Pharisees, the Sadducees rejected the innovation. For details of the Daniel links, see Brown, *Birth*, 270–271; Lincoln, *Born of a Virgin?* 50.

16   Tannehill, *Luke*, 44–45; Green, *Luke*, 74; on p. 73, he refers to a divine remembrance motif; God remembers and acts on behalf of certain people (see Gen 30:22; 1 Sam 1:11, 19–20). Marshall, *Luke*, 56, thinks it unlikely that Zechariah was praying for a personal request at that time, though he may have done so at other times; prayer for the salvation of Israel was associated with the evening sacrifice. Brown, *Birth*, 260, takes the opposite view. Carroll, *Luke*, 30, implies both. Amy-Jill Levine, *Short Stories by Jesus* (New York: HarperOne, 2014), 98, believes that the text suggests that Zechariah had prayed for a child.

17   The same is true later with the name Jesus. Carroll, *Luke*, 30, notes how the hymns of Zechariah and Mary make explicit what the giving of the name only implies.

18   Judg 13:4–14; Jer 35:1–11; Num 6:3; 1 Sam 1:9–15. Luke is linking John with Samuel and Samson. Abstinence from wine, cider and beer was associated with separation from normal life for a divine task, temporary (like officiating in the temple) or lifelong. Here it is indication of John's lifelong dedication to God. (See Green, *Luke*, 75). For Marshall, *Luke*, 57, John is simply described as an ascetic. For Carroll, *Luke*, 31, he will live an ascetical life, and also be set apart for a special vocation in God's service.

19   See Samson in Judg 16:17; 13:7, and Jeremiah in Jer 1:5, 14. This is the first mention of the Spirit in Luke; the Spirit is active throughout the Infancy Narrative, and then into the ministry of Jesus, and, in Acts, in the mission of the church.

20   Carroll, *Luke*, 33.

21   Mal 2:7; 3:1; 3:23; 4:5. In the original text the "Lord" refers to God; it probably does here, since Gabriel has not yet announced the coming of Jesus. Brown, *Birth*, 273–274, notes how the language of these verses anticipates the descriptions of John found in the ministry (3:1–3; 7:27–28; 7:33; 20:6), an ascetical prophet calling upon Israel to repent. Fitzmyer, *Luke*, 1:327, observes that, contrary to the view of many, in pre-Christian literature Elijah is not presented as precursor of the Messiah.

22   This phrase is found in Mal 2:6 LXX; 3:24 and Sir 48:10 regarding Elijah. The influence of Malachi on the text is significant, and communicates the coming of the end time. Carroll, *Luke*, 32–33, observes that in Jesus, family undergoes radical redefinition. Perhaps there is a hint in Gabriel's words of surprising reversals, as the structures of power within the family (fathers) are turned upside-down (they return to their children, not vice versa).

23   Brown, *Birth*, 278–279, interprets this difficult parallelism as the fathers/ancestors are the disobedient; the (unexpected) children of Abraham, the gentiles, find the Wisdom of God in Jesus (see 7:31–35). Marshall, *Luke*, 60, favours the meaning of the restoring of good family relationships. Green, *Luke*, 77, notes the image of God in the Gospel as a father caring for his children, and similar references to human fathers.

24   Johnson, *Luke*, 35.

25   His question is the same as that of Abraham (Gen 15:8).

26   Gabriel in Dan 8–9 is entrusted by God to reveal divine mysteries, which pertain to the end time. "Good news" recalls Isa 40–66, the coming final redemption.

27   Green, *Luke*, 79–80; Marshall, *Luke*, 60–61. Tannehill, *Luke*, 46, sees this as a punishment, but not a rejection; as an elder and priest Zechariah ought to have known the traditions of Israel concerning Abraham and other childless couples.

28   Brendan Byrne, *The Hospitality of God: A Reading of Luke's Gospel* (Collegeville, MN: The Liturgical Press, 2000), 22. The literary parallels with Daniel suggest dumbness as a sign. Carroll, *Luke*, 34, comments that the onset of his condition and its later reversal attest the reliability of the angel and the promises he delivers.

29   There are clear echoes of 1 Sam 1:19–20. Green, *Luke*, 63, observes that the spotlight shines brightest on Elizabeth: barren and disgraced at the outset, pregnant and restored to a position of honour at the close. On p 66, he comments that Elizabeth's having a child does not depend on Zechariah but on a miraculous intervention. The language of the text recalls Sarah's rejoicing (Gen 21:6), and Rachel's (Gen 30:22–23).

30   Brown, *Birth*, 282; Marshall, *Luke*, 62; Fitzmyer, *Luke*, 1:321.

31   McBride, *Luke*, 24.

32   Lincoln, *Born of a Virgin?* 102, describes the five stages as: a divine appearance (God or angel); a reaction of fear or amazement; a message; an objection or request for a sign; the giving of confirmatory sign.

33   Mary (Miryam) was a common name among first-century Jewish women. The word *parthenos* is twice used to describe her. It means a young unmarried girl. Johnson, *Luke*, 36, holds that there are no implications concerning sexual experience, but Marshall, *Luke*, 64; Green, *Luke*, 86; Fitzmyer, *Luke*, 1:343, maintain that, following the LXX, there are strong implications of virginity. Lincoln, *Born of a Virgin?* 101, refers to a young woman of child-bearing age who has not yet given birth to a child. Green, *Luke*, 85, and Marshall, *Luke*, 64, make a link with Isa 7:10–17. Brown, *Birth*, 300, does not find arguments making the link with the Isaian passage convincing. He notes that the Isaian terminology is found in other Old Testament annunciation stories. Borg & Crossan, *First Christmas*, 113–114, are also of the view that there is no evidence that Luke knows any connection between Mary's virginity and the Isaian text. Similarly, Fitzmyer, *Luke*, 1:336.

34   Brown, *Birth*, 287; Fitzmyer, *Luke*, 1:344.

35   Deut 22:23–24

36   Johnson, *Luke*, 39; Tannehill, *Luke*, 48. Byrne, *Hospitality*, 22, writes that we have moved from the centre to the margins.

37   See Brown, *Birth*, table X, 294, and table XI, 297. Johnson, *Luke*, 38, comments that because of the many parallels between this story and the previous angelic visitation, the points of difference are all the more striking: John is great before the Lord, Jesus is great and is Son; John will prepare the people, Jesus will rule them; John has a temporary role, Jesus' will last forever; John is a prophet, Jesus is Son; John is filled with the Spirit as a prophet, the Spirit overshadows Jesus and makes him the "Holy One". Green, *Luke*, 83–84, discusses the similarities and points of contrast between the two stories; also, Carroll, *Luke*, 43–44. Brown, *Birth*, 296, makes the point that the material not explained by the literary pattern requires attention: the (virginal) manner of conception, the

description of the future accomplishments of the child, and the portrait of Mary in vv. 34 and 38. Close adherence to the literary form raises a question about the historicity of the stereotyped features.

38   See Zeph 3:14–15; Zech 9:9; Joel 2:21.

39   See Gen 26:24; 28:15; Ruth 2:4; Judg 6:12; Jer 1:8, 19; 15:20. The phrase is a declaration, not a wish.

40   Barbara E. Reid, "Prophetic Voices of Elizabeth, Mary and Anna in Luke 1–2", in *New Perspectives on the Nativity*, ed. Jeremy Corley (London: T&T Clark, 2009), 38, understands this scene as Mary's prophetic call. Like the great prophets Moses and Jeremiah, she is full of questions and fear, but receives God's reassurance. Elizabeth A. Johnson, *Truly Our Sister. A Theology of Mary in the Communion of Saints* (London: Continuum, 2003), 248, maintains that the literary structure of the announcement of birth is the same as that of the commissioning of a prophet (Exod 3:1–14; Judg 6:11–24); she lists the same five elements as Lincoln above (n. 30). Carroll, *Luke*, 39, notes that Mary is troubled by the angel's greeting, not his appearance.

41   Hagar (Gen 16:11), Leah (Gen 30:13), the mother of Samson (Judg 13:24), and the mother of Samuel (1 Sam 1:20).

42   "Most High" is frequent in the LXX, and is used of God by Luke in 6:35 and 8:28; Jesus' origins and role transcend those of John.

43   As Brown points out (*Birth*, 310–311; *Coming*, 64), the parallels between vv. 32–33 and 2 Sam 7:9–16 are very close, (see Isa 9:7; Ps 89:3); Mary's child will be the Davidic Messiah; Lincoln, *Born of a Virgin?* 102, likewise notes the 2 Sam 7 background; the promises to David will be fulfilled. Green, *Luke*, 88, states that the connection with the expectation of a restored Davidic monarchy is unmistakable. Also, Fitzmyer, *Luke*, 1:348. Lincoln, *Born of a Virgin?* 102, believes that nothing in this suggests fulfilment by any other means than the normal way of conception.

44   Gen 46:27; Exod 19:3; Isa 8:17.

45   Byrne, *Hospitality*, 23.

46   Many explanations of a psychological nature have been put forward to explain Mary's question. The best explanation, however, is literary: it is a feature of the usual pattern and it allows the angel to explain more about the child's identity. Luke's message is Christological. For details, see Brown, *Birth*, 303–309; Fitzmyer, *Luke*, 1:348–350. Lincoln, *Born of a Virgin?* 103, notes the question of Abraham (Gen 17:17) and Sarah (Gen 18:12).

47   "The Holy Spirit" and "the power from the Most High" are synonymous. For Pentecost see Acts 1:8; see also Isa 32:15 and 1 Sam 16:13. Brown, *Birth*, 311–316, notes that the language here (v. 35) also has links with that used of the Davidic Messiah: the spirit comes upon the Davidic branch in Isa 11:1–2; the term "holy" is associated with the Davidic "shoot" in Isa 4:2–3; and there is a parallel between the "Son of God" and the "Son of the Most High" which echo the sonship of David in Ps 2:7 and 2 Sam 7:14. The terminology is not, however, primarily that of Old Testament prophecy, but that of New Testament preaching. The Spirit comes not on the Davidic king, but upon his mother. We are not dealing with the adoption of a Davidide by coronation as God's son, but the begetting of God's Son in the womb of Mary through God's creative

Spirit without human intercourse. We are dealing with early Christian formulations of Christology, in which Jesus is acclaimed as God's Son; this was linked originally with the resurrection (see Rom 1:3–4: "born of the seed of David, designated Son of God in power according to the Spirit through the resurrection"), moved backwards into the ministry (especially in the baptism and transfiguration scenes), and now moved further backwards to the Infancy Narrative. See also Fitzmyer, *Luke*, 1:340; Johnson, *Truly our Sister*, 252–53. Lincoln, *Born of a Virgin?* 103–4, is of the view that use of this Spirit and overshadowing language, also present in Isa, Exod, Acts, does not mean that the Spirit replaces any activity that humans would be expected to exercise. A Jew would not have considered it as a substitute for normal parenthood. However, talk of divine agency and of nothing being impossible to God has to be read as an explanation to Mary of how she will conceive shortly while she is still a virgin in her relationship with Joseph; a natural conception is thus not envisaged.

48   Gen 1:2; Exod 40:35; Num 9:18, 22; see Pss 91:4; 140:7.

49   Byrne, *Hospitality*, 24. McBride, *Luke*, 25–26, notes that a virginal conception has no precedent in Jewish thought. Such a conception through the power of the Holy Spirit points to Jesus' unique status. Caird, *Luke*, 52, points out that the Old Testament was familiar with the concept of divine fatherhood (Israel, David). In Jesus' ministry, he refers to God as "Father", expressing an intimate relationship of which he was aware. Luke is telling us that Jesus entered upon this status of sonship at his birth by a new creative act of the Spirit.

50   Levine, *Stories*, 99, maintains that "kinswoman" indicates Mary's priestly ancestry.

51   Gen 18:14. Lincoln, *Born of a Virgin?* 107–8, observes that if a barren woman can have a child, a virgin can conceive, even if unprecedented in Jewish scripture. Step parallelism would entail a greater miracle, but only Mary and the reader would be aware of a superior miracle. This is the traditional view. Mary's visit to Elizabeth emphasises her absence from Joseph. On pp. 108–115 he examines stories from the Greco-Roman world concerning miraculous conceptions so that the origins of subjects' future greatness can be traced to the gods, without a human father. Luke is aware of ancient biographical conventions. Lincoln also notes the significant differences.

52   Green, *Luke*, 91. Marshall, *Luke*, 71, notes that the term indicates a female relative, not necessarily a cousin; it may also suggest that Mary is of priestly descent. Also, Fitzmyer, *Luke*, 1:352, 344.

53   Reid, "Prophetic Voices", 39, stresses the risk involved when a prophet says "yes". With Mary, there is an undercurrent of upheaval and scandal, the problem of local suspicions, gossip, whisperings. Carroll, *Luke*, 43, writes: "Mary provides an authentic model of trust and obedience in response to God's initiative, anticipating her later role among the disciples of Jesus." Johnson, *Truly Our Sister*, 247, emphasises that Mary is a disciple in the existential sense that she heard the word of God and acted upon it.

54   Brown, *Birth*, 316–319, is of the opinion that Luke's portrait of Mary in this episode is shaped by his account of her in the ministry, and is consistent with it, as in the case of John the Baptist in the previous episode. Similarly, Fitzmyer, *Luke*, 1:341.

55   Johnson, *Truly Our Sister*, 250, who sees this episode as a prophetic vocation

story of a Jewish girl and her God, set within the traditions of her people struggling for freedom.

56   McBride, *Luke*, 27.

57   Fitzmyer, *Luke*, 1:335.

58   Johnson, *Truly Our Sister*, 254; on p. 258 she refers to an encounter in the solitude of one's heart before God, and a courageous response.

59   Johnson, *Truly Our Sister*, 254–256, discusses the problematic nature of "handmaid" (female slave) terminology in feminist and womanist theology. Mary is independent of patriarchy; her decision is a self-determining act of personal autonomy.

60   "Do not be afraid" introduces the message of the angel to the women at the empty tomb (Matt 28:5).

61   Green, *Luke*, 92.

62   Brown, *Birth*, 331, 341. The phrase can also be translated as "with eagerness".

63   The phrasing recalls 2 Sam 2:1. It was highly unusual for a young woman to wander round her own town unaccompanied, let alone make a lengthy journey. The idea of a journey is an important Lukan theme; journeys are often related to the fulfilment of God's purpose. See Green, *Luke*, 95; Nicholas King, "The Significance of the Inn for Luke's Infancy Narrative", in *New Perspectives*, ed. Jeremy Corley (London: T&T Clark, 2009), 71–73.

64   1 Sam 1:1.

65   Gen 19:14; 22:3.

66   For Eugene LaVerdiere, *Luke* (Dublin: Veritas, 1980), 23, in Mary the New Testament reaches out to the Old, transforms it, and gives it its ultimate significance. Johnson, *Truly Our Sister*, 259, notes that a conversation between two women is rare in the Bible; this story is gynocentric. Later, p. 263, the *Magnificat* is the longest passage put on the lips of a female speaker in the New Testament.

67   Gen 25:22

68   McBride, *Luke*, 29; Byrne, *Hospitality*, 25; Johnson, *Luke*, 41; Brown, *Birth*, 341.

69   Carroll, *Luke*, 46, maintains that Elizabeth is playing the part of a prophet.

70   The word used here is *eulogēmenos*, which is used to invoke on human beings the blessing of God; here the blessing has already been granted. (See Brown, *Birth*, 333). The fact that it is Elizabeth who blesses Mary indicates Jesus' superiority over John. Fitzmyer, *Luke*, 1.364, reminds us that for the Jewish mind a woman's greatness was measured by the children she bore; Mary therefore surpasses all others. Carroll, *Luke*, 46, observes that by pronouncing a blessing on Mary, Elizabeth assumes the posture of one higher in status (apt for an older and married woman), yet she does so only to give Mary the higher honour, as mother of Elizabeth's "Lord".

71   Jdt 13:18: "Blessed are you, daughter, ... among all women on earth"; in Judg 5:24, the prophet Deborah says: "Blessed among women be Jael"; in Deut 28:4, Moses tells the people: "Blessed shall be the fruit of your womb." Elizabeth speaks likewise as a prophet; Mary too has a salvific role. (See also Reid, "Prophetic Voices", 40).

72   2 Sam 6:9.

73   2 Sam 24:21. Green, *Luke*, 96, notes that in Mary's travelling to visit her relative, and in greeting her first, social conventions are turned upside-down, for she is the greater

one. This foreshadows the way in which her son, though recognised as "Lord", will live and serve. Carroll, *Luke*, 46, notes the irony of status reversal here, where the narrative pivots on the encounter between two women and the words they exchange,

74   Fitzmyer, *Luke*, 1:358.

75   Johnson, *Truly Our Sister*, 262, suggests that Elizabeth nurtures Mary, nourishing her confidence; they support each other. "The figure of Elizabeth stands as a moving embodiment of the wisdom that older women can offer younger ones, who, brave as they are, are just starting out on their journey through life."

76   Exod 3:5.

77   Tannehill, *Luke*, 53, observes that lowly Mary responds with praise, whereas Zechariah, a priestly man of status was tongue-tied, until later. The issue is one of faith. Johnson, *Truly Our Sister*, 263–64, notes Mary's connection with Miriam (Exod 15:2–21), Deborah (Judg 5:1–31), Hannah (1 Sam 2:1–10) and Judith (Jdt 16:1–17) who sang dangerous songs of salvation, victory songs of the oppressed. Similarly, Green, *Luke*, 101. In this way God's activity is extended into the past; what is happening in Mary's case is in continuity with what has gone before.

78   The Latin for "glorifies" or "magnifies". Some scholars have suggested that this canticle is more appropriate on the lips of Elizabeth; but the manuscript evidence overwhelmingly favours Mary. See McBride, *Luke*, 30; Caird, *Luke*, 56; Johnson, *Luke*, 41; Green, *Luke*, 96; Marshall, *Luke*, 78; Fitzmyer, *Luke*, 1:365–366. Brown, *Birth*, 334–336, provides a detailed treatment of the issues involved. Carroll, *Luke*, 48, believes that the narrative's structure requires a response from Mary to the praise expressed in Elizabeth's greeting, not a second statement from Elizabeth.

79   Tannehill, *Luke*, 54–55, discusses the two strophe poetic structure (personal part and social part), parallelism, alliteration, contrast, rhyme, and other poetic aspects of the hymn. Carroll, *Luke*, 48, opts for two strophes; the first refers to the singer, the second to Israel; each concludes with a reference to God's mercy.

80   1 Sam 2:1–2; see also Hab 3:18; Sir 51:1; Ps 35:9. For details of Old Testament background, see Brown, *Birth*, Table XII; Fitzmyer, *Luke*, 1:356–357; Levine, *Stories*, 100.

81   Carroll, *Luke*, 47, writes: "Drawing language from Jewish scripture, Mary celebrates the power and faithfulness of God, who has brought help to Israel, fulfilling ancient promises. ... Mary pictures divine deliverance as a dramatic reversal of power and fortune."

82   2:11; 2:30. Jesus later tells Zacchaeus: "today salvation has come to this house" (19:9).

83   See Acts 13:26; 28:28.

84   Fitzmyer, *Luke*, 1:367. Johnson, *Truly Our Sister*, 264–65, stresses that Mary is a peasant woman, one of the poor and lowly, a member of an oppressed people who experience redemption.

85   See Leah in Gen 29:32; 30:13 and Hannah in 1 Sam 1:11.

86   Fitzmyer, *Luke*, 1:367.

87   1:35, 37. See Zeph 3:17. Acts 2:22; 10:38 recognises such power at work in Jesus' ministry.

88   Acts 3:14; 4:27, 30.

89 See Hannah's canticle in 1 Sam 2:7–8. McBride, *Luke*, 30, refers to the hymn of a Cinderella people. Brown, *Birth*, 357, refers to Mary as the spokeswoman of the *anawim*, the faithful remnant of Israel who put their trust and hope in God. Carroll, *Luke*, 51, highlights the balanced series of six divine acts of either judgement or mercy. On p. 53 he maintains that Mary's song proclaims a social revolution and inverts conventional roles; it presents a charter of social transformation that Jesus will embrace in his ministry.

90 Green, *Luke*, 104. Reid, "Prophetic Voices", 40, observes that it is on Mary's lips that Luke first articulates a vision for a new world order.

91 Johnson, *Truly Our Sister*, 267, quotes Dietrich Bonhoeffer, "This is not the gentle, tender, dreamy Mary whom we sometimes see in paintings; this is the passionate, surrendered, proud, enthusiastic Mary who speaks out."

92 The normal aorist tense refers to the past; a 'prophetic' aorist refers to the future; a 'gnomic aorist' refers to the present.

93 Caird, *Luke*, 55. Marshall, *Luke*, 84, suggests that what God has now begun to do, and Mary regards prophetically as already having come to fruition, is described in terms of what God actually did in Old Testament times, as expressed in Israel's praise there.

94 Brown, *Birth*, 363. Luke is anticipating here the beatitudes and woes of the sermon on the plain (6:20–26). Throughout his Gospel he includes the teaching of Jesus which emphasises that wealth and power are not the true values (see 12:16–19; 16:25–26; 21:1–4). Green, *Luke*, 100, points out that the images of God's saving work are set within the larger narrative world of foreign occupation and religio-political oppression; Mary's vision of redemption should not be spiritualised as though unconnected with the social realities of daily existence. Also Marshall, *Luke*, 85; Brown, *Birth*, 363.

95 Mention of Abraham may suggest that God's saving presence could extend beyond Israel (see 3:8).

96 Johnson, *Luke*, 42, translates v. 54 as: "he has taken Israel his child by the hand, remembering his mercy." On p. 43, he notes that Mary has a representative and symbolic role for Israel.

97 Reid, "*Prophetic Voices*", 39, notes that it is not only a question of Mary helping Elizabeth; Elizabeth, the older woman who has lived with integrity and faithfulness despite the anguish and shame of being childless, also supports Mary like a wise mentor in these difficult days for her.

98 Brown, *Birth*, 346, stresses that literary structure is far more important than the psychology of the characters involved; we are not dealing with family history but the dramatisation of the theology of salvation history; Fitzmyer, *Luke*, 1:362. Carroll, *Luke*, 53, notes that Luke avoids cluttering a scene with characters; after focussing on the encounter between Mary and Elizabeth, he wishes to rivet attention on Elizabeth and Zechariah.

99 Brown, *Birth*, 346–355.

100 Noted without agreement by McBride, *Luke*, 28–29.

101 Borg & Crossan, *First Christmas*, 213, see the hymns as pre-Lukan Christian canticles. Fitzmyer, *Luke*, 1:357 holds that the *Magnificat* is from a pre-Lukan Jewish Christian source. Johnson, *Truly Our Sister*, 268, notes that an alternative view suggests

that the milieu of origin was not the religious life of the Jerusalem community, but the political struggle of the people of Palestine against their oppressors. The verbs denote strong action. The spiritual themes of the *Magnificat* have real economic and political resonance.

102   Brown, *Birth*, 352.

103   Brown, *Birth*, 354.

104   Reid, *"Prophetic Voices"*, 41. Johnson, *Truly Our Sister*, 269, notes how people in need in any society hear a blessing in this canticle (single parents, discarded elderly, abandoned youngsters, the homeless ...). On pp. 272–74, she explores some of the implications of the hymn for women seeking full participation in governance and ministry in the Church.

105   With regard to the Baptist the emphasis is on the naming; with Jesus, it is on the birth.

106   The description echoes Rebecca in Gen 25:24; the rejoicing recalls Sarah in Gen 21:6.

107   Circumcision was the sign of faithfulness to the covenant made by God with Abraham (Gen 17:9–14). It was enshrined in the Mosaic Law (Lev 12:3). The elderly couple are obedient.

108   The tense of the verb could be simple imperfect rather than conative ("they were trying to call").

109   Leonard J. Maluf, "Zechariah's 'Benedictus': A New Look at a Familiar Text", in *New Perspectives on the Nativity*, 50 ed. Jeremy Corley (London: T&T Clark, 2009), sees the neighbours as clinging to the patterns of their past. The parents embrace what is new and heaven-inspired. Reid, *"Prophetic Voices"*, 42, notes that Luke does not say how Elizabeth knew the name; she is attuned to God, and this is a prophetic word. Carroll, *Luke*, 55, n. 18, notes biblical precedent for the mother's naming of the child (Gen 19:37–38; 29:32–35; 30:6; 38:3–5).

110   Tannehill, *Luke*, 57; making signs to the father suggests he is deaf as well as mute.

111   Amazement and fear are typical reactions to the supernatural in Luke.

112   Zechariah will answer this question to some extent in the *Benedictus*.

113   Exod 6:1; 13:3; Acts 10:38; 11:21.

114   Green, *Luke*, 115, notes that the gift of the Spirit was often bestowed for the purpose of prophecy, which provided God's perspective on events. Carroll, *Luke*, 58, observes that the canticle offers praise to God and a reliable interpretation of the events being narrated; he is a reliable speaker, whose message can be trusted.

115   Marshall, *Luke*, 90. Tannehill, *Luke*, 58, notes that Zechariah's hymn focuses on the Messiah rather than John, and presupposes all that we have been told in the Infancy Narrative so far.

116   Byrne, *Hospitality*, 27, is of the view that this canticle offers the best summary of the theology of the Gospel. Green, *Luke*, 111, observes that Mary's canticle is linked with Elizabeth's response, and Zechariah's with those of the angels, shepherds and prophets. Brown, *Birth*, 379, links Zechariah's blessing with the earlier one of his wife; this scene, like the previous one, moves to termination with a canticle proclaiming what

God has done.

117   See Brown, *Birth*: introduction 68a; body 68b–77 (subdivided: 68b–71; 72–75; 76–77); conclusion 78–79. The insertion (vv. 76–77) is probably a Lukan addition to the original hymn. Some (McBride, *Luke*, 33; Marshall, *Luke*, 86) consider verses 76–79 to be a birthday hymn in honour of the child (a *genethliakon*). For a list of the Old Testament background, see Brown, *Birth*, Table X111, 386–389. Fitzmyer, *Luke*, 1:382, speaks of a canticle or hymn of praise; like Brown he sees its origin in a Jewish Christian context, whereas the earlier narrative is from a Baptist source. Maluf, *"Zechariah's 'Benedictus'"*, 49, holds that the passage is more a "prophetic proclamation" than a hymn. He divides the text into two sections: 68–75, and 76–79. He maintains that Luke himself composed the passage precisely for the context in which it appears. Carroll, *Luke*, 60, affirms "Zechariah's song, like Mary's, centres on God and God's ways with Israel."

118   Ps 41:14; 72:18; 106:48. Maluf, *"Zechariah's 'Benedictus'"*, 60, sees Exod 18:10 and 1 Kings 1:48 as more pertinent.

119   For judgement, see Exod 32:34; for saving, see Gen 21:1; Exod 4:31; Ruth 1:6; Ps 105:4. The NRSV translation ("looked favourably") loses this nuance. Tannehill, *Luke*, 59, comments that although God's inspection could result in judgement on a guilty people, the word often means that God is taking careful note of their need and responding to it. Carroll, *Luke*, 58, maintains that visitation and redemption express one idea: God has visited the people for the purpose of redeeming them. Zechariah envisages a divine visitation to save. Lincoln, *Born of a Virgin?* 53, adds Jer 29:10. For "redemption", he suggests Exod 15:13; Lev 25:8–55; Deut 7:8; Ps 111:9; Isa 43:1; 48:20.

120   1:78; 7:16; 19:44; Acts 7:23; 15:14.

121   Marshall, *Luke*, 90. Fitzmyer, *Luke*, 1:383, writes that Zechariah's words could refer to the past, but the Christological thrust of the first part of the canticle makes one realise that Zechariah is praising God for what He has done in the conception and coming birth of Jesus. Green, *Luke*, 116, refers to the experience of Sarah, and to the exodus, the paradigmatic act of deliverance from enemies (see Ps 106). Maluf, *"Zechariah's 'Benedictus'"*, 50, challenges the view that this is a messianic hymn. For him the text moves from a consideration of Israel's past, represented by the fathers of Israel (and father Zechariah), to a prophetic glimpse of Israel's future, represented by the child John, the forerunner of Christ, and prophet to a new generation of Israel at the dawn of the messianic age. The past tenses refer to past events in Israel's past as the primary focus. He concludes, p. 68, that the terms in vv. 68–75 never go beyond the Old Testament hope; they invoke the story and notion of salvation current in the Old Testament.

122   See Ps 18:3; 1 Sam 2:10; Ezek 29:21. Maluf, *"Zechariah's 'Benedictus'"*, 50–51, comments that the almost universally accepted view that vv. 68–75 refer to Christ and his saving mission stems from the interpretation of the "horn of salvation" as messianic, referring to Jesus. He, however, sees these verses as referring to Israel's past, and its traditional understanding of salvation.

123   Brown, *Birth*, 371. Maluf, *"Zechariah's 'Benedictus'"*, 51–59, claims that this phrase is not an allusion to Jesus; the image of brute strength and aggressive military might hardly fits the Messiah of compassion and peace. It is a reference to David and his house, through whom God provided protection and salvation for the people. Carroll, *Luke*, 59,

detects the replaying of notes sounded by Gabriel to Mary.

124   Tannehill, *Luke*, 59, maintains that it refers to the powerful king who will ascend David's throne, that is, the Messiah. Carroll, *Luke*, 59, n. 20, sees it as a messianic image in Hannah's prayer (1 Sam 2:10; Ps 131:17). Maluf, *"Zechariah's 'Benedictus'"*, 61, on the other hand, sees this as referring to salvation brought by God to David and his house later in Israel's history.

125   See this theme in Acts 1:16; 3:18; 4:25; 15:7. Carroll, *Luke*, 59, writes: "The salvation that Zechariah celebrates is the culmination of a story that began long ago."

126   See Ps 106:10; 18:18. Carroll, *Luke*, 59, says that salvation is a multivalent term, one that has both socio-political and religious dimensions.

127   Gen 22:16–18. See Acts 3:25; Gal 3:6–18. See Johnson, *Luke*, 46. With regard to God's "remembering", Lincoln, *Born of a Virgin?* 53–54, refers to Micah 7:20; Ps 106:45; Exod 2:24; Jer 11:5.

128   Fitzmyer, *Luke*, 1:384.

129   See Wis 9:3; Josh 24:14. There are echoes of exodus here.

130   Green, *Luke*, 117; Fitzmyer, *Luke*, 1:385; Brown, *Birth*, 372 (Exod 3:12; Deut 11:13). Maluf, *"Zechariah's 'Benedictus'"*, 65, reminds us that worship was part of the story of exodus and David, and a feature of the story of Joshua: "Israel worshipped the Lord all the days of Joshua and all the days of the elders ..." (Josh 24:29). Tannehill, *Luke*, 62, states that Zechariah's interpretation of the promise to Abraham is not narrow nationalism but a hope for religious freedom so that Israel can shape its own identity as the worshipping people of God.

131   Carroll, *Luke*, 60.

132   For Maluf, *"Zechariah's 'Benedictus'"*, 63, 66, the salvation-type of Israel's past history (especially the exodus and David's monarchy) took the form of the destruction of enemies. Now, by contrast, a new form of salvation is envisaged, consisting in forgiveness, reconciliation and peace.

133   Green, *Luke*, 118. This phrasing recalls Isa 40:3 (Mal 3:1, 23) and the Elijah figure spoken of in Mal 4:5; but it also anticipates the Gospel proper. Fitzmyer, *Luke*, 1:385, maintains that "Lord" here refers not to Yahweh, but to Jesus.

134   3:4; 7:27; 16:16.

135   3:3; 3:10–14. The phrase is first used in Mark 1:4.

136   4:18; 5:20,24; 7:48–49; 11:4; 17:4; 23:34; 24:47; Acts 2:38; 5:31; 10:43; 13:38; 26:18.

137   The word used here (*splangchna*) refers to one's innermost being; it can mean bowels, womb, guts.

138   The word is *anatolē*. The shoot of Jesse is found in Isa 11:1; a branch is found in Jer 23:5–6; Zech 6:12; and the star of Jacob in Num 24:17; see Matt 2:2, 9. Fitzmyer, *Luke*, 1:387, prefers shoot or scion with a messianic meaning. Jesus is the Davidic Scion sent by God. Tannehill, *Luke*, 62, believes this seems to be a designation for the Davidic Messiah, which means that verses 78–79 are no longer referring primarily to John the Baptist.

139   Marshall, *Luke*, 94; Johnson, *Luke*, 47; Maluf, *"Zechariah's 'Benedictus'"*, 56, n. 18; Fitzmyer, *Luke*, 1:388; Carroll, *Luke*, 57, favour the manuscript evidence for the future

tense; Brown, *Birth*, 373; Evans, *Luke*, 187, the past. Fitzmyer refers to the switch from past tenses earlier in the canticle to the eschatological future here. Carroll, *Luke*, 62, believes that the dawn that will come is probably the Messiah, whom God will send. The action and the purpose are God's.

140   Ps 106:10, 14 LXX. Green, *Luke*, 119, notes that "darkness" and "shadow" represent an arena of existence ruled by cosmic forces in opposition to God, a domain into which the light of God's redemptive presence is made to shine by the advent of God's agent, the "Dawn". Lincoln, *Born of a Virgin?* 54, notes that "dawn" is the term for the messianic heir to the throne of David (see Isa 60:1–3).

141   Ps 107:9–10; Isa 42:6–7; 9:2; 59:8. Evans, *Luke*, 188, speaks of an existence marked by wholeness and fullness of life. Tannehill, *Luke*, 62, says that the term refers to a social condition of harmony, prosperity and happiness, and would include salvation from our enemies, freedom of religion, and forgiveness of sin. As Carroll, *Luke*, 62, points out, however, it remains to be seen whether all the people will follow him on this road.

142   Green, *Luke*, 114–115, notes the bringing together of two concepts of salvation in this canticle: social/political and religious.

143   Brown, *Birth*, 383. He believes that the hymn was composed by Jewish Christians. They would be conversant with the martial language of their forebears; they see salvation as already accomplished through Jesus; they have the *anawim* mentality; the Christology is Jewish and early; in vocabulary and prophetic spirit there is a link with Luke's Jerusalem community in Acts.

144   Isaac ("the child grew up": Gen.21:8), Samson ("the child became mature, and the Lord blessed him; and the spirit of the Lord began to go with him": Judg 13:24–25 LXX), and Samuel ("and the child waxed mighty before the Lord": 1 Sam 2:21, 26).

145   Brown, *Birth*, 376–377.

Chapter Two
Bethlehem and Jerusalem

This chapter, which follows the sequence of Luke's original narrative, can be seen as a tale of two cities: Bethlehem, the city of David; and Jerusalem, the Holy City.

Bethlehem (2:1–21)

We have been reflecting on the first chapter of Luke's Gospel: the annunciation to Zechariah and then to Mary; the visitation, with the *Magnificat* canticle; and finally, the birth and naming of the future Baptist, concluding with the *Benedictus*. The latter forms a second diptych with the story of Jesus' birth and naming. The broad sequence of the two birth narratives is the same: birth, circumcision, naming. But whereas the narrative about John centres on the naming of the child, this second narrative focuses on the birth of Jesus. However, the main point of interest in the story is, in fact, the third angelic annunciation; in the subsequent final scene the various protagonists or characters (Mary, Joseph, the child, the shepherds and other folk) are brought together, and Luke dwells on their responses to what has taken place.[1]

The complete text reads as follows:[2]

In those days, a decree went out from Emperor Augustus that all the world should be registered. This was the first registration and was taken while Quirinius was governor of Syria. All went to their own towns to be registered. Joseph also went from the town of Nazareth in Galilee to Judea, to the city of David called Bethlehem, because he was descended from the house and family of David. He went to be registered with Mary, to whom he was engaged and who was expecting a child. While they were there, the time came for her to deliver her child. And she gave birth to her firstborn son and wrapped him in bands of cloth, and laid him in a manger, because there was no place for them in the inn.

In that region, there were shepherds living in the fields, keeping watch over their flock by night. Then an angel of the Lord stood before them, and the glory of the Lord shone around them, and they were terrified. But the angel said to them, "Do not be afraid; for see—I am bringing you good news of great joy for all the people: to you is born this day in the city of David a Saviour, who is the Messiah, the Lord. This will be a sign for you: you will find a child wrapped in bands of cloth and lying in a manger." And suddenly there was with the angel a multitude of the heavenly host, praising God and saying, "Glory to God in the highest heaven, and on earth peace among those whom he favours!"

When the angels had left them and gone into heaven, the shepherds said to one another, "Let us go now to Bethlehem and see this thing that has taken place, which the Lord has made known to us." So, they went with haste and found Mary and Joseph, and the child lying in the manger. When they saw this, they made known what had been told them about this child; and all who heard it were amazed at what the shepherds told them. But Mary treasured all these words and pondered them in her heart. The shepherds returned, glorifying and praising God for all they had heard and seen, as it had been told them.

After eight days had passed, it was time to circumcise the child; and he was called Jesus, the name given by the angel before he was conceived in the womb.

The Setting and Birth (2:1–7)

The Census (1–5)

Luke begins this stage of his story with an elaborate setting,[3] that of an imperial census ordered by Augustus (emperor from 30 or 27 BCE to 14 CE) and conducted by Quirinius, the governor of Syria, the main Roman province of the region. This affects Joseph in that he is obliged to return from Nazareth in Galilee, where he is living, to his ancestral city, Bethlehem.[4] It is while he is there that Mary, who has accompanied him, gives birth to Jesus.

The census, which is mentioned four times, thus makes it possible for Jesus to be born in Bethlehem, the place of promise. But the setting has other purposes. It provides a solemn beginning for the story of Jesus, emphasising the cosmic and universal significance of his birth. His birth is an event that touches the whole world, not simply Israel, as in the case of John. Through his edict, the emperor is unwittingly serving God's plan, as Cyrus did in the Old Testament; Augustus is subservient to a greater purpose and sovereignty.[5] Later, the new religion inaugurated by Jesus will spread to the confines of the empire and beyond. Perhaps Luke saw it as significant that Jesus was born in the reign of Augustus, the emperor who finally brought an era of peace after a century of war (the *pax romana)*. He was popularly called the "saviour of the world", and accorded honours appropriate to the divine.[6] Luke challenges this statement. It is the child whose birth he is about to describe who brings real peace and is the world's true saviour, as the *Benedictus* celebrated.

From a historical point of view, there are problems with this introduction.[7] There is no other evidence that Augustus ordered a census of his world. He did, however, accumulate a lot of statistics for taxation purposes, possibly as a result of more local provincial censuses. A census was a symbol of Roman overlordship, a reminder that Israel was a conquered people. Quirinius, the Roman legate in Syria, was indeed responsible for a census in Judea, probably for taxation purposes, but that was ten years later, coinciding with the deposing of Archelaus and the annexation of Judea. It did not apply to Galilee.[8] This problem seems to have no definitive conclusion. Scholars tend to take the census as a Lukan literary device to explain the presence of Mary and Joseph in Bethlehem and consider it to be based on "confused memory". Nor had the evangelist access to the relevant information available to the contemporary historian. "We are dealing, not with a scientifically determined chronology, but with purposeful storytelling".[9] The Roman system did not demand enrolment in one's ancestral city but one's place of residence.[10] It is not clear why Mary had to go as well, and it is uncertain whether she was required to register. Joseph may have wished to secure her protection, given the nature of her pregnancy, and was afraid to leave her alone at home in Nazareth; he wanted them to be together for the birth.[11]

Luke, according to most manuscripts, uses the term "betrothed". This is probably intended to suggest that the marriage had not been consummated, though presumably they were now living together. It indicates subtly that Joseph is not the child's father, which links with the earlier narrative. His Davidic descent and his roots in Bethlehem are emphasised.[12]

The Birth of Jesus (6–7)

The vastness of imperial Rome and the biblical context of the Royal House of David are in strong contrast with the humble event of this child's birth. God reverses normally accepted values, as we saw in the *Magnificat*.

The "fulfilment of the days" refers both to the gestation period and the angelic announcement as God's plan unfolds.[13] There is no indication of the length of time spent in Bethlehem prior to the birth of Mary's child, but a period of time is implied. The evangelist simply and soberly states the fact that "while they were there, she gave birth to a son".[14] The child is said to be her "firstborn", fulfilling the angel's announcement. Some take this to imply that she had other children later, the "brothers and sisters" referred to during the ministry. But the word "firstborn" does not demand this. What is important for the evangelist is that Jesus, as the firstborn, must be presented in the temple and consecrated to God, and that he should receive the position and privileges that tradition gave to the firstborn: the birthright and Davidic inheritance.[15]

Mary performs two actions for the newly born child: she "wrapped him in swaddling clothes" and she "laid him in a manger". Swaddling consisted in wrapping linen strips like bandages around the child's limbs to ensure that they would grow straight, and was a normal expression of parental care. Rather than an indication of poverty and lowliness, as some suggest, the detail is probably intended to recall the description of Solomon's swaddling in the book of Wisdom,[16] and so is not incompatible with the child's royal Davidic background. The word translated "manger" (*phatnē*) can refer to an open feeding area or a trough for feeding cattle, which could be movable or be a cavity shelf in the rock. It can also mean a stall where cattle are tied up. Many scholars see this as an indication of poverty and humility: at his birth, Jesus had to accept the habitation of animals. The detail of the manger probably holds symbolic significance, for it is repeated three times and is referred to as a sign. One suggestion is that it recalls Isaiah 1:3: "The ox knows its owner and the donkey its master's crib; Israel does not know, my people do not understand." This situation is partly reversed or repealed by the later coming of the shepherds, as Israel begins to find its way back to God, and begins to know the manger of the Lord, but the challenge remains.[17] Incidentally, there is no specific mention of the animals in Luke; given the situation described, it can be presumed. Their appearance at the crib is a later, longstanding and not inappropriate development.

Luke makes an explanatory comment that there was no room for them in the *katalyma*. This word is open to a variety of interpretations, and precision is difficult to achieve. It can indicate a place where a traveller lays down his baggage when stopping over while on a journey. Its basic meaning is a guest room.[18] Traditionally, it has been taken to be an inn, like a khan or caravansary, where large numbers found shelter under one roof. There were two levels: one for people and one for the animals. The traditional view is that Luke's idea would be that the hostel was full, presumably because of the influx of travellers caused by the census. Maybe because of overcrowding, courtyard space normally kept for the animals was brought into use. So, some vague word like living space or lodging is probably best.[19]

Kenneth Bailey is critical of this traditional view.[20] He notes that Joseph was returning to his village of origin. In the Middle East, historical memories are long, and the extended family, with its connection to its village of origin, is important. Joseph could have appeared in the village and told people he was son of Heli, son of Matthat etc., and most homes would have been open to him. He was also from the family of King David, and the village was known locally as the city of David. Being of the Davidic family, Joseph would have been welcome anywhere in town.

In every culture, a woman about to give birth is given special attention. Rural communities always assist their women in childbirth, regardless of the circumstances. The Bethlehem community would have sensed its responsibility to find adequate shelter and provide the care needed. To turn away a descendant of David in such circumstances would be an unspeakable shame on the village. Mary also had relatives in a nearby village. If Joseph had been unsuccessful in Bethlehem, they would have gone to Zechariah and Elizabeth. Joseph had time to make necessary arrangements. The text does not indicate that the child was born the night they arrived. This myth dates from the Protoevangelium of James, who was not a Jew, did not understand Palestinian geography or Jewish tradition, and wrote 200 years after the birth of Jesus.

In traditional Middle Eastern villages, simple village homes had two rooms. One was for guests, which would be attached to the end of the house or on the roof.[21] The main room was the family room in which the entire family cooked, ate, slept and lived. The end of the room next to the door was either a few feet lower than the rest of the floor or blocked off with heavy timbers. Each night, into that designated area, the family cow, donkey and a few sheep would be driven. And every morning those same animals were taken out and tied up in the courtyard of the house. The animal stall would then be cleaned for the day. Such homes traced back to the time of David and up to the mid-twentieth century (3,000 years). The peasant wants the animals in the house for warmth in winter and because they are safe from theft. The mangers, perhaps two of them, were dug out of the lower end of the living room; this was sloped in the direction of the animal area, which aids sweeping and washing. If a cow is hungry at night, it can stand up and eat from a manger. Mangers for sheep were made of wood and placed on the floor of the lower level.[22]

Current popular tradition demands an inn with a "no vacancies" sign! But the Greek does not refer to a room in an inn; it simply means "space" in the *katalyma*. This is not the ordinary word for a commercial inn, which is *pandocheion*, as in the story of the Good Samaritan, meaning "receive all"; *katalyma* is simply a place to stay. Later in Luke's Gospel it is a guest room, upstairs, used for the Last Supper.[23] So, Luke says that Jesus was placed in a manger in the family room because in that home the guest room was already full.[24]

The Annunciation to The Shepherds (2:8–14)

The Message and Sign (8–12)

The second half of the episode centres around the angelic annunciation to the shepherds, an incident of role reversal.

Shepherds were not too highly regarded at the time. They were peasants, poor and marginalised. Rabbinic traditions label them as unclean, possibly because flocks ate private property.[25] In post New Testament times they were on lists of proscribed trades; perhaps such ideas were alive in Jesus' time. They were close to the bottom of the social scale in their society. They had a reputation for petty theft; they were partial to pasturing their sheep on other people's land; they tended to be neglectful of religious observance; they were not permitted to function as legal witnesses.[26] They would therefore be classed among the lowly ones, forerunners of the many ordinary folk who will encounter Jesus later during his ministry, the "poor" to whom the Gospel will be preached.[27] From the outset, Jesus is part of their world, and in this way his mission is anticipated. They gather to see the descendant of David, who in the tradition was the shepherd of the flock of Israel; his messianic successor was also to be a shepherd-leader.[28] The shepherds are also outside the circle of Jesus' family. The contrast with the emperor and powerful is strong; the Good News comes to poor shepherds not the rulers or urban elite.

In the narrative, a group of such shepherds are keeping night guard over their sheep in the fields, probably watching in shifts.[29] More importantly, the darkness stands in contrast with the coming light of God's glory, the sign of God's presence.[30] Some scholars note that their being out in the open suggests that winter is over; others point out that the place traditionally associated with the shepherds' fields is below the snowline. Really there is nothing in the narrative to indicate clearly the time of year.

There follows a third angelic annunciation, structured according to the basic pattern, though here it concerns a birth that has already taken place. An angel, probably Gabriel again, stands over the shepherds, and the glory of the Lord shines round about them.[31] The term "glory" usually refers to God's presence in majesty, sometimes considered visible in the form of a bright light.[32] The initial reaction of the shepherds is, as is to be expected, intense terror. The angel bids them to lay aside their fear, substituting it with great joy, which is also a feature of Chapter One, as we have seen. He then proceeds to impart joyful news for them and for all the people. Many think that "people" here probably refers only to Israel; others, however, maintain that it has a universalist meaning.[33] This joyful news[34] is densely expressed: "Today in the town of David a Saviour has been born to you; he is Christ the Lord."

"Today" can be taken literally, but may also have an eschatological ring: it denotes the long-awaited day of salvation, on which are fulfilled the hopes of centuries. Luke frequently emphasises the 'now' of God's deliverance. The term "Saviour" is rare in the New Testament and is found only here in the Synoptics and twice in Acts (5:31; 13:23). At the time, gentiles were looking for a saviour, and the term was applied to the emperor and other Hellenistic rulers and was used in the mystery cults. The Jewish background, however, is strong: the Jews longed for a king to liberate them from oppression. In the Old Testament, it is God who is the saviour. Luke believes that God is now acting through Jesus in order to save.[35]

The child is given the titles "Messiah" and "Lord", an unusual combination without the article. In the Septuagint "Lord" is used of God. Luke uses it frequently of Jesus during the ministry. In Isaiah 9:1–7, the interpretive context, we find the Good News that a child is born to the people, a son given; a list of names or titles follows: wonderful counsellor, everlasting father, prince of peace. For these titles, Luke substitutes titles from the Christian kerygma: Saviour, Christ, Lord, titles usually associated with the resurrection.[36] At this stage, the full meaning and implications of these titles is not evident.

Without their asking, a normal item in annunciation narratives, the shepherds are given a sign. Paradoxically, the child proclaimed in such exalted terms is to be found in extremely lowly conditions. They will recognise him by the swaddling clothes and manger. The discovery will point to the validity of what has been said about his significance for the future of the people.[37]

Initially, the shepherds were afraid of the angels. Then, because they were asked to visit the child, they expected to be rejected by the parents if he was the Messiah.[38] The angels tell them that they would find him in an ordinary peasant home like their own, not in a governor's mansion. The manger was a sign for lowly shepherds. They must have found the family in perfectly adequate accommodation, otherwise they would have moved them to their own homes. The honour of the village rested on their shoulders. They obviously felt that they could not offer better hospitality than had already been made available.

The Angels and their Canticle (13–14)

At this point, the annunciation pattern is disrupted by the appearance of an immense throng of the heavenly hosts, army or entourage.[39] They sing the praises of God. The *Sanctus* canticle in Isaiah probably served Luke as an antecedent. "Glory" in 2:9 referred to the visible manifestation of God's majesty; here it means the honour which angels and men pay to God in recognition of his majesty, transcendence and gracious mercy.[40] On earth it is the gift of peace that the angels celebrate. Peace here does not mean the cessation of violence, a peace of the kind introduced by Augustus. It means the full sum of blessings associated with the coming of the Messiah, as prophesied by Zechariah, scriptural *shalom*, which indicates peace with justice, universal healing.[41] In particular, it connotes the healing of man's estrangement from God, the forgiveness of sins, the establishment of a loving relationship between God and humankind, which introduces inner harmony and better human relationships. This promise of peace and well-being is offered to those favoured by God, those with whom God is pleased, those on whom God's redemptive mercy has been bestowed. Some understand this as suggesting the universal implications of Jesus' coming, since the Good News is for "all people", not just Israel.[42] God's mercy is inclusive; *shalom* is for the cosmos. Again, there is the sense of God's saving freedom and choice.

There is an echo of this hymn on the disciples' lips later in the Gospel when Jesus enters the city of Jerusalem: "Peace in heaven and glory in the highest heavens!"[43]

The Reactions (2:15–20)

The final part of Luke's narrative provides us with various responses to what has taken place. There is the initial response of the shepherds to the angels' message, and then a threefold response: from the crowd, from Mary, and from the shepherds again.

The Shepherds (15–17)

On the return of the angels to heaven, which brings the annunciation structure to its conclusion, the shepherds express their belief that they have received a revelation from God through the angel, and they respond positively in obedience by going over to Bethlehem with haste, like Mary earlier.[44] The 'little ones' are open and responsive. No details of their search are provided, but there they find Mary and Joseph (in that order, which is significant in that culture) and the cradled child. What was promised is now fulfilled. They tell their story to the couple and, as we learn shortly, to others around, informing them of what has happened and what the angel has told them. The shepherds were made welcome at the manger; the unclean were judged to be clean; the outcasts became honoured guests; the song of the angels was sung to the simplest of all.[45]

Three Further Responses (18–20)

Luke then provides three reactions to the revelation of God's saving mystery in the child: the response of the audience, of Mary, and of the shepherds. In parallel with the relatives and neighbours in the earlier Baptist story, the others present at the birthplace, who hear what the shepherds have to say, react with wonder and astonishment. A similar reaction has occurred at the circumcision and naming of John. Here, however, there is no indication of further interest; amazement is not faith, nor is it a guarantee of real understanding.

Mary, who stands in pivotal position at the centre of this threefold structure, treasures these things and ponders them in her heart, as had Elizabeth's neighbours at John's naming. This phrase about pondering in her heart, which is again applied to Mary in the later episode in the temple,[46] is an expression found frequently in revelation and apocalyptic contexts in the Old Testament as a response to something mysterious, which is beyond human comprehension and control. Mary does not fully understand what God is doing in her life; she reflects in order to grasp the full meaning of it all; she is open to God's action and awaits the developments of God's purposes in God's time. She alone appears in the later ministry period, where she is presented by Luke as a believer and as a disciple, a form of response that she has already initiated. Things will become clearer only with the coming of the Spirit at Pentecost.[47]

The shepherds leave and return to their flocks, praising and glorifying God, their part in the story completed, rather like the Magi in the Matthaean story. They have linked what they have heard with what they have seen and have made known to others what was made known to them, thus being in a sense the first evangelists. They represent for Luke the future believers, who will likewise praise God for what they have heard and seen, an earthly praise which echoes that of the angels in heaven.

Circumcision and Naming (2:21)

Observing the pattern of events followed in his treatment of the story of John the Baptist, Luke next mentions the circumcision of the child Jesus eight days later, which underlines his solidarity with the human situation and his identification with his people.[48] The evangelist's main emphasis, however, is not on the circumcision but on the naming of the child in accordance with the command of the angel to Mary. Jesus' name is thus given by God. The obedience of Mary and Joseph to God's word is also illustrated. It comes as a surprise that the meaning of the name Jesus, 'Yahweh saves', is not explicitly underlined, in spite of that role being mentioned earlier and the fact that it is a key Lukan theme.

Reflections

A newborn child is a source of wonder and joy and is also the epitome of human dependency and need. As we gaze at the manger and the swaddled babe, taking in the atmosphere of the place in Bethlehem where Earth and heaven meet, we are overwhelmed by a God of such bewildering humility and self-giving love. Like Mary, we are confronted with so much to ponder in our hearts, encouraged to reflect at length about the meaning of it all. Unlike the youthful mother Mary, we, centuries later, know in advance what the outcome will be when her child becomes a man. In Domenico Ghirlandaio's nativity in the Church of Santa Trinità in Florence, the babe lies in a sarcophagus filled with hay. "The one laid in a manger at his nativity is destined to be laid in a tomb ... , a tomb that will become the gateway to life."[49] At his final meal with his disciples, Jesus will take a loaf of bread, give thanks to the Father, break it and give it to his disciples, with the words: "This is my body, which is given for you." And as the disciples subsequently argue as to which of them is the greatest, Jesus will say with emphasis: "I am among you as one who serves."[50] Cradle and cross are closely linked; the humility, generosity and self-giving love witnessed in the manger reaches a climax on Calvary's hill. But for Mary in Bethlehem, there is the immense joy of now being a mother. We can never thank her enough for having brought Jesus into our world.

As we ponder Luke's Christmas scene in gratitude and wonder, we cannot escape the stark invitation to embrace Jesus' humble servant, self-giving lifestyle, which is his revelation of the self-giving servant God. In almost every section of the Infancy Narrative, we have seen how Luke's God turns our human expectations, attitudes and presuppositions upside-down. A God of compassion and faithful love, he is a God of freedom and surprises. The greatest surprise remains the depth of God's love for us, his reaching out to draw us into his embrace.

The hillside shepherds in the storyline, on recovering from their initial shock at the angel's message of revelation, make their speedy journey to Bethlehem to find the child. They tell their story to Mary and Joseph and the others who are present. They are bearers of the "good news" brought by the angel. Like them, we are called to leave the crib and journey on to make known to others the ongoing, daily significance of the Christmas event. Our lives are meant to be "good news" for those we encounter in the wide variety of circumstances of a typical day. We take with us the joy of knowing God's unfathomable love and offer of salvation in Jesus. Another journey begins, the journey into mission, midwife-like, helping the birthing of Jesus in people's lives.

Jerusalem (2:22–52)

For the next two episodes that we shall consider, the scene changes from Bethlehem, the place where Jesus was born and given his name, to Jerusalem and its temple, the heart of Israel, some five miles (8 km) away.[51] The temple was understood as the locus of the presence of God with Israel, the centre of Israel's piety and nationhood. The temple has already featured in Luke's narrative as the place where the angel appears to Zechariah and announces the birth of the forerunner of Jesus. It is the place where our story begins. Twelve years later, the Nazareth family will visit the temple again, and this occasion will be the topic of our second reflection. The temple will later serve as the context for Jesus' preaching in the days before his death and will remain as a focal point for the nascent Christian community after the resurrection and the gift of the Spirit.

The Presentation of Jesus in The Temple (2:22–38)

The storyline reads as follows:

> When the time came for their purification according to the law of Moses, they brought him up to Jerusalem to present him to the Lord (as it is written in the law of the Lord, 'Every firstborn male shall be designated as holy to the Lord'), and they offered a sacrifice according to what is stated in the law of the Lord, 'a pair of turtle-doves or two young pigeons.' Now there was a man in Jerusalem whose name was Simeon; this man was righteous and devout, looking forward to the consolation of Israel, and the Holy Spirit rested on him. It had been revealed to him by the Holy Spirit that he would not see death before he had seen the

Lord's Messiah. Guided by the Spirit, Simeon came into the temple; and when the parents brought in the child Jesus, to do for him what was customary under the law, Simeon took him in his arms and praised God, saying,

"Master, now you are dismissing your servant in peace,
according to your word;
for my eyes have seen your salvation,
which you have prepared in the presence of all peoples,
a light for revelation to the Gentiles
and for glory to your people Israel."

And the child's father and mother were amazed at what was being said about him. Then Simeon blessed them and said to his mother Mary, "This child is destined for the falling and the rising of many in Israel, and to be a sign that will be opposed so that the inner thoughts of many will be revealed—and a sword will pierce your own soul too." There was also a prophet, Anna the daughter of Phanuel, of the tribe of Asher. She was of a great age, having lived with her husband for seven years after her marriage, then as a widow to the age of eighty-four. She never left the temple but worshipped there with fasting and prayer night and day. At that moment she came, and began to praise God and to speak about the child to all who were looking for the redemption of Jerusalem.

When they had finished everything required by the law of the Lord, they returned to Galilee, to their own town of Nazareth. The child grew and became strong, filled with wisdom; and the favour of God was upon him.

The episode divides into four sections: the setting, the meeting with Simeon, the prophecy of Anna, the return to Nazareth.

The Setting (22–24)

Joseph and Mary have already complied with Roman law in making the journey to Bethlehem for the census. Now, after the circumcision of their son, as pious Jews they seek to fulfil the requirements of the Law of Moses. The evangelist stresses their obedience.[52] "Here we glimpse Mary, a young daughter of Israel, now decidedly part of a married, parenting couple, growing into the long line of mothers in Israel, celebrating her childbirth in accordance with prescribed ritual."[53]

First, the parents were required to present their firstborn son to the Lord. Since God's sparing of the firstborn of Israel at the time of the exodus, firstborn boys were considered to belong to God, the source of all life (see Exod 13:1, 11–16). The firstborn of the flock or herd had to be offered in sacrifice. The firstborn male child was to be dedicated to God. The tribe of Levi fulfilled this requirement, and the other tribes were allowed to ransom or redeem their children by paying to a priest an amount of money: five shekels (Num 8:15–16). This could, in fact, be paid without bringing the child to the sanctuary, and this seems to have been the normal custom.[54]

Secondly, the mother was deemed ritually unclean after childbirth. After a week's strict segregation leading up to the child's circumcision, she spent a month (thirty-three days to be exact) unable to participate in religious services (Lev 12:1–8). After these forty days, she was expected to present herself to the priest at the Nicanor Gate of the Court of the Women, and offer for her purification a yearling lamb and a turtle dove or pigeon as burnt offering and sin offering. For the poor, the lamb could be commuted to a second dove or pigeon (Lev 12:6–8). In his narrative, Luke seems to have conflated or confused the two ceremonies; he was probably unaware of Jewish legal intricacies.[55] He speaks of "their" purification, though the Law referred only to the mother. The parents of Jesus make the required offering of the poor; "their very offering reveals their social location at the insignificant lower ranks of society."[56] No mention is made of any ransom for Jesus; probably, Luke intends us to understand that Jesus is now totally consecrated to God, dedicated to God's service; he is "holy", according to the angel's earlier message (1:35).

Again, there are strong echoes of the story of Samuel, which Luke is using as a model. After his conception and birth, Hannah brings him to the sanctuary at Shiloh and offers him for the Lord's service. The aged Eli blesses them. There is also a reference to women ministering at the door. The episode concludes with the growth refrain (1 Sam 1:24–28). [57]

The Encounter with Simeon (25–35)

The main thrust of Luke's narrative is to be found in the meeting between the family and Simeon, an event reminiscent of the story of Hannah, Elkinah and the child Samuel (1 Sam 1:24–28). Simeon is described as upright or righteous, like Zechariah and Elizabeth (1:6) and Joseph (Matt 1:19), and devout or careful about religious observance. He "looked forward to the consolation of Israel."[58] Simeon is typical of the faithful poor of Israel, steeped in God's promises to his people; he "personifies faithful and expectant Israel."[59] He is a man profoundly open to the Holy Spirit. The Spirit is said to "rest on him", and the presence of the Spirit finds threefold expression. First, the Spirit has revealed to him that he will not see death until he sets eyes on "the Christ of the Lord".[60] Secondly, it is through the Spirit's prompting that he comes to the temple area (*hieron*) that day.

And thirdly, on taking the child in his arms and recognising in him the fulfilment of his dreams and of God's promise, he bursts forth in prophecy.[61]

Simeon's words fall into two parts: the brief canticle *Nunc Dimittis* (29–32), and his prophecy concerning the future of the child with its implications for the mother (33–35).[62] Like the other hymns that we have considered, the *Nunc Dimittis* is heavily influenced by the Old Testament, especially Isaiah (40:1–5; 42:6; 46:13; 49:6; 52:9–10; 56:1; 60:1).[63] It begins implicitly with praise and then rehearses the motives for this. Simeon's message is rooted in God's purpose expressed in scripture, especially the Isaian vision of divine restoration and healing; it emphasises the universalistic outreach of God's salvation, and it points to the image of the Isaian Servant of Yahweh as a fundamental scriptural metaphor for interpreting the mission of Jesus as a whole.[64] Before pronouncing his hymn, Simeon blesses Mary and Joseph.[65]

The initial "now" of the canticle is emphatic, an indication that the time of salvation has dawned. Simeon uses the language of Master and servant (or slave: *doulos*), which expresses his dependency and allegiance, his fundamental poverty of spirit.[66] He recognises in a moving expression of faith that God has fulfilled his word of promise, a theme so typical of Luke. In joyful acknowledgement of God's faithfulness to him personally, and the realisation of his dreams, Simeon is content to be dismissed, to be released from service; he is ready to die. The phrasing combines the sentiment of joy experienced by the watchman with the feelings of one about to die (Gen 15:15), like Israel when he sees his long-lost son (Gen 46:30).[67] As one of those favoured by God, he experiences that deep peace of which the angels sang (2:14) and Zechariah spoke (1:79) and for which the prophets longed (Ps 72:7; Zech 8:12; Isa 9:5–6). He is aware that the child in his arms is the embodiment of God's salvation. Later, Jesus will say: "Blessed are the eyes which see what you see" (10:23). At another level, Simeon is speaking in a representative role on behalf of all that has gone before, the whole long economy of the Old Testament, the hopes of his people articulated for centuries. God's history has now reached its turning point, the past can now recede in peace, and a new era is beginning.

This salvation God has made ready "in the sight of the nations" (Isa 52:10), a term which here means both Israelites and gentiles, widening the vision. His thought reaches out beyond his own personal joy to proclaim the child's significance for the wider world, a pattern observed in the other canticles that we have seen. The child will bring deliverance not only to the people of Israel, as in Zechariah's canticle (1:68), but, surprisingly, he will be a light, a source of revelation also to the gentiles. And through this action of God, Israel will be vindicated and brought to the glory of her national destiny.[68] Simeon here mentions the gentiles before Israel; "there is a note of reversal, boundaries being extended, salvation widely cast."[69]

The response of the parents to these words about the child is one of wonder, typical of this kind of story.[70] This wonder probably includes the revealing of the significance of the child for the nations. "The Holy Spirit enables prophets to discern the ways of God, but it is sometimes difficult for even faithful, devout persons to comprehend."[71] The old man then blesses them, and looking prophetically into the future, he addresses Mary in words that cast a deep shadow across the joy of all that has preceded.[72] The child is destined "for the fall and for the rise" of many in Israel; he will be a sign that will be opposed. His presence will be the occasion for conflict. This will produce a twofold result: the secret thoughts of many will be laid bare, and Mary's own soul will be pierced by a sword.[73] The comment about Mary seems inserted as a parenthesis interrupting the flow of Simeon's warning.

While the falling and rising can be understood of the same persons in sequence,[74] which will be the experience of the disciples, and perhaps other members of the Jewish people, the statement most probably implies two groups of people. Some will respond to Jesus positively; others, the majority in fact, will find his message and style challenging and unacceptable, and will reject him and the God in whose name he comes, and later the Christian mission. He is a sign from God, a sign which will be contradicted.[75] Jesus will meet with opposition. The way in which people respond will reveal their inner thoughts and dispositions.

Mary herself, as a member of her people, will "also" be caught up in this drama and experience its pain. A sword will pierce her soul, her whole being (Ezek 14:17). The salvation that her child will bring demands openness to God's ways. She has already shown such openness, but more will be required of her. She will know anguish at the struggle of her son and the experience of contradiction, opposition and rejection that he will endure. She will have to cope with uncertainty and puzzlement in her journey of faith, her journey into discipleship. Like all members of the natural family of Jesus, she will have to pass the test of hearing God's word and doing God's will (8:19–21), she cannot be spared the sword.[76] There is perhaps also the special anguish caused by having to let her son go, recognising that the Father has prior claims, a pain first encountered in the next scene.[77] Like Mary, the reader is left puzzled, mulling over Simeon's words, wondering how this opposition will unfold.[78]

The Prophecy of Anna (36–38)

The atmosphere and mood again change as the elderly Anna arrives on the scene, and the negative note recedes. For her, like Zechariah, "vibrant hope coincides with long experience of delay in the fulfilment of God's promises."[79] Luke again pairs a man and a woman. She is a prophetess (like Sarah, Miriam, Hannah, Deborah, Esther and a few others in Israel's past). Her arrival "just at that moment" is, implicitly, divinely inspired. It is not clear whether she is eighty-four years old or eighty-four years a widow, which would make her 105 years old.[80] In either case, her advanced age brings respect and is understood as a sign of God's favour. She is described as spending all her time in the temple area; while perhaps hyperbolic and not to be taken too literally, this is clearly a sign of her dedication to God and as devoting herself night and day to fasting and prayer, which are the classic indications of deep Jewish piety (see also Acts 26:7).[81] She is thus open to God's Spirit, and with prophetic insight she breaks into praise of God in parallel with Simeon (and perhaps as the second official and valid witness to the significance of Jesus as required by Deut 19:15) and the Bethlehem angels. She recognises the significance of the child, and, like the shepherds earlier, proclaims publicly her insight about the child to all awaiting the messianic deliverance of Jerusalem, which means in effect the whole of Israel (Isa 52:9).[82] Along with Simeon, Anna is a symbol of the people of God that welcomes Jesus. From such as these he will gather a new people—those in Israel who will "rise".

As one who embodies the ideals and piety of the *anawim*, Anna is also to be seen as a forerunner of the Jerusalem community as it is described in Acts, where it is characterised by prayer and daily attendance in the temple (Acts 2:42, 46), and the Antioch community, noted for fasting, and the presence of the Spirit (Acts 13:2). Together with Simeon, she anticipates the atmosphere of Acts and Pentecost (see Acts 2:17). Widowhood was an ideal in the early Christian communities, as witnessed by Acts 6:1; 9:39, 41. Many of the aspects of widowhood mentioned in 1 Tim 5:3–16 match the situation of Anna. While Luke may have been influenced by contemporary Christian widowhood, he may also have drawn on some Old Testament background. Judith (in the second century BCE) did not remarry when her husband died. She observed the Law and fasted. After delivering Israel from its enemies, she expressed her thanks to God in a hymn of praise and lived on to the age of 105.[83]

As well as echoes of the Old Testament, there are echoes of earlier themes evident in the Infancy Narrative (like exemplary piety, the presence and inspiration of the Spirit, hope for deliverance, joy and praise, peace, saviour), but the clearest emphases are the universal reach of God's salvation and the opposition to the mission of Jesus which will ensue.[84]

The Return to Nazareth and Growth Refrain (39–40)

Having fulfilled their religious obligations, the family now returns to Nazareth in Galilee, which will be the place from which Jesus will begin his saving ministry in later life. This detail parallels the ending of the John the Baptist narrative (1:80). The faithful obedience of Mary and Joseph and the centrality of God in their lives provide the context in which the child will grow up.[85] In Nazareth, Jesus grows to maturity, a motif found in the Old Testament concerning Isaac, Samson and Samuel.[86] He is filled with wisdom, which in Jewish thought is akin to being filled with the Spirit (see 11:49); and the favour of God rests with him (4:22). This verse technically brings the Infancy Narrative to an end, since the next episode concerns the boy Jesus.[87]

Reflections

Luke's story began with an elderly couple, who were good, prayerful people burdened with the pain and shame of being childless. God's gracious and dramatic intervention changed that. The Infancy Narrative proper ends with two more elderly people, also prayerful, burdened with the pain of waiting and longing for the coming of Israel's salvation. Simeon, "righteous and devout" as he is, is sensitive to the promptings of the Spirit. He is guided by the Spirit to go to the temple around the time that Mary and Joseph were visiting in order to fulfil the Law of Moses. Earlier, the Spirit revealed to him that he would not see death until he had seen the Messiah. His burden had thus been lightened; a fresh hope filled his mind and heart. Anna too, no doubt similarly prompted by the Spirit, also arrives in the temple precincts on cue.

Our world is a strange world. The media of all genres vaunts physical beauty and athleticism; many seek to preserve their youthful vigour at some cost. Elderly people can easily be sidelined and judged to be 'past it'. And yet grandparents are playing a greater role than ever in helping their children by caring for grandchildren and doing the school run. Often it is the grandparents who, as persons of faith, seek to help grandchildren go to church when parents are too busy. This episode in Luke's Gospel highlights the wisdom of the elderly, their sensitivity to God's presence and purposes, their faith and trust, their broad vision and outreach. This can, I believe, be a source of great encouragement for elderly followers of Jesus; they still have so much to offer because of their experience of discipleship and life. Their wisdom, humour and compassion can be such a help and inspiration to the young.

Simeon must have been so thrilled to hold this child in his arms, this child who was the long-awaited salvation of his people. At last! God really has been faithful to promises made. But Simeon also realises the significance of this child for those beyond the confines of Israel. He senses the wider dimensions of God's love. He is also aware the child's future will be marked with conflict, that not everyone will accept him. In warning Mary and Joseph of this, even as he blesses them, he introduces new themes to the infancy story, themes that alert the reader to what lies ahead. Wonder and realism come together, as Simeon contentedly surrenders to his own future, ready to move on, mission accomplished. Anna cannot hold back her enthusiasm and joy as she reaches out to share with others the exciting news of this child's coming.

Elderly people can still be used by God in the service of the Good News. There are still areas of mission for which they are well equipped, and needs that they can meet, encouragement and affirmation which they can provide, rich experience which they can share, sensible perspectives on life which they can promote, deep humanity which they can reveal.

The Finding of The Child Jesus in The Temple (2:41–52)

The next episode in Luke's story of Jesus also takes place in the Jerusalem temple some twelve years later.[88] It forms a transitional bridge between infancy and ministry and offers a preview of what is to come later.[89]

> Now every year his parents went to Jerusalem for the festival of the Passover. And when he was twelve years old, they went up as usual for the festival. When the festival was ended and they started to return, the boy Jesus stayed behind in Jerusalem, but his parents did not know it. Assuming that he was in the group of travellers, they went a day's journey. Then they started to look for him among their relatives and friends. When they did not find him, they returned to Jerusalem to search for him. After three days, they found him in the temple, sitting among the teachers, listening to them and asking them questions. And all who heard him were amazed at his understanding and his answers. When his parents saw him they were astonished; and his mother said to him, "Child, why have you treated us like this? Look, your father and I have been searching for you in great anxiety." He said to them, "Why were you searching for me? Did you not know that I must be in my Father's house?" But they did not understand what he said to them. Then he went down with them and came to Nazareth, and was obedient to them. His mother

treasured all these things in her heart. And Jesus increased in wisdom and in years, and in divine and human favour.

This is the only glimpse provided by Luke to his readers of the process of Jesus' growth and development over the years between infancy and full adult maturity.[90] We are left to fill in the gaps through our own efforts by becoming more conversant with peasant life in the villages of Galilee, the extended family relationships, the rhythm of the seasons, the struggle for survival, the deeply religious context and sense of God—such a rich tapestry of factors that played a part in influencing the mind, heart and personality of the growing Jesus.[91] Clearly, the Nazareth household observed Torah carefully. There were three annual pilgrimage feasts in the Jewish liturgical calendar: Passover, Weeks (Pentecost) and Tabernacles. Ideally, folk travelled for the celebrations every year, especially at Passover. The text intimates that this was the case for Joseph and Mary in keeping with their deep piety; Jesus clearly shares their temple piety.[92] However, many of the poorer peasants of Galilee would probably not have been able to make the journey each year, given the time involved and the survival demands of their lives.[93] The journey from Nazareth or Galilee to Jerusalem anticipates the journey in the ministry that takes Jesus to the temple at Passover time.[94]

Some scholars hold that as a twelve-year-old adolescent, Jesus becomes *bar mitzvah*, a son of the Law, assuming the responsibilities and obligations incumbent on a Jewish male. Others strongly maintain that this is not the case; this would have taken place a year later.[95] It is at this time that he accompanies his parents to the temple for the great pilgrimage feast of Passover. Like adolescents everywhere, he has his own agenda, which proves problematic for them.[96] Instead of leaving the city with them and their Galilean caravan of kinsfolk and friends, he stays behind on his own, obviously fascinated by what he is seeing and hearing and by the temple itself. His parents assume that he is with other members of the party, and it is only in the evening when it is time to set up camp that they realise that their boy is missing. Deeply concerned, they retrace their steps to the city. It is not difficult for us to imagine their angst. After three days of searching for him around the city, they find him in the temple.[97] There, he is sitting among the teachers, listening, asking and answering questions, showing amazing understanding of the Law. The effect he has on the audience is one of astonishment; they are impressed by his precocious insight. This is, of course, a foretaste of what is to come.[98]

His parents, naturally, are deeply distressed, and Mary tells him so, asking him reproachfully why he has done this to them and informing him of their anxious search.[99] His reply, his first words in Luke's Gospel story, is very significant and highlights the central issue of the episode. "I must be about my Father's affairs" or "in my Father's house."[100] There are two fathers in the story; the issue is to clarify to which one Jesus owes primary allegiance.[101] This his mother ought to have known.[102] It is the God to whom he refers as "Father" who is at the centre of his life. "Into their tranquil family life bursts a sharp reminder of Jesus' true status and destiny."[103] Already all that concerns the Father is the absorbing interest of his existence; the "must",[104] used here for the first time, betrays an awareness of a relationship and an agenda that will determine his life.[105]

The parents do not understand Jesus' remarks. His blunt riposte, expressive of his disappointment, must have been a painful shock for them both, unsettling, disconcerting, puzzling.[106] It must have opened the gaping wound of uncertainty about the future, reminding Mary of Simeon's words about the piercing sword. It is always difficult for parents to let their children go. This experience was perhaps the first wrench of many until the final separation. The immediate outcome, however, is that Jesus returns with them to Nazareth and obediently lives a normal life under their authority.[107] There, over the years, he will increase in wisdom and in physical stature, and he will grow in favour with God and also with people.[108] Mary, characteristically, "stored up all these things in her heart." She had much to ponder.[109] The reader, too, is left pondering how what has been said throughout the Infancy Narrative concerning Jesus' mission and the response of the people will unfold.[110]

Reflections

This is a fascinating story, deeply human, profoundly moving. We see a family united in their journey to Jerusalem and the temple for the celebration of Passover. We can imagine their excitement as they draw near to the city with their neighbours and friends, singing the traditional psalms. As they head back home after the festival, the mood suddenly changes as they discover that Jesus is missing. It is not difficult for us to enter into their initial panic and then their dismay as reality dawns. Their Jesus is lost. They leave the caravan and rush back to the city. The hours must have seemed like months, until they finally come across him in the temple, engaged in theological discourse.

The relief and joy of finding him cannot mask their deep concern and distress; Mary's words have a reproachful tone: "Why have you done this to us?" Sometimes young people, focused on the present, fail to realise the impact that their actions can have on others. Jesus, in responding, seems surprised and disappointed at their lack of awareness and understanding. But his answer must have pained them, making them more aware that their child was special and different, that he did not fit normal parameters, that there was another dimension to his person and future. But they went home together; Jesus "was obedient to them"; for a while, life unfolded in a normal way. But they had been left with much to ponder, a pondering which, despite their trust in God, must have been unsettling.

In different ways, many a parent has experienced this kind of heart-rending loss, anxious searching and inexpressible relief in the finding. Sadly, for some that loss has not been made good, and an anguished void remains. As the years pass, parents have to cope with the questioning and growing independence of their children. It can be very difficult when a son or daughter opts for values, a lifestyle or career that is different from parental mores or dreams for their future. Selfless love and letting go is demanded. Jesus' choice of celibacy, his decision to leave home in search of the Baptist, his embarking on his prophetic ministry, the excitement and opposition surrounding him, must have been an alarming puzzle for Mary and the wider family, as Mark's story implies (3:21, 31–35).

Prior to this temple incident, others have spoken about the identity and role of this child: Gabriel, Elizabeth, Zechariah, shepherds, and Simeon and Anna. Now Jesus himself articulates to his parents his growing understanding, as he refers to God as his Father and sees the centrality of attending to that Father's business. Later, the baptism and transfiguration scenes will underline and clarify this relationship and mission. The reader will be well prepared for this. But, historically, it is only after the resurrection that it all becomes clear for Mary, for the disciples and for Christians over the centuries.

We leave Luke's Infancy Narrative aware of the rich Old Testament background to his story and the strong sense of promises fulfilled. We have encountered the God whom Luke proclaims, a God of surprises, a God who is compassionate and faithful. We have been enlightened about the identity of Jesus as Davidic Messiah, Saviour and Lord, as the holy Son of God. We have been introduced to many themes, which will thread their way through the coming narrative of Jesus' ministry, culminating in his passion, death and resurrection: the pervading presence of the Spirit, the atmosphere of praise and joy, the journey motif, the role of women, the importance of Jerusalem and the temple, God's preference for the poor and lowly, the idea of reversal.

Before we move on into the ministry of Jesus, it is important that we take stock of what we have learned and that we ponder our responses. What is my image of God; does it coincide with the God Luke proclaims? Am I aware of the Spirit's presence and prompting in my life? Who is Jesus for me; has my understanding of him and my relationship to him grown? Am I open to the new and unexpected, the challenging and uncomfortable? Am I a person who ponders and prays, who is an active and generous contemplative? Do I recognise my poverty of being, my neediness, and can I genuinely place my trust in God and God's faithful care? Can I surrender my life to the Father's will, constantly reiterating my "yes", wherever that may lead me? What is my attitude to the poor, the lowly, the marginalised in my locality and wider world, and to the forms of control, injustice and oppression which abound in society? The depth of Luke's spirituality, so artfully presented in these two chapters, is quite amazing and so enriching.

Notes

1   For details see Brown, *Birth*, 408-412.

2   Brown, *Adult*, 15, notes that nothing that happens in this second chapter of Luke presupposes what happens in the first; it was probably originally independent. The focus in Matthew 2 and Luke 2 is the divine proclamation to an audience (the magi and the shepherds respectively).

3   The structure which I am following is that of Brown, *Birth*, 410.

4   Marshall, *Luke*, 105, suggests that Joseph may have had property in Bethlehem; also, Evans, *Luke*, 196. Fitzmyer, *Luke*, 1:405, maintains that there is no hint of this. In Matthew Bethlehem is the place where Joseph and Mary live; Jesus is born at home. The census recalls that instigated by David (2 Sam 24:1–9); see also Ps 87:6.

5   Carroll, *Luke*, 64, observes the irony in that Caesar calls the shots, but it is God who is directing the action.

6   On the imperial cult, see Green, *Luke*, 122–123; Brown, *Adult*, 18. The Myrian inscription reads: "divine Augustus Caesar, son of a god ... saviour of the whole world." Lincoln, *Born of a Virgin?* 56–57, notes that Luke both echoes and contradicts imperial propaganda about Augustus.

7   Brown, *Adult*, 17, refers to "formidable historical difficulties". For a full discussion see Marshall, *Luke*, 99–104; Fitzmyer, *Luke*, 1:399–405. Johnson, *Luke*, 49, states that Luke simply has the facts wrong. Carroll, *Luke*, 65, maintains that it is impossible to salvage historical accuracy for Luke's report; within the narrative it advances the plot.

8   For a detailed discussion of issues connected with the census, see Brown, *Birth*, 413–418, and Appendix VII, 547–555; also, Lincoln, *Born of a Virgin?* 139–140.

9   Johnson, *Luke*, 51–52; see Fitzmyer, *Luke*, 1:393; Johnson, *Truly Our Sister*, 275. As Lincoln, *Born of a Virgin?* 55, says, the census serves as the means for securing Jesus' birth in Bethlehem, city of David.

10   The terminology used, "going up", and "city of David", normally refers to Jerusalem.

11   Kenneth E. Bailey, *Jesus through Middle Eastern Eyes* (London: SPCK, 2008), 46. Borg & Crossan, *First Christmas*, 147–148, maintain that the Roman system focused on where a person lived; Mary would not have been obliged to register; also, McBride, *Luke*, 36.

12   Note the links with Gabriel's earlier message (1:27, 32–33) and Mic 5:2. Fitzmyer, *Luke*, 1:406, asserts that Luke knows of no Davidic connection for Mary.

13   Green, *Luke*, 128. King, *"Significance of the Inn"*, 74–75, makes some interesting comments on Luke's subtle use of indicators of time; usually, God's time is also involved. This phrase "the days arrived" is found in 1:57; 2:6, 21, 22. For Carroll, *Luke*, 66, this shows that there is purposeful pattern to these events on two levels: the divine plan and obedient human participation in it.

14   Johnson, *Truly Our Sister*, 276, describes childbirth in that part of the world at that time, with its anxiety, pain and stress. Rejecting later views in the church which sought to make the birth miraculous, she comments that "real blood was shed at this delivery by a poor woman of peasant society far from home, labouring in childbirth for the first time. And it was holy." See also Brown, *Birth*, 437, n. 23.

15   Johnson, *Luke*, 50; Marshall, *Luke*, 106; Green, *Luke*, 128; Evans, *Luke*, 199; Fitzmyer, *Luke*, 1:408; Brown, *Birth*, 398. See Exod 4:22–23; 13:2, 12; 34:19; Num 3:12–13; Deut 21:15–17; Jer 31:9. Carroll, *Luke*, 66, recalls the story of Samuel (1 Sam 1–2).

16   Wis 7:4–5: "nursed with care in swaddling clothes."

17   Green, *Luke*, 136: the sign "lays bare God's gracious act to embrace anew, through this child, his people." See Brown, *Adult*, 20. Johnson, *Luke*, 53, wonders whether the three details: "wrapped ... placed ... no place" perhaps anticipate the threefold rhythm of the burial scene (23:53). See also Green, *Luke*, 124. Ian Boxall, "Luke's Nativity Story: A Narrative Reading", in *New Perspectives on the Nativity*, ed. Jeremy Corley, (London: T&T Clark, 2009) 33-34, upholds the link between cradle and grave; he also sees a link between the angelic annunciation of Christ's birth to the shepherds, and the proclamation of the resurrection to the women at the tomb (p. 32). Carroll, Luke, 67, notes that the link between manger and Messiah is disorientating for Luke's audience.

18   Green, *Luke*, 128; Brown, *Birth*, 399–401. Borg & Crossan, *First Christmas*, 150, suggest a caravansary: an open courtyard surrounded with doorless, covered rooms; the rooms were all gone, so Jesus is born among the animals in the courtyard, and laid in a feeding trough. Likewise, Byrne, *Hospitality*, 31. Fitzmyer, *Luke*, 1:408, too opts for a public caravansary where groups of travellers would spend the night under one roof.

19   King, *"Significance of the Inn"*, 67–69, defends the traditional view, preferring to translate the term as "inn". He sees this in the wider context of Luke-Acts as a whole, in which no human agency or setback is going to thwart the divine project. Johnson, *Luke*,

52, sees Mary and Joseph as "transients", like the homeless of our contemporary cities. There are echoes of the Samuel story: 1 Sam 1:18.

20   Bailey, *Jesus Through Middle Eastern Eyes*, 25–37.

21   See 1 Kings 17:19 concerning Elijah.

22   See 1 Sam 28:24; Matt 5:14–15; Luke 13:10–17. Bailey, *Jesus*, 31, quotes W. Thompson from 1871: birth took place in an ordinary house of some common peasant, and the baby was laid in one of the mangers; also E.F.F. Bishop, before 1950. For more than 100 years, scholars resident in the Middle East have understood Luke 2:7 as referring to a family room with mangers cut into the floor at one end. Green, *Luke*, 128–9, concurs; he comments that there was probably no commercial inn in Bethlehem, since it stood on no major roads. Marshall, *Luke*, 107, also suggests a room in a private house. Tannehill, *Luke*, 64, refers to either the main room of a simple home or an attached room used for guests. On p. 65, he assumes a one-room farmhouse where the family quarters might be separated from the animal quarters only by being on a raised platform. Levine, *Stories*, 101, believes that Luke gives no indication that residents rejected the family.

23   22:10–12. The verbal form (*kataluein*) is used in 9:12 and 19:7, meaning to find lodging, or be a guest.

24   The word is used in 2 Sam 7:6 LXX as the dwelling place of God's presence during the journey in the desert. In 1 Sam 1:18, it is used of the place where Hannah and her husband stay at Shiloh. See also Jer 14:8.

25   Bailey, *Jesus Through Middle Eastern Eyes*, 35; Brown, *Birth*, 420–424; Caird, *Luke*, 61. Green, *Luke*, 130, speaks of peasants, located toward the bottom of the scale of power and privilege; also, Johnson, *Truly Our Sister*, 276, who suggests that they may have worked the estates of the priests, supplying livestock for temple sacrifice. Tannehill, *Luke*, 65, is doubtful about the view that considers them as sinners.

26   McBride, *Luke*, 40, observes that shepherds may have had a place of importance in the folklore of the Israelite people, but they had no place of importance in their society at the time of Jesus.

27   Levine, *Stories*, 101, on the contrary, states that Jews at the time did not view shepherds as outcast or unclean; there are numerous positive images of shepherds in Israel's scriptures.

28   1 Sam 16:11; 17:15; 2 Sam 5:2; Jer 3:5; Ezek 34:11–12; Mic 5:4. Brown, *Birth*, 421–424, believes that a midrashic reflection on Mic 5:1 and Gen 35:21 underlies Luke's narrative; Fitzmyer, *Luke*, 1:396, disputes this; he maintains (p.395) that the shepherds are introduced because of the association of Jesus' birth with the town of David.

29   Wisdom 18:14–15 may have suggested the choice of night-time by Luke: "When all things were in quiet silence, and the night in its course was half spent, Your all powerful word leaped down from heaven's royal throne."

30   Green, *Luke*, 132; the closing line of Zechariah's canticle is recalled.

31   Green, *Luke*, 131, notes that God's glory is normally associated with the Jerusalem temple, not a farm. Luke is (proleptically) suggesting the coming of a new world.

32   See Exod 13:21; 16:10; 24:17; Ezek 43:2.

33   Johnson, *Luke*, 50, believes that "people" refers only to Israel; Carroll, *Luke*,

69. Green, *Luke*, 133–4, compares it with the universalist references concerning Augustus, claims now being countered. Marshall, *Luke*, 109, considers a wider reference possible. Borg & Crossan, *First Christmas*, 153–161, discuss "saviour, Lord, peace" as counterpropaganda. Tannehill, *Luke*, 66, mentions a "counterclaim for another ruler". Not all would agree.

34   As well as in Isaiah, especially chapters 40–66, the term was used in the pagan world. Green, *Luke*, 123, notes that this sets Jesus in opposition to the emperor. Also, Borg & Crossan, *First Christmas*, 158–167, concerning "good news" and "peace". Carroll, *Luke*, 69, is of the view that the angel's message makes both theological and political claims. Byrne, *Hospitality*, 33, discounts any hostility to Rome in this.

35   "Saviour" is used of God in 1:47; in 1:69 Jesus is designated as "horn of salvation". See also 2:30. Carroll, *Luke*, 69, writes: "Jesus enters Israel's history as the agent of divine deliverance (salvation) and as the anointed ruler (Messiah) who has received sovereign authority from God."

36   See Isa 52:7; 61:1; Brown, *Birth*, 425. In Luke 2:9 "Lord" refers to God; in 2:11 to Jesus (as in 1:38 and 1:43). Acts 2:36 reads: "Therefore let the entire house of Israel know with certainty that God has made him both Lord and Messiah." See Phil 3:20. For Fitzmyer, *Luke*, 1:397, "Messiah" and "Lord" are early kerygmatic titles, stemming from the Jewish Christian community in Palestine. Most scholars prefer the manuscript reading: "Christ the Lord".

37   Boxall, "Luke's Nativity Story", 35, sees the shepherds as being commissioned like Moses (Exod 3) and Gideon (Judg 6); they become bearers of the Gospel. He also sees a parallel between 2:20 and 24:52–53.

38   Bailey, *Jesus Through Middle Eastern Eyes*, 35–36.

39   See 2 Chr 33:3; Neh 9:6; Jer 8:2. Green, *Luke*, 131, notes that it is a farm not the temple which is the locus of God's presence; a radically new world is beginning.

40   Brown, *Birth*, 403.

41   Marshall, *Luke*, 112; Green, *Luke*, 137; Evans, *Luke*, 207. Fitzmyer, *Luke*, 1:411, maintains that the correct translation reads: "Glory in highest heaven to God; and on earth peace for people whom he favours." It does not mean "men of good will". Thus, our liturgical *Gloria* at Mass is an incorrect translation. In 1:397, he maintains that this hymn is a Lukan composition. Brown, *Birth*, 403–405, is similar; also, NRSV, New Jerusalem Bible. Carroll, *Luke*, 68, 70, suggests that the grammatical ambiguity allows both interpretations: peace will come to human beings who are recipients of God's good pleasure, and who have the capacity to embrace the gift.

42   Green, *Luke*, 131, 137; Borg & Crossan, *First Christmas*, 158.

43   19:38. Some note that in contemporary Jewish literature are to be found hymns of praise for creation. And the Qumran community composed hymns for angels to sing. They also evinced a sense of being chosen and favoured by God. Brown, *Birth*, 427, suggests that the canticle could feasibly have been composed by a community of Jewish Christian *anawim*. Borg & Crossan, *First Christmas*, 166, note that Roman peace is peace through victory, the peace of Jesus comes through justice.

44   1:39. The angel speaks of the "city of David"; the shepherds of "Bethlehem" (rather than Jerusalem). Carroll, *Luke*, 71, observes that the shepherds recognise that the

word they have heard, and the event it puts into language (*rhēma* in its dual meanings), is God's word, God's action.

45 Bailey, *Jesus Through Middle Eastern Eyes*, 37.

46 2:51. The verb means to throw together, discuss, debate. See Gen 37:11; Dan 7:28; 8:26; 12:4, 9; see also the sapiential tradition: Prov 3:1; Ps 119:11; Sir 39:1–3. King, "Significance of the Inn", 76, translates the verb as "watching".

47 See Acts 1:14; 2:36. Carroll, *Luke*, 72, writes: "The need of Jesus' mother to ponder these events reminds Luke's audience that God's activity in the world, in its mystery and surprise, sometimes requires discernment that is achieved only with difficulty, even among those specially favoured by God."

48 Green, *Luke*, 140. Fitzmyer, *Luke*, 1:418, and Carroll, *Luke*, 73, include the circumcision with the following episode, the presentation of the child Jesus in the temple, which includes a Spirit-inspired canticle; in this way, the parallelism is better maintained. Brown, *Birth*, 407, includes it here.

49 Boxall, "Luke's Nativity Story", 24.

50 Luke 22:19, 27.

51 Some scholars, (Caird, Johnson, McBride, Marshall among them) choose to begin this scene at verse 21, the circumcision and naming of Jesus. Green, *Luke*, 140, sees circumcision, naming, purification, presentation, consecration as the normal flow of events following the birth of a firstborn son in a Jewish family. I prefer to see that verse as the conclusion of the previous scene, in parallel with that of the Baptist (see Evans, *Luke*, 209; Brown, *Birth*, 436).

52 There are five references to the Law in this passage. Brown, *Birth*, 452, suggests that Luke is underlining that this story which centres on the future greatness of Jesus is made possible through obedience to the Law of Moses.

53 Johnson, *Truly Our Sister*, 279. Brown, *Birth*, 436, notes that it was childbirth not conception that rendered a woman ritually impure.

54 Tannehill, *Luke*, 69, maintains that there is little evidence to show that this was the requirement or custom.

55 Johnson, *Truly Our Sister*, 279; Brown, *Adult*, 27, suggests that as a gentile convert and perhaps a proselyte, Luke would have "only a book knowledge" of the customs. Luke (according to the best manuscripts) mistakenly includes Joseph in this purification; Lincoln, *Born of a Virgin?* 52. In *Birth*, 448, Brown suggests that Luke has either misunderstood a tradition or created a setting from an inaccurate reading of Old Testament laws; he favours the latter view.

56 Johnson, *Truly Our Sister*, 280.

57 Brown, *Birth*, 450. In *Adult*, 28–29, he notes the parallel between Zechariah and Elizabeth and Simeon and Anna: pious people, the temple setting, the presence of the Spirit, the hymn of praise. Both pairs have their biblical foreshadowing in Elkanah and Hannah, both in their longing for a child, and their presenting the child in the temple. The textual parallels are very close (1 Sam 1:24–28). Here the link has shifted, and lies between the parents of Samuel and the parents of Jesus. Similarly, Lincoln, *Born of a Virgin?* 51.

58 Echoes of Isaiah are strong. The wording recalls Isa 40:1 LXX: "console

my people; speak to the heart of Jerusalem"; 66:12–13 LXX: "as one whom a mother consoles ..."; 52:9 MT: "the Lord has consoled his people; he has redeemed Jerusalem." Carroll, *Luke*, 76, notes that many of the images in Luke 1–2 are packed into a single verse in Isa 49:13.

59   Green, *Luke*, 144; similarly, Brown, *Birth*, 452, who sees them as the embodiment of the piety of the *anawim*.

60   For the phrasing see Ps 89:48; 16:10; John 8:51.

61   Carroll, *Luke*, 75, comments that God's Spirit orchestrates the encounter. Green, *Luke*, 145, believes that Luke is attempting to portray Simeon in prophetic terms borrowed from Isaiah 66:1: "The Spirit of the Lord is upon me." God's purpose in "consoling" Israel is realised in the coming of Jesus.

62   Brown, *Adult, 30,* notes that such doubling has already occurred twice: Elizabeth's praise followed by the *Magnificat*, and the angel's annunciation to the shepherds followed by that of the heavenly host. In those cases, it seemed that the second part was a Lukan addition. Here, he feels that the first oracle of the *Nunc Dimittis* is the Lukan addition. There is a smooth transition from 27–34, so the canticle was probably added. It is of a general nature; it does not refer particularly to the conception or birth; it could apply to the crucifixion. It refers to the whole work of salvation as something already accomplished (like the *Magnificat* and *Benedictus*.) The second oracle is specific, as in the second part of the *Benedictus*, and concerns the future of the child. See more fully in *Birth*, 454–456.

63   Brown, *Adult*, 31, n. 52, refers to a "cento or pastiche technique of composition" which is characteristic of the hymnology of early Judaism, and visible also in the Dead Sea Scrolls. Also, *Birth*, 458.

64   Green, *Luke*, 147.

65   Johnson, *Truly our Sister*, 281, notes the use in the whole episode of "they" and "parents" and "father and mother" concerning Mary and Joseph. "The two are bonded in marriage, adjusting to the care of a new baby, and divine favour is invoked upon 'them' as such." Brown, *Birth*, 438, maintains that there is nothing in the Lukan account to favour the idea that Simeon was a Levitical priest.

66   The term "Master" as an address for God is unusual, and is found only here and in Acts 4:24. Brown, *Birth*, 439, notes that the term "Master" is used again in Acts 4:24 in the prayer of the Jerusalem community, "a community that may have been the ultimate source of this hymn as well."

67   Brown, *Birth*, 457.

68   According to Brown, *Birth*, 459, the universalism of Isaiah is subordinated, in the sense that the nations must come to Jerusalem, for Israel is God's people. But 2:31 has reinterpreted Isaiah to mean that the gentiles too are God's people. It is interesting that both Matthew and Luke anticipate in their Infancy Narratives the future of the Gospel "by already bringing into the birth story the theme of gentiles who are attracted by the light of God's son." Tannehill, *Luke*, 71, sees this as Luke's text for Epiphany. "In the sense that it presents God's saving purpose through Jesus in its broadest scope, the *Nunc Dimittis* is the climax of the Lukan infancy narrative." N. Tom Wright, *Luke for Everyone* (London: SPCK, 2002), 26, points out that the true glory of Israel is to have

been the bearer of promise, the nation in and from whom the true world ruler would arise.

69   Byrne, *Hospitality*, 35. Brown, *Birth*, 440, notes that revelation for the gentiles and glory for Israel are two equal aspects of the one salvation and light that God has made ready.

70   After the earlier annunciation, and the message of the shepherds, this is perhaps a little surprising. Perhaps it is an indication of separate pre-Lukan traditions. McBride, *Luke*, 45, suggests that it could be a Lukan device to underline something of supreme importance not hitherto revealed, namely, the significance of Jesus for the gentile world. Marshall, *Luke*, 115, thinks the wonder is due to the fact that a stranger recognises the significance of the child. Brown, *Birth*, 440, maintains that an astonished reaction to divine revelation is stereotypical.

71   Carroll, *Luke*, 78.

72   Marshall, *Luke*, 123, comments that Mary is singled out to the exclusion of Joseph not because of the virgin birth or because Joseph died before the sad experience of Jesus' crucifixion, but because of the parallel with Hannah. Brown, *Adult*, 25-26, notes that Luke's introduction of the theme of opposition and contradiction, pointing to the passion, parallels Matthew's story about Herod and the killing of the innocents. In *Birth*, 460, he calls this oracle a prophetic woe on Israel, like those of the prophets of old.

73   *Dialogismoi kardion* is always pejorative, so the thoughts are negative (doubting, unbelieving, hostile).

74   Marshall, *Luke*, 122, understands it in this way; also Caird, *Luke*, 64, who sees this as the theme of suffering leading to glory. Evans, *Luke*, 218, thinks this unlikely; Brown, *Birth*, 461, "certainly wrong".

75   Tannehill, *Luke*, 73, notes several Old Testament passages which connect sign and gentiles; see Isa 11:10-12 LXX, which refers to the "root of Jesse", "in him will the gentiles hope"; the Lord "will raise a sign for the gentiles." Johnson, *Luke*, 57, sees Simeon's prophecy as programmatic for the entire subsequent narrative.

76   Brown, *Birth*, 462-466, lists many interpretations which he considers implausible. He refers to the sword of discrimination and spiritual discernment. See 8:19-21; 12:51-53; Mark 3:31-35.

77   Carroll, *Luke*, 79, notes that Simeon's prayer and prophetic oracle define the narrative programme for the rest of the story. Johnson, *Truly Our Sister*, 280, notes that Luke did not believe Mary was present at Calvary, so the sword does not refer to this. Brown, *Adult*, 36, observes that the physical fact of motherhood gave Mary no special status according to the values Jesus preached. She is remembered as a mother in the Christian community because she believed the Lord's word in a way that gave her preeminent membership in his true family of disciples (1:41; 8:21)

78   Green, *Luke*, 149-150.

79   Carroll, *Luke*, 80.

80   Judith was 105; both women did not marry again, and devoted themselves continually to serving God through fasting and prayer. Green, *Luke*, 151, suggests that Anna's fasting may be an expression of her hope, a form of prayer entreating God to set

things right. James L. Resseguie, *Spiritual Landscape: Images of the Spiritual Life in the Gospel of Luke* (Peabody MA: Hendrickson, 2004), 57, notes that her fast is a visible expression of her spiritual hunger, a plea for God to usher in the promised redemption of Israel (Ezra 8:21–23; Dan 9:3; 6:16–24).

81   Brown, *Birth*, 453, sees her as the forerunner of the Jerusalem Christian community and its daughter community in Antioch (Acts 2:42, 46; 13:2); she lives out the ideals of the *anawim*.

82   Israel and Jerusalem are synonymous. Tannehill, *Luke*, 70, notes that she speaks publicly, which was unusual for a woman in that society, whereas Simeon speaks only to Mary and Joseph. Brown, *Birth*, 442, notes the similarity with Simeon's description in 2:25.

83   Brown, *Birth*, 465–466.

84   Green, *Luke*, 144.

85   Matthew too has Jesus go to Nazareth, though for different reasons; and it is not "their own city".

86   Gen 21:8, 20; Judg 13:24; 1 Sam 2:21, 26. Both verses of the conclusion echo the story of Samuel, and are echoed and complemented in 2:51–52. Evans, *Luke*, 221, refers to "idealised and conventionally biblical terms."

87   Brown, *Birth*, 479, notes that 2:39–40, prepares for Jesus coming from Nazareth to begin his ministry, but Luke does not move there directly, adding the next scene. Now v. 40 is a transition to the present story, and v. 52 to the ministry.

88   Tannehill, *Luke*, 75, sees the scene as an elaborate pronouncement story. Brown, *Birth*, 483, calls it a biographical apophthegm (a short story centred around a saying). In *Adult Christ*, 37, he notes that this story may at one time been a narrative quite independent of the infancy sequence which precedes it. It spoils the symmetry of the previous diptychs. It is read more easily as an independent unit: Joseph is called the father of Jesus; Mary and Joseph do not understand Jesus when he refers to God as Father. Luke probably appended this once independent story to his Infancy Narrative; it does not depend on what now precedes it. These points he discusses more fully in *Birth*, 479–481. Lincoln, *Born of a Virgin?* 115–124, maintains that Luke's annunciation story is best interpreted as intending to present Jesus' conception as miraculous and as bypassing any involvement on the part of Joseph. However, knowledge of such a conception has no impact on the understanding of any of the characters later in the narrative; the narrator's own depictions, even in chapter two, show no awareness of this earlier announcement. The stress on Joseph's Davidic descent in chapter two makes little sense if he had no part in his betrothed's pregnancy. In 2:27, 33, the narrator refers to "parents" and to Joseph as "father"; throughout this second visit to the temple, the two are referred to as "parents", and Mary refers to Joseph as "father". There seem to be two traditions and perspectives. In ancient biographies, natural and miraculous traditions are often juxtaposed. Lincoln believes that it was possible for Luke and his first readers to entertain simultaneously the notions that Jesus was Joseph's son and was son of God whose conception was miraculous. Earlier (21–33), he examines Paul (Gal 4:4; 3:16, 19; Rom 1:3; Phil 2:7), who assumes Jesus' full humanity in his birth. Acts, also written by Luke, has a "seed of David" tradition (2:30; 13:23, 32–37). Mark seems unaware of a tradition suggesting an

extraordinary occurrence concerning Jesus' birth. The same is true for John.

89   Green, *Luke*, 153, notes how the summary statements of 2:40, 52, form an "inclusion" around the account of the visit to the temple. Both note Jesus' relationship to God ("favour") and mention his wisdom. Both these points are central to the story of the visit to the temple. Brown, *Birth*, 484; *Adult*, 43, accepts these "framework statements" in his structure for the episode.

90   Carroll, *Luke*, 83, observes that in biographies of great men, it was customary to portray them already as children displaying the character they manifest as adult heroes. Similarly, Tannehill, *Luke*, 75; Johnson, *Luke*, 60; Marshall, *Luke*, 125; Brown, *Birth*, 481–482; *Adult Christ*, 40–47. In addition to stories from world literature (concerning Buddha, Osiris, Cyrus, Alexander, Augustus, Josephus), he includes legends concerning Moses, Samuel and Daniel. The idea is that the child must have been what the man was known to be. So here Jesus has begun his activity in the temple; he places priority on God's demands over family; he proclaims God as Father (anticipating the voice at his baptism). Three key points which Luke makes are Jesus' piety, wisdom and the anticipation of the priority of God's claim.

91   See, for instance, Johnson, *Truly Our Sister*, 137–206; Joel Kauffman, *The Nazareth Jesus Knew* (Nazareth, USA: Nazareth Village, 2005), 8–43; Bargil Pixner, *With Jesus through Galilee According to the Fifth Gospel* (Rosh Pina: Corazin Publishing, 1992), 49–64; James Martin, *Jesus, A Pilgrimage* (New York: HarperCollins, 2014), 65–91; John P. Meier, *A Marginal Jew: Rethinking the Historical Jesus* (London: Doubleday, 1991), vol.1, 205–371; José A. Pagola, *Jesus: An Historical Approximation* (Miami: Convivium Press, 2011), 31–73.

92   Such piety was also a characteristic of the early Christians (Acts 2:46; 3:1; 5:12).

93   Brown, *Birth*, 472, notes that many Palestinian Jews may have gone to Jerusalem only once a year.

94   Brown, *Birth*, 485.

95   Marshall, *Luke*,126, and Evans, *Luke*, 224, maintain that this took place when a boy was 13 years old. Brown, *Adult Christ*, 44; *Birth*, 473, maintains that Jesus' visit at the age of 12 has nothing to do with *bar mitzvah*, which was a much later custom. The general Talmudic principle is that a child reaches manhood at his 13th birthday. Amy-Jill Levine, "Luke: Introduction and Annotations" in *The Jewish Annotated New Testament*, eds. Amy-Jill Levine and Marc Zvi Brettler (New York: Oxford University Press, Inc., 2011), 103, states categorically that this is not Jesus' *bar mitzvah*.

96   Johnson, *Truly Our Sister*, 284–85, notes that the boy went off to chart his own course; his parents did not understand. "When children are precocious, navigating the waters of parental love and responsibility becomes ever more complex." She also points out the number of times that "they" is used in this passage; Mary and Joseph are partners in parenting. The source behind the story was probably unaware of the annunciation story in the previous chapter, and the implication that Joseph was not the biological father of Jesus.

97   Marshall, *Luke*, 127, notes that they discovered him on the third day, the first two days being spent in travelling from and back to the city; similarly, Brown, *Birth*, 474. Evans, *Luke*, 224, comments that three days is too conventional an expression to permit

calculation of how much time was spent in journeying or searching.

98   Green, *Luke*, 155, refers to Jesus' "scriptural acumen". Jesus teaches in the temple throughout his final days in Jerusalem (19:47-21:37). Brown, *Adult*, 45, notes comments of amazement concerning Jesus' teaching in the ministry (4:22; 4:36; 19:47): "Jesus is already showing the wisdom in sacred teaching which will mark his career as a man, and the people are reacting in the same way they will react during the ministry." As a child Jesus does not experience the hostility which he will encounter later, nor is he hostile to them, as later; Luke refers to Jesus' interlocutors as "teachers" rather than "scribes". Brown, *Birth*, 489, notes that the child's "understanding" is an illustration of his wisdom mentioned in vv. 40 and 52. In *Adult*, 46, he suggests that the tone of reproach is best understood if this was once an independent story. See Mark 3:31; John 23; "where a demand is placed on Jesus in the name of family obligations, his response shows that his priorities are with God rather than with his earthly family."

99   Johnson, *Truly Our Sister*, 283-284, notes both the parental joy of relationship as children grow, and the accompanying fear that harm may befall them; both are facets of love. In the story, the parents are overwhelmed with sadness and anxiety. On finding Jesus, Mary's words carry a tone of rebuke as well as relief. "She corrects him, scolds him, complains about his behaviour."

100   Both translations of the Greek (*en tois tou patros mou*) are possible. The word "house" does not occur here (as in John 2:16). Carroll, *Luke*, 83, suggests "domain", which captures something of the ambiguity, and can refer to house and activity. As Tannehill, *Luke*, 76, puts it, Jesus is indicating not only where he can be found, but why. Johnson, *Luke*, 61, prefers activity to place; Marshall, *Luke*, 129, prefers place. Brown, *Birth*, 490, maintains that Jesus "is saying that his presence in the temple and his listening to the teachers is indicative of where his vocation lies, namely, in the service of God who is his Father, and not at the beck and call of his natural family." This is a Christological statement which identifies Jesus as God's son. On p. 476 he suggests it is equivalent to the French *chez*.

101   Green, *Luke*, 156. In n. 14 he notes that Mary says, "Your father and I", not out of courtesy but as a point of emphasis.

102   In Greek Jesus' question expects a positive answer, and is gently reproachful; he is disappointed that his parents have understood him so poorly. Johnson, *Truly Our Sister*, writes, 284, "Intellectually curious about matters religious and enamoured of the whole temple experience, this is a village boy discovering his vocation." Brown, *Birth*, 481, observes that so far there have been revelations about Jesus (the angels and Simeon), now it is Jesus himself. "The Christological moment here occurs in Jesus' youth when he is old enough to express in word and in work his self-consciousness."

103   Byrne, *Hospitality*, 37. Carroll, *Luke*, 84, stresses that this is the family to which Jesus ultimately belongs, "the one that defines his identity and vocation and claims his allegiance." Normal family ties are relativised.

104   The Greek word for "must" (*dei*) is used by Jesus several times in during his ministry (4:43; 9:22; 13:32–33; 17:25; 22:37; 24: 7, 26); many of these concern his suffering.

105   Caird, *Luke*, 66, says: "Besides becoming a *bar mitzvah* he had become intensely

aware of being Son of God, and henceforth he was to live his life not merely under the Law but under the higher authority of his filial consciousness."

106   McBride, *Luke*, 48, comments that, given the earlier stories of the annunciation and the shepherds, and Simeon's prophecy, one would have expected less misunderstanding on the part of Jesus' parents. Consequently, some scholars view this story as a separate pre-Lukan piece of tradition. In fact, no one in the Gospel narrative really understands until after the resurrection. Marshall, *Luke*, 128, does not see any conflict with their earlier knowledge of his destiny. As the story stands, suggests Brown, *Birth*, 489, the amazement of the parents is at the way in which the already known vocation and identity have begun to be expressed; on p. 492 he adds that this is especially because of his being called away from family obligations. Johnson, *Truly Our Sister*, 285, notes the likelihood that Luke received this temple story, in which Joseph appears straightforwardly as Jesus' parent, from a source that knew nothing of the annunciation story or its implied point that Joseph was not the biological father of Jesus. Brown, *Birth*, 484, notes that Mary's lack of understanding (v. 50) is for Luke only an instance of the standard misunderstanding that greets a parabolic revelation or a prophetic statement. "It is a stylised reaction in Gospel literature and tells us nothing historical about Mary's psychology."

107   Now Jesus is the subject of the verb, whereas earlier it was his parents. (In fact, "they" occurs eight times in the narrative.) Brown, *Adult*, 49, observes that this comment about Jesus' return to Nazareth and normal obedience to his parents shows that this moment of self-assertion is unique, and that his townsfolk would never suspect that God was his father (4:22). In *Birth*, 493, his obedience also serves the piety motif.

108   In parallel with 1:80, concerning John the Baptist. Reference to Jesus' growth in wisdom and favour is made also in 2:40; these echo the story of Samuel. Here there is a new term, "maturity"; the Greek *hēlikia* can mean age or stature. Both are probably implied. In v. 40 the verb was "filled", in this verse it is "increase". Johnson, *Truly Our Sister*, 286, notes that the summary statements about Jesus' growth cover over the enormous amount of mothering and the fathering he received, without which he would not have reached adulthood physically, emotionally and spiritually as the person he became.

109   Mary's response is similar to 2:19. Later, in 8:19–21, Mary is included in Jesus' new family because she hears God's word and carries it out. Brown, *Birth*, 494, comments that though Mary may have been amazed at what Jesus did, and failed to understand what he said about himself, and may have reproached him, she is not unresponsive to the mystery which surrounds him; she keeps the events in her heart; this is a preparation for later understanding (Acts1:14). It is only after the resurrection that the Christology of Jesus as God's son was understood. Johnson, *Luke*, 61–62, notes how the episode anticipates Jesus' resurrection (empty tomb story and Emmaus).

110   Brown, *Birth*, 483, writes: "The present setting and saying are no less and no more historical than are the divine voice and its setting at the baptism of Jesus. Jesus was baptised; Jesus had a boyhood—those are historical facts. But in Luke those historical reminiscences serve as the occasion for the articulation of a revelation apprehended by post-resurrectional faith, namely, the divine sonship."

Chapter Three

Beginnings: Jesus

In this and the following chapter, I would like to explore beginnings: the beginning of the mission of Jesus and the beginning of discipleship. Many Lukan scholars take 3:1–4:13 as a single narrative unit, comprising the ministry of the Baptist and then the baptism, genealogy and testing of Jesus.[1] This is then followed (4:14–9:50) by a section devoted to Jesus' ministry in Galilee, before the clear indication in 9:51 that Jesus is embarking on his journey to Jerusalem. In this chapter, I plan to deal with what I would entitle "The Beginning of Jesus' Mission", and after the temptation scene, include Jesus' initial preaching and his visit to Nazareth (4:14–30). I believe that in this block of material, the evangelist further clarifies the identity and role of Jesus, so that the reader is able better to appreciate what is really taking place as the rest of the narrative concerning Jesus' deeds and words unfolds.

The Coming of The Baptist (3:1–20)

As a prelude to the ministry of Jesus, now a grown man, Luke, like the other evangelists, describes briefly the ministry of John, likewise an adult.[2] For this he provides an elaborate setting, situating the precursor of Jesus on the world stage, "in the fifteenth year of Tiberius Caesar's reign", and in the political and religious context of Palestine, "when Pontius Pilate was governor of Judea, and Herod was ruler of Galilee … , during the high priesthood of Annas and Caiaphas."[3] In this context "the word of God came to John in the wilderness."[4] God, too, is clearly a player on this world stage, and conflict is inevitable. A link with the Infancy Narrative is made by the reference to John as the son of Zechariah. After his birth and naming, the reader was informed that "he lived in the desert until the day he appeared openly to Israel" (1:80). His role as forerunner, mentioned by Gabriel to Elizabeth (1:17), and outlined by Zechariah in the *Benedictus* (1:76), is recalled and highlighted by the quotation from Isaiah (40:3–5), which Luke introduces into the narrative (3:4); prophecies are reaching fulfilment:

The voice of one crying out in the wilderness:
"Prepare the way of the Lord,
  make his paths straight.
Every valley shall be filled,
  and every mountain and hill shall be made low,
and the crooked shall be made straight,
  and the rough ways made smooth;
and all flesh shall see the salvation of God."

John operates in the desert area around the Jordan river, which recalls Israel's earlier exodus journey and symbolically suggests a fresh entrance into the land of promise; it is a threshold experience.[5] As well as baptising, the prophet John conducts an extended and powerful ministry of the word, "proclaiming a baptism of repentance for the forgiveness of sins"; this also echoes the words of Gabriel and Zechariah (1:17, 77). Baptism and proclamation stand in tandem. John explains in harsh, urgent and challenging terms to those who come to him, no doubt conscious of their Abrahamic ancestry, what they must do to show their repentance, their change of mindset, heart and lifestyle. His demands to the people in general, and then to the tax collectors and the soldiers, have to do with wealth and possessions: sharing food and clothing with those in need, no extortion or blackmail, being content with one's wages.[6] The cleansing and accompanying repentance lead to forgiveness of sins, and this outside the temple system; it must also lead to committed action and concrete changes that would involve social renewal and a reformed way of life in keeping with the purposes of God.[7] It is significant that Luke's quotation from Isaiah concludes with the concept of salvation for everyone ("all flesh"), echoing the words of Simeon (2:20–22). "John's ministry may be more narrowly directed towards Israel, but it is part of God's larger project of bringing redemption to all humanity."[8]

In the atmosphere of growing expectancy and speculation about whether he might be the Messiah, he openly directs his hearers' thoughts to one more powerful, who is to come, whose sandals he is unworthy to untie (the task of a slave) and "who will baptise with the Holy Spirit and with fire". His description of the role has a strong tone of severity and imminent, discriminating judgement, with winnowing fork and fire. Finally, before Jesus arrives personally on the scene, Luke informs his readers that Herod, rebuked by the prophet for his adulterous and unacceptable marriage to Herodias, "added a further crime to all the rest by shutting John up in prison" (3:20). Response to God's prophet is thus both positive and negative, a presage of things to come also for Jesus, as Simeon foretold. In this way, the Baptist, his prophetic role fulfilled, leaves the stage free for the "coming one".[9]

The Baptism of Jesus (3:21–22)

Each of the Gospels, with different nuances, describes the baptism of Jesus by John. Luke's description reads as follows:[10]

> Now when all the people were being baptized, and when Jesus also had been baptized and was praying, the heaven was opened, and the Holy Spirit descended upon him in bodily form like a dove. And a voice came from heaven, "You are my Son, the Beloved; with you I am well pleased."

The narrator observes first of all that all the people were receiving baptism. He situates Jesus in the midst of his people, a people needing to be changed in mind and heart, and through the ritual, indicating their openness and basic orientation to God.[11] Jesus, in coming forward for baptism, identifies with them. Without mentioning John's name, Luke notes almost in passing that Jesus, too, has been baptised. Jesus is one with his people in responding to the Baptist's call for renewal. The focus of Luke's narrative is, therefore, not the baptism itself, but the twofold revelation that follows.

Jesus is at prayer, as he will be in so many crucial moments in the unfolding of the Lukan narrative.[12] As he prays, an expression of openness to God's presence and action, heaven opens, which in scripture is usually an indication that a revelation from God is imminent (see Isa 63:19; 64:1; Ezek 1:1; 2:2). Luke's language is less dramatic than Mark's graphic "torn open". From the open heaven, the Holy Spirit descends upon Jesus. Luke underlines the reality of what is taking place by objectifying the Spirit, observing that the Spirit descended "in physical form, like a dove", implying materiality and visibility. The same objectifying tendency and spatial movement are found in the Pentecost scene (Acts 1:8–11; see also 2:1–4).[13] The Spirit has, of course, been active earlier in the story (1:15, 35, 41, 67; 2:25, 26). The coming of the Spirit here is to be understood as Jesus' anointing for messianic mission (see Isa 42:1, quoted later in Nazareth in 4:18). The Spirit, involved creatively in the conception of Jesus, is the creative and empowering source of his mission.[14] The coming of the Spirit also fulfils the promise of the gift of the Spirit in a new creation (Isa 42:1–5; 11:1–3; 61:1; 63:10–14).

This somewhat puzzling dove imagery, "at once evocative and obscure",[15] is perhaps intended to evoke the Spirit's hovering over the waters of chaos at the dawn of creation (Gen 1:2) or to recall Noah's dove at the time of the flood (Gen 8:8). It may be, however, that rather than seeking the meaning of the dove in biblical precedents, we should recall the annunciation (1:35) and the angelic song (2:14). The Spirit comes down and the child will be called Son of God; the power will "overshadow" Mary. Later the heavens open, and peace is declared to people who enjoy God's favour. Perhaps the dove hovering in baptism is the symbol allowing "the reader's imagination to pull these elements into a single focus."[16]

A voice then speaks from heaven directly to Jesus. The reader is thus drawn into Jesus' deeply personal experience and "is provided access to an empowerment and declaration that takes place between God and Jesus in the communication that is prayer."[17] The wording in most manuscripts is identical to Mark's version and indicates the significance that the evangelists saw in the event. There can perhaps be discerned a distant echo of God's words to Abraham concerning his only son, Isaac (Gen 22:2). But most commentators see them as a fusion of two Old Testament texts, Psalm 2:7 and Isaiah 42:1.[18] Jesus is addressed in words similar to the coronation formula: "You are my son, today I have become your father."[19] These words were applied to the new king at the moment of his anointing, when he was considered to become God's son in a special way. In the Psalm, the words are adapted to the future messianic king. The other source passage refers to the Servant of Yahweh, called and ordained by the Spirit's anointing to a saving mission: "Here is my servant whom I uphold, my chosen one in whom my soul delights. I have endowed him with my spirit that he may bring true justice to the nations." Luke would see this as the restatement and confirmation of an existing status (1:35; 2:49).[20] The word translated "beloved" (*agapētos*), when applied to a son or daughter, usually means "only".[21]

Jesus, then, is anointed by the Spirit as the kingly Messiah, anointed for mission, "a task expressed in terms of the mission of the servant."[22] He is also designated as the only Son, with a uniquely personal relationship with God. "He is divinely empowered and divinely authorised for the work he will do."[23] God's voice provides "an unimpeachable sanction of Jesus with regard to his identity and mission" as agent of redemption.[24] Denis McBride views the scene as Jesus' formal recognition by the Father and his anointing for his task by the Spirit, an investiture, an initiation into a new life of ministry.[25]

Having sought the significance that the evangelist saw in the episode, there are some further issues to be addressed. The fact of Jesus' baptism by John is not seriously put into question. The incident seems to have caused some embarrassment to the early Church, particularly in dealing with the Baptist's disciples, who sought to establish John's superiority. Matthew's changes reflect this situation. In the light of Jesus' subsequent teaching, his receiving of baptism cannot have been an empty ritual. Its significance perhaps lay in his wishing to be identified with his people in response to the Baptist's preaching of repentance.

It seems safe to say that Jesus probably had some strong religious experience in connection with his baptism that changed his life, an experience of the Spirit in some ways rather like a prophetic call.[26] Our information is inadequate to clarify whether this experience was something unexpected, a new revelation about himself, or whether it "represented the end of a long development, of deepening appreciation of the divine fatherhood and his own filial responsibility, of growing insight into his mission and the world's need, of meditation on the meaning of the Scriptures and their application to himself."[27] This position seems to be in keeping with the later part of Luke's Infancy Narrative. Jesus' convictions concerning his relationship with God and his mission must have crystallised at some point in his life, and tradition links this with the Jordan baptism. Perhaps Jesus alluded to the experience and its importance, and this formed the basis for the post-resurrectional elaborations, so rich in Old Testament imagery, found in the Gospel narrative. Alternatively, during his ministry it became clear that Jesus experienced a close relationship with God and was deeply committed to mission, and was convinced of the power of the Spirit working through him. This made an impact on his disciples; as they later remembered it, they linked it with the event with which his active ministry began, using Old Testament texts to describe it.[28]

The Genealogy of Jesus (3:23–38)

After the baptism, Luke provides a genealogy of Jesus. Genealogies are not uncommon in the Old Testament; they are a way of establishing one's belonging to a particular tribe or clan, or to a priestly or noble family, with the status and rights and security that such identity brings. Luke introduces his genealogy with the statement that at the beginning of his ministry Jesus was "about" thirty years old, clearly a round number. David happened to be that age when he began to reign as king. Thirty was regarded as the age of mature manhood, and was the minimum age for public preaching.

The evangelist then traces Jesus' ancestry from his putative father Joseph back through David (thus re-emphasising his Davidic status and claims), on through Abraham to "Adam, son of God." This is the climax of the genealogy and echoes the voice from heaven at the baptism. Johnson maintains that the baptism and genealogy should be read together "as making a single emphatic statement."[29]

Luke's version of Jesus' genealogy is thus quite different from that of Matthew, who works in the other direction, building up to Jesus, and who begins with

Abraham. Matthew lays stress on the fact that Jesus is son of David and son of Abraham, and his format is more consciously structured.[30] Luke's concerns are different. By taking the genealogy back to Adam, Luke wishes to highlight the universal significance of Jesus, his being one with the whole of humanity. Some scholars believe that Jesus is being presented as the second Adam, whose obedience will reverse the disobedience of the first. There may also be an allusion to a new creation, especially when one considers the role of the Spirit in the narrative so far. By placing the genealogy after the baptism of Jesus rather than at the beginning of the Gospel, as does Matthew, Luke shows that Jesus is more than an heir to a long biblical history; his human ancestry is subordinated to his divine sonship.

The Testing of Jesus (4:1–13)

Luke picks up the thread of his narrative after the genealogy by introducing the fascinating theme of the testing or temptations of Jesus; it concerns the discernment of vocation and mission.[31] It is introduced early in each of the Synoptic Gospels. Mark's version is quite brief. It states the simple fact and provides us with no information about the possible content of the experience. The versions of Matthew and Luke offer a much fuller description. Their format is very similar and takes the shape of a mini three-act drama. For there are three separate temptations in different locations, and in each a creative suggestion is made by Satan and a scriptural rebuttal is offered by Jesus, quoting a text from the Greek version of the book of Deuteronomy. The view generally held among biblical scholars is that these two evangelists were basing themselves on a written source to which they both had access. It is usually referred to as 'Q', a document no longer extant.

There are slight differences in the way each handles this source, particularly in the order of the second and third temptations. Matthew has a liking for mountains, and the high hill of the third temptation with its worldwide vista links well with the concluding scene of the Gospel when the risen Jesus encounters the disciples on a mountain in Galilee and gives them a universal mission. The third temptation in Luke takes place in Jerusalem. Jesus' journey to Jerusalem is a major Lukan theme in the body of the Gospel, and it is in Jerusalem that the risen Jesus appears and the Holy Spirit later descends upon the disciples.[32] Luke ends the whole temptation episode in a different way from Matthew. Luke's version reads as follows:

Jesus, full of the Holy Spirit, returned from the Jordan and was led by the Spirit in the wilderness, where for forty days he was tempted by the devil. He ate nothing at all during those days, and when they were over, he was famished. The devil said to him, "If you are the Son of God, command this stone to become a loaf of bread." Jesus answered him, "It is written, 'One does not live by bread alone'."

Then the devil led him up and showed him in an instant all the kingdoms of the world. And the devil said to him, "To you I will give their glory and all this authority; for it has been given over to me, and I give it to anyone I please. If you, then, will worship me, it will all be yours." Jesus answered him, "It is written, 'Worship the Lord your God, and serve only him'."

Then the devil took him to Jerusalem, and placed him on the pinnacle of the temple, saying to him, "If you are the Son of God, throw yourself down from here, for it is written, 'he will command his angels concerning you, to protect you', and 'On their hands they will bear you up, so that you will not dash your foot against a stone'."

Jesus answered him, "It is said, 'Do not put the Lord your God to the test'." When the devil had finished every test, he departed from him until an opportune time.

The opening reference to the Jordan river explicitly links this episode with that of Jesus' river baptism by John. There, the Holy Spirit descends upon him, anointing him for mission. The voice from heaven proclaims him as the "Beloved Son". Before proceeding further, Luke comments that "Jesus was about thirty years old when he began his work". It would seem that Luke views the temptation experience as Jesus' first foray into mission.[33]

The action begins with two references to the Spirit. Jesus is described as "full of the Spirit". The Spirit which fills his being now leads Jesus in (not "into") the wilderness. The verb has a gentler ring than Mark's "drove him".[34] The implication seems to be that Jesus moves away from the Jordan and wanders through the desert area for a period of forty days and is led throughout by the Spirit.[35] During this time, he eats nothing and is subjected to testing by the devil. The desert period culminates in the threefold detailed temptations.

The desert or wilderness can operate as a symbol recalling the place of Israel's privileged encounter with God during the lengthy period of wandering from Egypt to the land of promise. It was also popularly regarded as alien to God, a place of insecurity, devoid of comfort, the haunt of demons and wild beasts.[36] The verb which is translated as "test" is used in the Old Testament of God testing the faith and obedience of Israel[37], and also of human beings testing God by doubting God's goodness and power.[38] Israel is referred to in Hosea as

God's "son".[39] The duration of the fast, "forty days", perhaps recalls the fasting of Moses and Elijah prior to their inaugurating their respective missions,[40] and the fast of Moses on the Sinai mountain.[41] More clearly, it is a reminder of the forty-year exodus experience of Israel in the wilderness. The testing occurs at the end of this period. Jesus recapitulates the experience of testing of God's "son" Israel in the wilderness; Jesus gives God the trust and obedience that Israel failed to give.[42]

In the first temptation, Jesus' opponent, the devil,[43] approaches him and says: "If you are Son of God, tell this stone to turn into a loaf." In this and the third temptation, the devil's opening gambit refers to the issue of divine sonship proclaimed in the scene of Jesus' baptism.[44] He probes its meaning, suggesting that Jesus should prove the authenticity of his sonship by solving his immediate hunger/starvation problem through the miraculous transformation of a stone into a loaf of bread. Matthew's form of the temptation uses the plural: stones and loaves. In the background is the situation, which occurred during Israel's wilderness wandering, when the people grew hungry. Comparing their condition with the copious food supply of their Egyptian days, fleshpots and bread, they complained bitterly against Moses and Aaron. They clearly doubted God's providential care. God responded by providing quails at twilight and manna in the morning.[45]

To the devil's proposal, Jesus replies in the words of scripture, which is a feature of his strategy each time: "Human beings live not on bread alone." This is the exact quotation of Deuteronomy 8:3 (Septuagint version). The writer sees the people's hunger as the way in which God is testing them in order to know what is in their heart, and whether or not they would keep his commandments. (Matthew, modifying 'Q', continues the quotation: "but by every word which proceeds from the mouth of God", which completes the verse). Jesus' view is that for quality human living, physical food is not enough. What really matters is to obey the word of God, "by walking in his ways and by fearing him".[46] Jesus understands sonship in terms of obedience and unconditional trust. The comment of Jesus to his disciples in John's Gospel is apposite here: "My food is to do the will of him who sent me and to complete his work."[47] Using divine power for his own ends in performing a miracle to alleviate his personal hunger in a moment of self-interest, cheating on his humanity,[48] would be a betrayal of his true identity. God will graciously provide.[49]

At this, the devil employs an alternative stratagem. Like a prospective house or land agent, he leads Jesus in what seems like a visionary experience to a high vantage point,[50] not a high mountain as in Matthew, and shows him "in a moment of time all the kingdoms of the world" (or possibly the Roman Empire),[51] saying: "I will give you all this power and their splendour, for it has been handed over to me, for me to give it to anyone I choose. Do homage, then, to me, and it shall be yours." That the devil exercised control over the world's kingdoms was not questioned in Jesus' day.[52] So he offers Jesus the instant power of empire and its concomitant glory and honour. But there is a condition: Jesus must switch allegiance and worship him. This suggestion Jesus absolutely refuses to entertain.

In replying, he again quotes a text from Deuteronomy (6:13): "You must do homage to the Lord your God, him alone you must serve." A few verses earlier in Deuteronomy, we read the *Shema*, Israel's creed and daily prayer, which opens: "Hear, O Israel; the Lord is our God, the Lord alone." Israel is commanded to "love the Lord your God with all your heart, and with all your soul, and with all your might."[53] This forms the topic in the discussion that Jesus holds with the lawyer later in the ministry prior to the parable of the Good Samaritan.[54] Idolatry, the allure of alien gods, proved a constant threat to the people of Israel, a temptation to which the people frequently succumbed.[55] Jesus is not interested in worldly power and glamour; God occupies the unassailable centre of his life. It is the reign of God that Jesus is sent to establish, and so in his ministry he will combat evil, setting captives free.[56] "The paths of this world do not lead to the Kingdom of God, and to pin one's faith in worldly wisdom or authority is to worship that which is not God. To worship God is to trust him and leave the results in his hands."[57]

The devil, changing tack, now moves on, and for the third, climactic test takes Jesus to Jerusalem and sets him on the royal colonnade of the temple, facing a drop of 450 feet (137 m) into the Kidron valley below. He challenges Jesus once again to prove his divine sonship in spectacular style, this time by leaping off to show his trust in God's saving intervention. The devil this time takes his cue from Jesus and himself cites the psalmist (91:11–12), who expressed his confidence in God's protection. "He has given his angels orders about you, to guard you; they will carry you in their arms in case you trip over a stone." The quotation is more complete than the version in Matthew, which omits "to guard you". Here we find the typical line of argumentation from the less to the greater. If God commands the angels to protect David from damage, how much more would God protect the Messiah, who is God's son, if he were to jump from such a height.[58] The temptation is for Jesus to prove the truth of God's promise by putting it to the test, which is a form of presumption.

In reply, Jesus returns to Deuteronomy (6:16): "Do not put the Lord your God to the test." At one point in their desert journey, near Rephidim, when suffering intense thirst, the people were on the point of stoning Moses because of their desperate situation. Moses interpreted this as a testing of God: "Is Yahweh among us or not?"[59] Moses called the place *Massah*, which means "testing" and *Meribah*, "quarrel". According to the version of the story in the book of Numbers,[60] Moses struck the rock, as God had commanded, and water gushed out. But he struck it twice, which God interpreted as a sign of lack of trust. But in Jesus' case there is no lack of trust; Jesus is successful where Israel of old failed. He does not betray his filial relationship with God; he does not attempt to force the Father's hand through a foolhardy venture; he needs no proof of God's choice and faithful care. His response is to trust without imposing conditions or making demands. Later in the story of Jesus there will be another testing in Jerusalem, where Jesus will refuse to save himself or demand that God do so.[61]

Luke then brings his narrative to a conclusion, without any mention of the ministering angels found in Matthew and Mark: "Having exhausted every way of putting him to the test, the devil left him, until the opportune moment." In observing that every possible form of testing has been exhausted, the evangelist brings out both the comprehensive nature of the assault on Jesus and the quality of his victory. "Jesus has demonstrated unequivocally his faithful obedience to God and thus his competence to engage in ministry publicly as God's Son."[62]

Luke leaves the reader wondering about the meaning of "the opportune moment" (*kairos*) when the devil is set to return. The phrase is usually taken to refer to the devil's powerful re-emergence at the time of the passion. In Luke 22:3, Satan is said to enter into Judas; in 22:31, Satan is said to have obtained his wish to sift the apostles like wheat; in 22:53, at the close of the arrest scene, Jesus affirms that the reign of darkness has arrived. Perhaps the most powerful struggle is the agony in the garden and his prayer (22:39–46). However, the conflict between the rival kingdoms of God and Satan, the cosmic struggle between the forces of evil and God's saving plan, continues in fact throughout Jesus' ministry,[63] and there are recurring temptation scenes, so some scholars prefer the translation "until an opportune moment" or "for a while" or "for the time being".[64]

Comments

Origen, one of the great theologians of the early Church, was of the opinion that this Gospel episode is not to be taken literally. This is a view that most contemporary scholars share. Satan's transporting Jesus to the pinnacle of the temple in the holy city, or to a high place from which he can view all the kingdoms of the world, has a distinctly mythical air, even if understood as a visionary experience. The dialogue between Jesus and Satan, the trading of scriptural quotations, which is the heart of the narrative, smacks of a rabbinic debate. It is not the record of a historical dialogue. Most likely, the story is the creation of a Christian teacher, reflecting on chapters 6–8 of Deuteronomy, and linking the story of the exodus, the testing of Israel and Israel's testing of God, with the tradition of the testing of Jesus. It is a literary device, a symbolic or parabolic reflection, a theological meditation on the nature of Jesus' sonship.[65]

Gerhard Lohfink writes: "Let us be plain about it: it is a fictional story. But it was this use of fiction that presented the possibility of telling something that was full to the brim with reality: Jesus was tempted more than once."[66]

In the Fourth Gospel, there is no temptation scene at the outset of Jesus' ministry. However, the substance of the Synoptic temptation narrative is found in different places in John's tradition.[67] In chapter six, Jesus takes a boat journey across the Sea of Galilee or Tiberias, and the crowds follow him by land. They are enthusiastic because of the signs that he has been working in curing the sick. Jesus is concerned for the crowds, and provides for them a banquet of loaves and fishes. Five thousand people partake. The story concludes: "When the people saw the sign that he had done, they began to say, 'This is indeed the prophet who is to come into the world.' When he realised that they were about to come and take him by force to make him king, he withdrew again to the mountain by himself" (6:14–15). The crowd's assessment links what has just happened with God's promise one day to raise up a prophet like Moses. Their messianic hopes fanned, the people determine to force Jesus to be their messianic king. He is clearly uncomfortable with this inadequate perception of his identity and role, misguided and dangerous as it is. He beats a hasty retreat, heading off to the hills.

Shortly afterwards, after Jesus and his disciples have crossed the lake again and returned to Capernaum, some of the same crowd meet up with him. To their enquiries about his coming there, Jesus replies: "Very truly I tell you, you are looking for me, not because you saw signs, but because you ate your fill of the loaves. Do not work for food that perishes, but for food that endures for eternal life which the Son of Man will give you" (6:26–27).

Jesus is well aware that they have failed to perceive the deeper meaning of what took place the previous day, and are interested only in ordinary bread. Jesus has come to offer them a form of bread that sustains life at a different level. Later in the dialogue, the people ask Jesus for a sign so that they can believe in him. They demand that he establish his messianic credentials in the style of Moses who provided manna in the wilderness. When Jesus again attempts to lift the conversation to another plane by stressing that it is the Father who is providing bread from heaven, a bread which gives life to the world, the people fail to grasp his meaning and remain at the level of their ordinary human needs, asking for copious and ongoing bread supplies: "Give us this bread now and always.'[68] The bread that Jesus is talking about is his word, the revelation he brings from God.

Some time later, as the Jewish Feast of Tabernacles draws near, the brothers of Jesus approach him with a persuasive suggestion: "Leave here and go to Judea so that your disciples also may see the works you are doing; for no one who wants to be widely known acts in secret. If you do these things, show yourself to the world" (7:3–4). They urge him to make the pilgrimage journey up to Jerusalem at a time when the city will be crowded to capacity for the weeklong celebration. That setting will enable him to make a public display of power for all to see further works and signs. He should capitalise on this golden opportunity to acquire a following no longer in the provincial backwoods but on the high stage of the thronging metropolis. But Jesus rejects their misguided idea and declines to accompany them.[69]

Returning to Luke's story of Jesus, it is clear that the temptation theme is not restricted to this wilderness scene at the outset of Jesus' ministry. Jesus continues to be tested throughout his ministry, though Satan is not the overt player. There are occasions, for instance, when he is pressed by the religious leaders to provide them with a sign to prove that he is genuine. "Others, to test him, kept demanding from him a sign from heaven" (11:16).[70] On another occasion Jesus states: "This generation is an evil generation; it asks for a sign, but no sign will be given to it except the sign of Jonah" (11:29). One of the most significant incidents takes place in the Gospels of Matthew and Mark after Simon Peter's profession of faith at Caesarea Philippi, when, in response to Jesus' question about the disciples' understanding of his identity, Simon Peter states: "You are the Messiah, the Son of the living God." Jesus goes on to speak about his journeying to Jerusalem, where he would suffer and be put to death; this is his first prediction of the passion. "And Peter took him aside and began to rebuke him, saying, 'God forbid it, Lord! This must never happen to you.' But he turned and said to Peter, 'Get behind me, Satan! You are a stumbling-block to me; for you are setting your mind not on divine things but on human things'" (Matt 16:21–23; Mark 8:27–33). Peter is uncomfortable with this new idea and its implications for Jesus and himself, and is seeking in strong language to deter Jesus from following what he understands to be the Father's will for his life and mission. Jesus' brusque reprimand links the disciple's stance with the role of Satan, and makes clear his own commitment to be faithful to the Father, even though this entails suffering and death.

The theme reaches a climax on Calvary's hill. After Jesus has been crucified and the two bandits with him, "Those who passed by derided him, shaking their heads and saying, 'You who would destroy the temple and build it in three days, save yourself! If you are the Son of God, come down from the cross'" (Matt 27:39–40). The chief priests, the scribes and elders also mocked him: "He saved others; he cannot save himself. He is the King of Israel; let him come down from the cross, and we will believe in him. He trusts in God; let God deliver him now, if he wants to, for he said: 'I am God's Son'" (Matt 27:41–43). In words and gestures that recall Psalm 22:7–8, and its commentary Wisdom 2:12–20, Jesus' adversaries play Satan's role. The nature of sonship, the issue of trust, the seeking of a sign and the question of salvation recur. As in the wilderness story at the beginning of the active ministry, Jesus is not interested in quick solutions, in spectacular signs, in power and glory. He shows that true sonship is a matter of trust in the Father and obedience to the Father's will, even in the face of failure, suffering and death.[71]

All this is not to deny that after his baptism, Jesus may indeed have spent some time in prayerful reflection in the wilderness near the Jordan, and he may have wrestled with the implications of his identity and mission. He may even have communicated this to his disciples, possibly in dramatic form. But it seems more likely that the Christian source behind the 'Q' narrative is responsible for focusing in concentrated and dramatic form in the wilderness scene, in a typically folkloric structure and using the biblical tradition, real moments of testing that punctuated the whole of Jesus' public life right up to the cross, as people, disciples and circumstances demanded that he clarify what faithfulness to God and to his mission entailed.[72]

Reflections

So, what has all this fascinating material got to do with us?

I believe that the theme of Jesus' temptations has two main aspects, which are closely connected. These are intimately linked with the baptismal scene, which precedes them in the Gospel narrative. Here, Jesus is anointed with the Spirit and is called "My Son, the beloved." The temptations all have to do with his relationship with the Father and with his messianic mission.

Israel of old had been called and commissioned to be in the world a people who gave honour to God, a people for whom God was central. They were called to love God with all their heart and soul and mind and strength. This was the core of their daily prayer, the *Shema*. But over the centuries and in so many different ways, Israel had been unfaithful, had wandered away and had served other gods.

With Jesus, it is different. The Father is utterly central to all he is and does. Jesus is completely caught up in God; he lives for God with uncompromising and unconditional determination. Jesus is totally devoted to the Father, and he is committed to his mission, to proclaim and make present and real the reign of God. His dream and passion is the Father's dream and passion. He searches for and surrenders to the Father's will, and he trusts unconditionally in the Father's love and providential care. This is what it means to be the beloved Son of God.

Through our baptism, we are anointed with the Spirit and are drawn into Jesus' relationship with the Father. We are children of God, sons and daughters of God, sharers in God's life now in the present. Each of us seeks to live out this relationship in a unique way in a particular moment and place in history. Our Gospel text invites us to ask ourselves whether we really do love God with the whole of our being, without reserve, nothing held back.

In the course of his ministry, Jesus found himself at odds with the various messianic expectations and presuppositions of the people, their leaders and even his disciples and family. Some were interested in a kind of social Gospel aimed at the amelioration of the material everyday conditions of life, which were particularly difficult and oppressive under Herod and Rome. Providing bread supplies would have been a welcome move. Though sensitive to these needs, this was not primarily what he was about. We today can become absorbed or bogged down by immediate concerns and lose the bigger picture. The secularised and consumer society bombards us. We can become anxious and preoccupied and want a quick solution to needs and problems. Plans and methodologies and targets can captivate us. We may find that we are not too interested in the word of God; it is left to linger on the back-burner. Or we can find ourselves using God for our own short-term ends.

Like people everywhere, the people Jesus encountered were open to the sensational and the flashing lights, enthusiastic about the extraordinary or wonderful. They wanted to see results. Many wanted tangible and absolutely clear proofs concerning Jesus' credentials, proofs on their own terms. We can be attracted subtly by the lure of success and the spectacular. We can find ourselves and our own interests and projects occupying centre stage. We can seek popularity and a touch of glory, a spot of stardom. We can find ourselves drawn to adopting methods not wholly consistent with the Gospel and its values. We can worship at other shrines; other idols can infiltrate or impinge. Sometimes occasions occur when we desperately want God to intervene, even dramatically, and show that he is really with us, that he loves us as his children, specially chosen and cared for. Trust in God can prove a tall order.

Most of the people of Jesus' day longed for a political, messianic leader who would rid them of the Roman eagle, the jackboot of pagan imperialism, and introduce an era of prosperity, splendour and greatness. The lure of power and control and influence and superiority lurked everywhere—the disciples weren't exempt. And this is still our world at all levels of society. We face the recurring danger of succumbing to false messianisms, forms of domination and oppression, power and control, rather than self-giving and service.

In the face of alternative messianic options, the lack of results and considerable outside pressure from all sides, Jesus is asked to trust unconditionally without demanding guarantees or proofs or verification—not only for his disciples and the authorities and the crowds, but also for himself—confirmation that God has chosen him, is faithful, is with him, and that his servant way really is the vehicle for the inbreak of the Kingdom. He is challenged to be true to the Father and to his deepest self.

And we, too, in response to events that occur, demands that are made on us, values that are challenged, pressures that can be imposed, are called to decide what it means to be true to our identity as disciples of Jesus and children of God. In the circumstances of our daily living, it is not always apparent what faithfulness entails, what love really demands, what the Father is asking of us. It can be difficult to discern what we need to do in the different areas of our lives to make the Kingdom dream come true and to see what being a child of God involves. Even when we know, there remains the challenge to accept and carry it out. But we are asked to be faithful to our God, to be faithful even when it costs, and costs a lot. This story speaks to us realistically in the midst of our daily lives and invites us to renew our love for the Father, to embrace more strongly Jesus' Kingdom dream and to trust in God's overwhelming love and providential care.[73]

Nazareth (4:14–30)

Nazareth was the place where Mary and Joseph lived prior to Gabriel's visit, and the village to which they returned from both Jerusalem visits. There, Jesus grew up.

Nazareth was a small town located on a hillside about 1300 feet (396 m) above sea level in Lower Galilee; it is not mentioned at all in the Hebrew Bible or the writings of the Jewish historian Josephus or early rabbinical literature.[74] The population was Jewish, probably descended from the house of David.[75] Its name is probably derived from the Hebrew word *netser*, which means a shoot or blossom.[76] The Mediterranean lies twenty miles (32 km) to the west, the Sea of Galilee fifteen miles (24 km) to the east. This stretch of water was also referred to as the Lake of Gennesereth, a name derived from the Hebrew word for a lyre or harp, a connection inspired by its shape.[77] Given the lack of real roads between the villages of the area, the town was rather isolated amid a beautiful, fertile landscape, though the north-south road from Jerusalem to the nearby city of Sepphoris ran fairly close to the town. The Gospels do not mention this cosmopolitan and affluent Greek-speaking city, though it was only four miles (6 km) from Nazareth. It had about 25–30,000 inhabitants, a large amphitheatre, houses with frescoes and mosaic floors, a bank and a fortress.[78] What an amazing contrast! Having been destroyed by the Romans in 4 BCE after an insurrection, Herod rebuilt it as his capital city. But the city of Tiberias, constructed on the western shore of the lake and named after the emperor, became the capital in 18 CE.[79]

Galilee was ruled by Herod Antipas, the son of Herod the Great, from 4 BCE to 39 CE; technically, he was a tetrarch rather than a king. Unlike Judea, Galilee was beautiful, green and fertile. It is usually divided into three areas: Upper Galilee, which is over 3,000 feet high (914 m), the source of the Jordan and sparsely inhabited; Lower Galilee, an area of lower hills, including Tabor and Hermon, and the fertile plain of Jezreel, containing numerous villages (maybe as many as 200), and the city of Sepphoris; and the Lake Region, which was densely populated, with a good fishing industry and the important cities of Capernaum, Magdala and Tiberias.

Estimates of Nazareth's population vary from 120 to 2,000.[80] Houses were built on the south, sunniest slope of the hill, probably tightly clustered groups of single or two-roomed buildings with a dirt floor around a central shared courtyard or patio, with a common oven and grindstone. Some would have had a cave as part of the living space or underground cisterns for water or storage. There was a good well at the northern end of the town; there were probably no public buildings, no market, maybe not even a proper synagogue.[81] The stone was mainly limestone, which was soft, and pleasantly bright and clean looking compared to the dark basalt of places like Capernaum. The roofing consisted of wooden beams covered with reeds, mud plaster and compacted earth.[82] Clothes, fruits and vegetables were dried on the roof; it also provided an extra place to sleep. Animals were penned in the courtyard or the house itself. Rubbish and sewage found their way into the alleys or streets, so the atmosphere could, at times, be unpleasant and was quite unhealthy!

There were vineyards and olive groves on the terraces, which had been laboriously constructed on the hillside; drainage was good and the soil was rich in calcium.[83] Wheat, barley and millet grew on the broad hillsides; fruit and vegetables, like dates, figs, pomegranates, melons, lentils, chickpeas, cucumbers, onions, garlic, in the shadier areas. The average temperature was about 11 degrees centigrade (51°F) in January, and 27 degrees (80°F) in July and August; so, Nazareth had quite a pleasant climate. Obviously, the women made bread; the villagers also ate fish (probably pickled by the lakeside), eggs, fowl, cheese, yogurt, lamb and, on special occasions, beef.[84] They ate two meals a day: in the late morning and evening. There was a common cistern, millstone, olive press and winepress.[85] It was customary for everyone to help out with the olives and grapes. Life expectancy was in the thirties; to reach the age of fifty was rare.[86] People suffered from iron deficiency, malaria, arthritis and tuberculosis.

In the villages, the families were closely knit, and the extended family or clan was a strong unity; there was a vibrant sense of community. People needed one another and supported one another for survival, especially in difficult times.[87] Upholding family honour was important. Jesus seems to have been uncomfortable with traditional patriarchy and with the situation of women.[88] Clothing was simple: the men wore a loincloth, a tunic, usually of cotton or wool with two vertical stripes, and a cloak or mantle and sandals. Women's dress was simple and plain. Women would weave and spin and sew, making and mending the clothes, as well as fetching the water and cooking. They would also work in the fields, and, of course, look after the children. Life was difficult. The taxes were severe: there was the temple tithe, and the impositions of Rome and of Herod. Some of the peasants had their own land, others were tenant farmers. Their existence was precarious; there was great fear of falling into debt.

The common everyday language of the people was Aramaic, as also in Jerusalem; Galileans had their own accent. Some Aramaic words have found their way into the Gospel text (*abba, corbona, talitha kum, cephas, raqa, rabbuni*).[89] Jesus probably knew some Greek also, which was necessary for business purposes. Greek was commonly spoken in the local city of Sepphoris. How much education Jesus would have received is debated. In Galilee, few people were literate; access to books, parchment or ink was minimal.[90] He probably knew Hebrew passages of the Bible by heart; some suggest that he may have been able to read and understand it. He was naturally very intelligent. His parents, especially Joseph, would have seen to his religious education. Some think Jesus did have education in scripture and became a 'scholar'.[91] John Meier writes that Jesus was able to read from the scriptures; his teaching is imbued with the outlook and language of the sacred texts of Judaism, which suggests his religious formation in his family was intense and profound, and included instruction in reading biblical Hebrew.[92]

After his Jordan baptism and subsequent time of testing, Jesus returns to Galilee, and there he embarks upon his ministry. Luke provides a brief transitional summary:

> Then Jesus, filled with the power of the Spirit, returned to Galilee, and a report about him spread through all the surrounding country. He began to teach in their synagogues and was praised by everyone.

Again, Luke emphasises the presence of the Spirit with Jesus. After receiving the Spirit at his baptism, his anointing for mission, and having in the Spirit's power been tested and proved true to God, Jesus moves into ministry "with the power of the Spirit in him", and his messianic ministry is initially one of teaching. Later summaries include healing as well.[93] Jesus makes a tour of the local communities, teaching in their synagogues.[94] No content of Jesus' preaching is provided, but from the outset his words create a widespread and profound impression, which will set a pattern for his early ministry. And the enthusiastic response is universal, for "everyone" sang his praises. This is a typical Lukan feature, but it is particularly significant here because of the contrast soon to follow.[95]

For Luke, Jesus' visit to the place where he was brought up, located by Mark and Matthew at a later stage in his ministry, signals the formal beginning of his ministry.[96] There are two parts to the scene: first, there is an account of his inaugural sermon; secondly, there is a description of two responses, the first positive, the second hostile and violent. The first part reads:

When he came to Nazareth, where he had been brought up, he went to the synagogue on the sabbath day, as was his custom. He stood up to read, and the scroll of the prophet Isaiah was given to him. He unrolled the scroll and found the place where it was written:

"The Spirit of the Lord is upon me, because he has anointed me to bring good news to the poor.

"He has sent me to proclaim release to the captives and recovery of sight to the blind, to let the oppressed go free, to proclaim the year of the Lord's favour."

And he rolled up the scroll, gave it back to the attendant, and sat down. The eyes of all in the synagogue were fixed on him. Then he began to say to them, "Today this scripture has been fulfilled in your hearing."

Nazareth (or *Nazara*) is described as the place where Jesus has been brought up; reference was made to it earlier in Luke's story (2:39–40, 51–52). On the Sabbath, he goes to the synagogue as usual. He is portrayed as a pious Jew, faithfully following the traditional mores of his people, as did his parents earlier in the story (2:42). Jesus is invited to read by the attendant, an important synagogue official who usually conducted the services. In the synagogue service after personal prayer, the reciting of the *Shema* took place, followed by some further prayers. The central part of the service consisted of the assigned readings from the Torah in Hebrew with Aramaic paraphrasing, a reading from the prophets, a prayer, a sermon and a blessing.[97] Most scholars believe that in Jesus' day the prophetic text did not follow a fixed lectionary. The text handed to him is the scroll of Isaiah, which may imply that Jesus requested it. This he unrolls and finds the extract he wants,[98] which reads:

The Spirit of the Lord is upon me, for he has anointed me to bring good news to the poor. He has sent me to proclaim release to the captives, and recovery of sight to the blind, to let the oppressed go free, to proclaim the year of the Lord's favour.

The text is a mixed citation from the Greek (the Septuagint) version of Isaiah 61:1–2; 58:5–7.[99] The reference to binding up the broken-hearted has been omitted, for reasons which are not evident, as has the concluding reference to "the day of vengeance", probably because of its negative connotation. "To let the oppressed go free" has been included, a phrase taken from Isa 58:5–7. The three uses of "me" link the anointing by the Spirit and the mission of Jesus. In his ministry, the accent will rest on God's gracious mercy and liberating generosity. After reading the text, Jesus rolls up the scroll and returns it to the assistant, then he sits down, the normal posture for preaching.[100] The eyes of everyone (the word is given emphasis by its position in the sentence) are riveted on him, and he begins to speak. It is a dramatic moment. Luke creates an atmosphere of suspense and expectancy as Jesus prepares to utter the first recorded words of his ministry. Jesus' opening statement is solemn and arresting, as the occasion demands: "Today this scripture has been fulfilled in your hearing."

The emphatic "today" conveys an intense sense of fulfilment. The long-awaited age of salvation has dawned, the scriptural dreams of centuries are coming true, and Jesus claims a central role in all this. Reference to "in your hearing" demands a response.[101] This text of Isaiah is clearly intended to communicate Jesus' programme of action; it summarises his mission (like a modern mission statement); it describes the kind of Messiah he will be. His mission stems from his anointing by the Spirit, which empowers him to act as God's eschatological representative and prophet. His role is spelled out in terms of proclaiming and making present the Good News of God's liberation and favour.[102] Like the Servant prophet of Isaiah, Jesus is sent to the poor. This is an important theme in Luke's Gospel; the word means those who are economically poor, struggling to survive, and also the marginalised, outcasts, people excluded from human fellowship.[103] "Blind" is to be interpreted physically and symbolically. The term for "release" (*aphesis*) is the same as that used for forgiveness (Zechariah in 1:77; the Baptist in 3:3) and is another significant word in Luke's vocabulary.[104] Mention of letting the oppressed go free, imported from a different Isaian text, which in the original context includes the idea of social justice, recalls the reversal theme of the *Magnificat* (1:51–53). "The year of the Lord's favour" alludes to the jubilee year, held every 50 years, when slaves were freed and debts cancelled.[105] This mission statement contains enormous potential and has far-reaching consequences, and sketches the contours of Jesus' future ministry.

The second part of the scene contains two responses to Jesus and his words:

> All spoke well of him and were amazed at the gracious words that came from his mouth. They said, "Is not this Joseph's son?" He said to them, "Doubtless you will quote to me this proverb, 'Doctor, cure yourself!' And you will say, 'Do here also in your home town the things that we have heard you did at Capernaum'." And he said, "Truly I tell you, no prophet is accepted in the prophet's home town. But the truth is, there were many widows in Israel in the time of Elijah, when the heaven was shut up for three years and six months, and there was a severe famine over all the land; yet Elijah was sent to none of them except to a widow at Zarephath in Sidon. There were also many lepers in Israel in the time of the prophet Elisha, and none of them was cleansed except Naaman the Syrian." When they heard this, all in the synagogue were filled with rage. They got up, drove him out of the town, and led him to the brow of the hill on which their town was built, so that

they might hurl him off the cliff. But he passed through the midst of them and went on his way.

Presumably, Jesus spends some time expounding this magnificent text, so pregnant with meaning, for the result is that he succeeds in winning the approval of his fellow townsfolk, who remain astonished by his "gracious" words. This may mean graciously delivered, grace-filled in content, or both.[106] But then the atmosphere changes quite suddenly, as the people begin to reflect that he is only the son of Joseph yet is making high claims for himself.[107] Jesus seems to sense the change of mood and takes the initiative, perhaps rendering explicit the crowd's incipient murmuring. With prophetic discernment[108] he suggests that they will go on to quote the common adage: "Physician, heal yourself", and bid him do in his own place what they have heard he has performed in Capernaum; he ought to start the ministry he has been describing at home, where culturally there are ingroup obligations, rather than elsewhere.[109] There are perhaps two implications to these words. First, with a touch of jealousy, parochial prejudice and provincial small mindedness, and a demand for preferential treatment, the people want Jesus to bring them the same benefits as the other places he has visited.[110] Secondly, he should provide some sign to guarantee the claims he has been making.[111]

Jesus continues by stating with solemnity "In truth I tell you"[112] (more solemnly than in Mark or Matthew) the adage that no prophet is ever accepted in his own country. He clearly sees himself as a prophet. The truth of the statement will soon be illustrated! He continues by recalling (with poetic parallelism) the days of the great prophets Elijah and Elisha (see also 7:1–16). During the prolonged drought and famine of Elijah's time, it was not to one of the many widows of Israel that the prophet was sent by God, but to a gentile widow from Zarephath near Sidon (1 Kgs 17:1–16). And it was not one of Israel's lepers that the prophet Elisha cured, but Naaman from Syria, also a gentile (2 Kgs 5:1–14). These examples indicate a rejection of a narrow, insider vision and exclusive claims, and hint at a wider understanding of Isaiah's words, even an opening to the gentile world.[113]

This plain-speaking attack of Jesus causes great indignation and resentment among his hearers. They have recourse to a type of lynch law and hustle him out of town, intending to throw him over the cliff of the hill on which the town was built, and perhaps then crush him with a boulder or batter him with stones, and this on the Sabbath. The prophet's words quickly come true! In fact, Nazareth was not built on the top of a hill, but there are cliffs nearby. Jesus, however, "passed straight through the crowd and went on his way" to continue the mission for which he was anointed. Later, in another place, there will be a greater rejection and a successful execution of this prophet.[114]

Luke, with great artistry, has set the scene for the rest of his story. This passage is a programmatic prophecy, a kind of manifesto; it sets a pattern for what is to come. Jesus is both Messiah and prophet. Luke explains something of the kind of Messiah Jesus will be as the Spirit guides and empowers him, a prophetic Messiah. The focus and nature of his ministry is outlined: to bring the Good News to the poor, blind, oppressed, captives. As the narrative proceeds, we will see this programme carried out. Later, John the Baptist, languishing in Herod's jail, having received information about what Jesus is saying and doing and how people are responding, sends two of his disciples to ask Jesus whether he is the one who is to come or should they await another. He is puzzled because there is clearly a discrepancy between his style and outlook and that of Jesus.

Jesus answers the messengers:

> Go back and tell John what you have seen and heard: the blind see again, the lame walk, those suffering from virulent skin diseases are cleansed, and the deaf hear, the dead are raised to life, the good news is proclaimed to the poor; and blessed is anyone who does not find me a cause of falling. (7:22–23)

The phrases of Jesus' reply echo the messianic expectations of the prophet Isaiah. The scriptural pedigree is strong, the evidence is clear. Jesus is inviting him to think again and not to be put off by his different approach and message.

At the same time in this episode at Nazareth, the theme of prophetic rejection, adumbrated in Simeon's words to Mary (2:34), is announced. Jesus' comment about the prophet being unwelcome in his own country is borne out by the subsequent action of the townsfolk. Simeon in his canticle (2:32) and the quotation from Isaiah used at the outset of the ministry of the Baptist (3:6) have already informed the reader that the salvation brought by Jesus would extend to all nations. His people hear this now, and they react with anger and provincial fervour, and so fulfil Jesus' statement.[115] As the narrative proceeds, this pattern of rejection will continue and will intensify. Jesus will create division, as Simeon foretold (2:34–35). The shadow of rejection hangs over his ministry from its inception. The same pattern will happen when Jesus visits the city of Jerusalem.

There, the people will respond positively, but the religious leaders will organise his death. "But in a true sense, through his resurrection and ascension, he will also 'pass through their midst'."[116]

Reflections

For some twenty years or more, mission statements have been fashionable in many areas of our lives. We have perhaps struggled to be creative and clear in articulating what we are really about. Some I have come across are pithy and catchy and clever, others somewhat pedestrian and laboured. In quoting Isaiah in the Nazareth synagogue, Jesus launches his mission in style; the contours are clear and strong, the vision exciting and hope-filled, the implications far-reaching but dangerous. He is embarking on an attempt to change the world, to turn accepted mindsets and ways of operating upside-down. For it is the reign of God that he is committed to establishing. Centuries of longing and dreaming are caught up in his mission. The possibilities are exhilarating. However, from the outset the response is not only ambivalent but violently negative, for change is always threatening, vested interests unmoving. The reader is drawn into a story of liberation and compassion but also of intensifying conflict.

As his followers, the episodes of this chapter can set our hearts on fire, as the presence of Jesus did for the Emmaus disciples. In our baptism, we have been anointed by the Spirit. We have been proclaimed by the Father as deeply loved sons and daughters, able to address God in familiar "Abba" terms. "Sealed" by the Spirit we belong to God in our deepest personal being (2 Cor 1:21–22; Eph 1:13; 4:30). Through that Spirit gift we have become "sent ones" (John 9:7), called to share the mission of Jesus, to make his Kingdom dream ever more real in our world, centuries later. The temptation story highlights some of the possible problems and pitfalls, suggesting the kind of challenges that will face us. Faithfulness to our true identity and our mission will not come easily.

The Nazareth incident provides us with clear guidelines as to what we are about in terms of compassion and liberation. It also makes it clear that we ourselves and our witness and message will not always be welcomed with interest, openness and enthusiasm. We must expect to be sidelined, opposed and rejected, even with violence. Recent events across our world make this limpidly clear. Each day we are invited by our God to utter our "yes", as Mary did, "yes" to who we are, "yes" to whatever God asks of us. We embrace our destiny humbly and with great trust in God's faithful love.

Notes

1   Carroll, *Luke*, 88; Green, *Luke*, 159; Marshall, *Luke*, 131. Tannehill, *Luke*, 77, goes as far as 4:44, Jesus' visit to the Capernaum synagogue.

2   For more details on the Baptist, see Michael T. Winstanley, *Jesus and the Little People* (Bolton: Don Bosco Publications, 2012), 12–16; Dunn, *Jesus Remembered*, 339–379; Meier, *A Marginal Jew*, 2:19–223; N. Tom Wright, *Jesus and the Victory of God* (London: SPCK, 2000), 160–162.

3   This setting is more elaborate than those in 1:5 and 2:1–2. Byrne, *Hospitality*, 39, notes the pattern whereby the "sacred" events of the life of Jesus interact with the ordinary flow of affairs; they do not run parallel or divorced from everyday life. Tiberias became emperor in 14 CE; Pilate governed until 36, Herod until 39. Annas was high priest from 6–15, Caiaphas, his son-in-law, from 18–36, though Annas seems to have maintained considerable influence. The date for the commencement of John's activity would probably be 28/29 CE. (See Carroll, *Luke*, 90; McBride, *Luke*, 50; Green, *Luke*, 167.) For further information about these characters, see Green, *Luke*, 168–169; Evans, *Luke*, 231–234. Luke is the only evangelist to situate the Gospel story on a world stage.

4   This introduction is similar to the call of the prophets of old (Isa 1:1; Jer 1:2–3; Hos 1:1; Jonah 1:1).

5   Resseguie, *Spiritual Landscape*, 11: "The Israelites crossed the Jordan, leaving behind the desert wandering for a new life in a new land; similarly, the new Israel crosses the Jordan once more in 3:7–17—a crossing that takes the form of baptism of repentance for the forgiveness of sins." Green, *Luke*, 170, notes that John remains apart from urban centres.

6   Luke's quotation from Isaiah, including the promise that everyone will see God's salvation (a key Lukan theme), is fuller than that in Mark and Matthew. Luke omits a description of John's clothing and diet, found in both. Mark has no reference to purifying "fire" or to John's dialogue with the crowd, tax collectors and soldiers; Matthew mentions only Pharisees and Sadducees. John's recommendations are in keeping with Luke's perspective. The imagery of Spirit and fire will recur in the description of Pentecost in Acts 2:3–4. The text originally referred to God; now it refers to Jesus ("Lord" and "his").

7   Carroll, *Luke*, 91; Green, *Luke*, 173.

8   Green, *Luke*, 172.

9   Luke tends to mention a character's departure before dealing with another character (see 1:56–57). Mark mentions John's imprisonment and death later in Jesus' ministry (6:17).

10   For Mark (1:9–11), see Winstanley, *Jesus*, 27–32, and the bibliography provided there. In Matthew, John objects to baptising Jesus, and Jesus has to persuade him to continue (Matt 3:13–17); in John, the baptism is implied rather than described; the Baptist witnesses to the descent of the Spirit, and testifies to Jesus' divine sonship (1:32–34). Evans, *Luke*, 245, prefers to speak of divine empowering rather than baptism in Luke's story.

11   Green, *Luke*, 185. Marshall, *Luke*, 152, understands that Jesus' baptism takes

place after the people have been baptised, and is the climax of the Baptist's work, though historically there was some later overlap.

12   3:21; 5:16; 6:12; 9:18, 28–29; 11:1; 22:41, 44–45; 23:46. This is the theme of chapter five.

13   Green, *Luke*, 185,187, considers the scene to be set in an apocalyptic world of which this is an element.

14   In Acts 10:38, Peter states: "God anointed Jesus of Nazareth with the Holy Spirit and with power." Tannehill, *Luke*, 84, makes the link with the Nazareth scene.

15   Johnson, *Luke*, 69.

16   Johnson, *Luke*, 71.

17   Johnson, *Luke*, 71.

18   Green, *Luke*, 187, stresses the importance of Abraham for Luke. He also refers to Isa 42:6; 49:6.

19   There are some manuscripts which give this complete verse, and the NJB adopts this alternative version, but it does seem to be secondary.

20   Marshall, *Luke*, 155.

21   Marshall, *Luke*, 156.

22   Marshall, *Luke*, 156.

23   Carroll, *Luke*, 97.

24   Green, *Luke*, 187.

25   McBride, *Luke*, 58.

26   Caird, *Luke*, 76. Evans, *Luke*, 245, thinks it unlikely that Jesus was the source (speaking to the disciples of himself as son of God). It is the result of theological reflection. Marshall, *Luke*, 151, believes that the case that Jesus' ministry was preceded by some kind of "call" experience is strong; the account may well express in concrete form the consciousness of divine calling with which he began his ministry; "historical study can scarcely go beyond this possibility." See Pagola, *Jesus*, 297–98. Marcus J. Borg, *Jesus: The Life, Teachings, and Relevance of a Religious Revolutionary* (New York: HarperOne, 2006), 120–122, 131–135, refers to a "vision" and a mystical experience.

27   Caird, *Luke*, 77: "Remembering Luke's story of the boy Jesus, we cannot suppose that all this now suddenly flashed upon him as a new and startling revelation, that up to this moment it had never occurred to him that God had singled him out for a special vocation."

28   Dunn, *Jesus Remembered*, 376. Meier, *A Marginal Jew*, 2:109, comments that we do not know whether the baptism was the cause, the ritual celebration or a step to a later decision.

29   Johnson, *Luke*, 70.

30   For reflections on Matthew's genealogy, see Winstanley, *An Advent Journey*, 102–106.

31   Carroll, *Luke*, 100, asks "Will Jesus wisely discern, and then faithfully obey, the vocation that God has set before him?"

32   See Fitzmyer, *Luke*, 1:507–508; he believes that Matthew retains the original order of 'Q'. In *Luke the Theologian*, (London: Geoffrey Chapman, 1989), 153–154, he also records other views, and dismisses them. The quotations which Jesus uses in

Matthew are in the reverse order of their Old Testament occurrence. Marshall, *Luke*, 167, also believes that Matthew's order is the original.

33 Johnson, *Luke*, 75, notes that Luke frames the temptation story by the genealogy and the Nazareth episode. Green, *Luke*, 191, views the story as an "episode of transition." Carroll, *Luke*, 101, n. 8, prefers to see Jesus' ordeal as a testing of his faithfulness. Marshall, *Luke*, 169, notes the illusion to Deut 8:2, where Israel was led in the wilderness to be tested by God.

34 Mark 1:12. Fitzmyer, *Luke the Theologian: Aspects of his Teaching*, (London: Geoffrey Chapman, 1989), 152, comments that Luke omits Mark's reference to the wild animals and angels, "the motif of Paradise Regained." There is no idyllic aspect to this episode in Luke.

35 Green, *Luke*, 191, observes that Jesus moves into an active role, but is not alone; he is God's agent. This special relationship and its implications lie at the root of Jesus' identity in Luke-Acts.

36 Lev 16:10; Isa 13:21; 34:14; Tob 8:3. See McBride, *Luke*, 59.

37 Exod 16:4; 20:20; Deut 8:2; 13:2.

38 Num 14:22; Pss 95:8; 106:14. See also Marshall, *Luke*, 169.

39 Hos 11:1; see Exod 4:22; Deut 14:1. Johnson, *Luke*, 76, lists the biblical symbolism.

40 Exod 24:18; 1 Kings 19:8. Matthew adds "forty nights".

41 Exod 34:28.

42 Evans, *Luke*, 256; Green, *Luke*, 193; Carroll, *Luke*, 102.

43 Luke uses "devil" in this episode, but tends to use "devil" and "Satan" interchangeably. His role recalls Job. For a brief note on the development of Israel's understanding of the devil, see Evans, 257.

44 "If" can also mean "since": (Evans, *Luke*, 258).

45 Exod 16.

46 Deut 8:6.

47 John 4:34.

48 A phrase of McBride's, *Luke*, 61; also: The devil "does not want Jesus to take his mission from the Father seriously, and accept the poverty of the human lot." Marshall, *Luke*, 170–171.

49 Green, *Luke*, 194, observes that the devil reinterprets sonship, wishing Jesus to use his power in his own way to serve his own ends. Jesus identifies with the starving people of God, while affirming his trust in divine provision. Similarly, Evans, *Luke*, 258.

50 Caird, *Luke*, 80, refers to Jesus being caught up into the air in "ecstatic and imaginative vision". Green, *Luke*, 194, speaks of "a visionary spectacle"; Marshall, *Luke*, 171, of "the visionary nature of Jesus' experience".

51 Johnson, *Luke*, 74, notes the use of *oikoumenē*, when he means the social or political order; it expresses Luke's perception of imperial arrangements. Carroll, *Luke*, 103, notes the political implications, especially with reference to Rome. Green too, *Luke*, 194, observes that in 2:1; 3:1, "all the world" was the Roman Empire; he refers to human and systemic agents opposed to God's plan who are manifestations of diabolic rule.

52   Caird, *Luke*, 80, acknowledges that "Jesus does not dispute his claim." Green, *Luke*, 194, refers to the promise of Psalm 2:8: "I will make the nations your heritage, and the ends of the earth your possession."

53   Deut 6:4–5.

54   Luke 10:25–28.

55   See 2 Kings 16: 3–4; Jer 7:31; Ps 106: 36–39.

56   Jesus' ministry is one of service and liberation, a different kind of kingdom.

57   Caird, *Luke*, 81. Jesus will achieve authority over the world, but through his fulfilling his mission by surrendering to suffering and death, a non-domination style; see Byrne, *Hospitality*, 42. Johnson, *Luke*, 75, notes that Luke sees the struggle between God and the powers of evil as one between two kingdoms.

58   Johnson, *Luke*, 74.

59   Exod 17: 1–7.

60   Num 20: 2–13.

61   Carroll, *Luke*, 104; also. Green, *Luke*, 195.

62   Green, *Luke*, 196.

63   Caird, *Luke*, 81, refers to "the insistent demands upon his compassion, the enthusiasm that would make him a national hero, the suspicion that demanded a sign from heaven." Green, *Luke*, 196, states that the three tests encapsulate all the tests Jesus would meet in the ministry, as Jesus encounters demons and forces hostile to God's purpose.

64   Carroll, *Luke*, 101, believes that the same phrase in Acts 13:11 suggests this translation.

65   For an insightful discussion see Fitzmyer, *Luke*, 1: 509–510. Marshall, *Luke*, 169, however, is of the view that it is likely that Jesus communicated something of his inner experience to his disciples; at the outset of his ministry he probably had to face up to the nature of his vocation.

66   Gerhard Lohfink, *Jesus of Nazareth: What He wanted. Who He Was*, trans. Linda M. Maloney (Collegeville, MN: Liturgical Press, 2012), 223.

67   See Raymond E. Brown, *New Testament Essays* (New York: Paulist, 1965), 203–207.

68   6:34.

69   The "brothers" of Jesus are referred to also in 2:12. Luke refers to them in 8:19–21, and Mark in 3:31–35, where sisters are mentioned too. In Mark 6:3 the brothers are named "James, and Joses and Judas and Simon". Paul in 1 Cor 15:7 refers to the appearance of Jesus to James. Three views have been proposed from the second century onwards: these were children of Joseph by an earlier marriage; they were cousins; they were natural children of Mary and Joseph. The two former views are generally held by Catholic scholars, the third view by non-Catholics. Meier, *A Marginal Jew*, 1:332, however, concludes that from a purely philological and historical point of view, the most probable opinion is that the brothers and sisters of Jesus were his siblings. This is probably the way Mark understood them. See M. Eugene Boring, *Mark. A Commentary*. (London: Westminster John Knox Press, 2006); Donahue and Harrington, *Mark*, 187–188: Francis J. Moloney, *The Gospel of Mark* (Peabody MA: Hendrickson, 2002), 112, n. 212. Pagola,

106

Jesus, 58, n. 11, comments that the Catholic Church has always assumed that texts are not referring to other sons of the Virgin Mary.

70   See Matt 12:38; 16:1–4; Mark 8:11–12.

71   The Passion of Luke is somewhat gentler than that of Mark or Matthew. The people do not mock Jesus; the leaders scoff just once (23:35); see Chapter Thirteen later.

72   See Michael T. Winstanley, *Come and See* (London: DLT, 1985), 57.

73   See also Heb 4:15; 5:2; 2:17 and John 12:27.

74   Pagola, *Jesus,* 56.

75   Kauffman, *Nazareth,* 17. Pixner, *With Jesus through Galilee,*14: Isa 11:1 writes "a shoot will come up from the stump of Jesse, from his roots a branch (*netzer*) will bear fruit." Rev 22:16b says, "I am the Root and Offspring of David". Pixner notes that Bartimaeus, when the people say that Jesus of Nazareth was passing by, says "Jesus, Son of David" (Mk 10:47). *Netzer* can also be used for a clan. He thinks the village got its name from a Davidic clan that came from Babylon around 100 BCE, when there was immigration from Babylon and Persia, at the time of John Hyrcanus, (134–104 BCE), Aristobulus I (104–103) and Jannaeus (103–76).

76   Kauffman, *Nazareth,* 17. In John's Gospel the term "The Nazarene" is used of Jesus only in the Passion narrative, for the inscription on the cross and twice during the garden scene in which Jesus gives himself up. "The Nazarene", it is maintained, can be understood as a messianic title. Isaiah speaks of the future spirit-endowed ruler as a "shoot" and as a "branch". The "branch" image is adopted by later prophets with a clearly messianic thrust. The name of the village where Jesus grew up, Nazareth, is derived from the Hebrew stem for "shoot", and its equivalent term "branch". Zechariah states that the future temple builder will be a man named "Branch". So, it is possible that John here intends Pilate to use two synonymous titles for Jesus: the Nazarene, and the King of the Jews. See M.L. Coloe, *God Dwells with Us: Temple Symbolism in the Fourth Gospel* (Collegeville, MN: The Liturgical Press, 2001), 171–174, for a strong case for the "branch" source; also, Pixner, *With Jesus through Galilee,* 14–19.

77   In John's Gospel, it is referred to as the Sea of Tiberias, which probably reflects a later designation linked with the Herodian city constructed on its shore.

78   Martin, *A Pilgrimage,* 80. Josephus called it "the ornament of all Galilee."

79   Donahue & Harrington, *Mark,* 64; Pagola, *Jesus,* 31–51.

80   Meier, *A Marginal Jew,* 1:301, suggests 1600–2000; Pagola, *Jesus,* 56, suggests a smaller population of about 500; the local guides prefer a lower figure too. Borg, *Jesus,* opts for 200–400, as does Martin, *A Pilgrimage,* 75. Kauffman, *Nazareth,* 16, opts for 400–1200. Pixner, *With Jesus through Galilee,* 15, suggests no more than 120–150; he thinks the hamlet belonged to the village of Japhia, a mile (1.5 km) away.

81   Pagola, *Jesus,* 65, states that probably in the small villages a simple house or a patio space served as a place of prayer and assembly. The larger towns probably did have synagogues (Magdala, Capernaum). Kauffman, *Nazareth,* 19, maintains that there was a multipurpose synagogue, probably facing Jerusalem. Carroll, *Luke,* 108, n. 1, quotes an article by Eric M. Meyers, stating the likelihood that the emergence of synagogues as separate buildings in Palestine was primarily a second century CE phenomenon; private houses were used previously.

82   See Kauffman, *Nazareth*, 26, for roofing details.

83   Kauffman, *Nazareth*, 8. Olive trees can last 1000 years; olive oil is used for cooking, medicine, anointing and cleansing, and for lamps; see also 38–39.

84   Jews did not eat pork, nor crab, lobster, clams, shrimps, mussels.

85   A winepress, hewn into the bedrock at the base of the terraces in Nazareth, has been discovered; it dates back to the time of Jesus. See Kauffman, *Nazareth*, 36–37.

86   Martin, *A Pilgrimage*, 77; Pagola, *Jesus*, 60, suggests that infant mortality was 30%; 60% died before the age of 16; few lived until 60.

87   Pagola, *Jesus*, 58, points out that they owned things in common, shared farm tasks, protected the family's goods and reputation.

88   Pagola, *Jesus*, 59, provides a good description of their plight.

89   Lohfink, *Jesus of Nazareth*, 100.

90   Pagola, *Jesus*, 68, observes that only the ruling classes, the Jerusalem aristocracy, the professional scribes and the monks of Qumran had access to a certain level of written culture.

91   Kauffman, *Nazareth*, 49.

92   Meier, 1:276.

93   For teaching, see 4:31–32; 19:47; 21:37–38. For both teaching and healing, see 4:40–42; 6:17–19; 8:1–3. Green, *Luke*, 205, insists that both aspects of his ministry are carefully balanced. Marshall, *Luke*, 176, suggests that the thought of power to do mighty works may be present, possibly present in some visible manner, leading to the spread of his fame.

94   Carroll, *Luke*, 108, observes that Luke seems to regard synagogues as buildings, whereas it would seem that the emergence of synagogues as separate buildings was a second century CE phenomenon. The word also means a "gathering" of people; presumably these took place in private houses. Johnson, *Luke*, 78, notes that the verb "was teaching" indicates repeated action. He views the synagogue as meeting hall, place of prayer, centre of education. Green, *Luke*, 209, suggests that anyone was allowed to speak who had something significant to say, and believes that Jesus frequently ("as was his custom") read and spoke in synagogue.

95   Byrne, *Hospitality*, 45, calls it "a significant backdrop to the drama at Nazareth."

96   Carroll, *Luke*, 108, writes: "Once at Nazareth, Jesus announces the focus, purpose and direction of his ministry—claiming the authorising power of God's own Spirit and marking the present as an era in which prophetic promise within the Scriptures comes to fulfilment."

97   Caird, *Luke*, 87. See also Green, *Luke*, 207, n. 17; Evans, *Luke*, 268; Marshall, *Luke*, 181.

98   Carroll, *Luke*, 111, notes the switch from passive verb to active: the scroll "was given" to Jesus, but he "found" the passage containing the message he wished to deliver.

99   Isa 61:1–2, in which the prophet announces his ministry to the exiles returning from exile, reads: "The Spirit of the Lord is upon me, because he has anointed me; he has sent me to bring good news to the poor, to bind up the broken-hearted, to proclaim release to the captives and recovery of sight to the blind; to proclaim a year of acceptance on the part of the Lord and the day of vengeance of our God."

108

100　Byrne, *Hospitality*, 46, suggests a chiastic structure (ABCDcba): stands; receives, unrolls, reads the scroll; rolls up, hands back the scroll; sits down. He maintains that this pattern lends maximum solemnity to the text which Jesus reads. Carroll, *Luke*, 110, sees two sets of gestures, over which Luke lingers, which slow down the action and highlight the words which follow.

101　Green, *Luke*, 214.

102　Luke often uses this verb *(euangelizesthai)* to describe the preaching of Jesus (4:43; 7:22; 8:1; 9:6; 16:16; 20:1).

103　Green, *Luke*, 211, maintains that "poor" should not be "defined merely in subjective, spiritual or personal, economic terms, but in the holistic sense of those who are for any number of socio-religious reasons relegated to positions outside the boundaries of God's people."

104　Tannehill, *Luke*, 92, suggests three groups: those imprisoned for debt; those suffering from physical ailments or the devil's oppression; and those needing forgiveness. Green, *Luke*, 212, adds that forgiveness implies restoration to the community. Release from debts is linked to the Jubilee legislation, but Isaiah and other texts employ Jubilee themes to signify the eschatological deliverance of God, with its profound social implications. "This interpretive tradition encourages a reading of Luke 4:18–19 as the announcement of the eschatological epoch of salvation, the time of God's gracious visitation, with Jesus himself presented as God's anointed herald."

105　Deut 15:1–18 insists that every seventh year the land should lie fallow, debts should be remitted and slaves released. Lev 25 decreed the jubilee year every fifty years, which entailed the release of slaves and the return of alienated land to the original owner. Here the word used is *dektos*, which means "acceptable"; some translate the phrase "to proclaim an acceptable year of the Lord." The word is also used (advisedly) in 4:24.

106　Carroll, *Luke*, 113.

107　The reader recalls that Jesus is also Son of God (1:32, 35; 2:49; 3:22). Mark 6:3 includes other family names: "Is not this the carpenter, the son of Mary, and brother of James and Joses and Judas and Simon, and are not his sisters here with us?" Green, *Luke*, 215, argues that the people's initial response is one of admiration, claiming Jesus as one of their own, and expecting to be beneficiaries.

108　Carroll's phrase (*Luke*, 114). Green, *Luke*, 216, observes that such knowledge is frequent in Luke and is a characteristic of a Spirit-endowed prophet.

109　Luke has not yet recorded any miraculous activity of Jesus in Capernaum; perhaps they are meant to be included in the earlier summary. In Mark, where the episode comes later, this is not the case. Wright, *Luke*, 47, notes the similarity with the Calvary taunt (23:35).

110　McBride, *Luke*, 64–65.

111　Marshall, *Luke*, 178, 187.

112　"Amen" usually came at the end of a sentence or prayer to denote agreement. Jesus characteristically used it at the beginning of a statement in a distinctive way, to stress the importance of what was to follow. Johnson, *Luke*, 80, calls this "an unmistakeable sign of prophetic consciousness."

113　Carroll, *Luke*, 115–116, notes that Elijah and Elisha worked primarily within the boundaries of Israel; Jesus will do the same. His words prefigure the later Church. However, his ministry to outsiders and marginalised in the community connects his ministry with that of the two prophets. See also Green, *Luke*, 218.

114   Green, *Luke*, 217, observes that he who was anointed to proclaim the year of the Lord's favour, fails to receive the favour of his own townsfolk. Wright, *Luke*, 47, notes the irony, linking this with the third temptation, where the devil invites Jesus to throw himself down from the pinnacle of the temple, trusting in God's protection. Marshall, *Luke*, 180, suggests that Jesus is threatened with the fate of a false prophet.

115   Johnson, *Luke*, 81–82.

116   Byrne, *Hospitality*, 52; similarly, Green, *Luke*, 219.

Chapter Four
Beginnings: Disciples

Having considered the beginnings of the ministry of Jesus, his launching into mission, I would now like to address the beginnings of discipleship. This is clearly a fundamental topic, as Jesus seeks to gather followers who will embrace his Kingdom message and values and share his mission. Each of the evangelists approaches this theme in his own way. For Luke there are, I suggest, two phases. First, there is the call of Peter (5:1–11) and then of Levi (5:27–32) early in the ministry, calls which receive a positive response. Secondly, there is a call sequence early in the journey narrative that involves three separate individuals in which the outcome is unclear (9:57–62), and later, towards the journey's end, the invitation extended to the rich ruler (18:18–23), which is not accepted. Taken together, these stories highlight the radical nature of discipleship.

The Call of Simon Peter (5:1–11)

After his rejection by the people of his native Nazareth, Jesus goes to the lakeside town of Capernaum. There, he teaches in the synagogue on the Sabbath and makes a profound impression on his hearers because of his authoritative style (4:32). While in the synagogue, he dramatically casts out an unclean spirit, which leads to even greater amazement among the people. After this, Jesus goes to the house of Simon, whom as readers we have not yet encountered, and cures his mother-in-law, who is sick with a high fever. As the sun sets, marking the close of the Sabbath, many of the townsfolk bring along their friends who are suffering from diseases of one kind or another; Jesus responds by healing and exorcising. Next morning, when Jesus has found a deserted place, the crowds follow him, wishing to prevent him from leaving them. He answers: "I must proclaim the good news of the Kingdom of God to other towns too, because that is what I was sent to do." And he departs to proclaim his message "in the synagogues of Judea."

In this sequence of events, Luke is following Mark's outline. However, he has omitted Mark's description of the call of the first disciples prior to the synagogue episode. He now gives his own version, which seems to be an expansion of the Markan narrative, into which he weaves an account of a miraculous catch of fish and focuses on Simon.[1] The text reads:

> Once while Jesus was standing beside the lake of Gennesaret, and the crowd was pressing in on him to hear the word of God, he saw two boats there at the shore of the lake; the fishermen had gone out of them and were washing their nets. He got into one of the boats, the one belonging to Simon, and asked him to put out a little way from the shore. Then he sat down and taught the crowds from the boat. When he had finished speaking, he said to Simon, "Put out into the deep water and let down your nets for a catch." Simon answered, "Master, we have worked all night long but have caught nothing. Yet if you say so, I will let down the nets." When they had done this, they caught so many fish that their nets were beginning to break. So, they signalled to their partners in the other boat to come and help them. And they came and filled both boats, so that they began to sink. But when Simon Peter saw it, he fell down at Jesus' knees, saying, "Go away from me, Lord, for I am a sinful man!" For he and all who were with him were amazed at the catch of fish that they had taken; and so also were James and John, sons of Zebedee, who were partners with Simon. Then Jesus said to Simon, "Do not be afraid; from now on you will be catching people." When they had brought their boats to shore, they left everything and followed him.

Luke's story unfolds in three stages: the preaching of Jesus, the catch of fish and the ensuing dialogue. Jesus has returned to the lake, locally known as Gennesar but called Gennesaret by Luke.[2] This area to the south of Capernaum on the north-west shore was a fertile plain and well populated. By now Jesus seems to be well known and is surrounded by an attentive crowd as he stands to preach God's word to them.[3] The phrase "word of God" is Luke's way of referring to the message of Jesus, the Good News. Jesus catches sight of two boats at the water's edge. After the night's work, the fishermen are washing their nets. The type of net referred to is the dragnet, used at night in deep water, rather than the casting net, which was used from the shore or in shallow water. At that time, there was a thriving fishing industry in the area; some of the fish were pickled and exported, even as far as Rome. Many of those involved in fishing were men of some means and standing in the community. Jesus gets into Simon's boat and asks him to pull out a little from the shore. Simon complies, and Jesus sits down, as rabbis were wont to do, and continues to teach the crowds from the boat. The reader gets the impression that Jesus and Simon Peter are already acquainted, as is implied by the earlier cure of his mother-in-law.

After Jesus has finished speaking to the crowd, the narrative moves on, and the crowd no longer features. He tells Simon to move out into deep water and let down the nets for a catch. The second of these verbs is in the plural, which suggests that Simon has others with him in the boat. With a touch of realistic common sense, the experienced fisherman replies: "Master, we worked hard all night long and caught nothing, but if you say so, I will let down the nets." The address, "Master" (*epistata*), is typical of Luke; he tends to use it on the lips of people, disciples or near-disciples, who submit to Jesus' authority or seek his help, as an equivalent of "teacher" (the term used by people who are not disciples) or "rabbi" (a word that Luke avoids).[4] Laying aside his practical common sense, Simon places his trust in Jesus' word; he is already on the way to discipleship.[5] The result of his compliance is an enormous catch of fish, so numerous that the nets begin to tear under the strain, and to avoid disaster "they" have to signal for help to their "companions" or business associates in the other of the two boats mentioned earlier, probably still moored by the shore. They respond positively and both boats are filled to sinking point.[6]

The third phase of the narrative consists in dialogue between Jesus and Simon, who is here referred to as Simon Peter, the name which Jesus will later bestow on him when appointing The Twelve (6:14) but which Luke does not use again. On seeing what has taken place, Simon falls at the knees of Jesus,[7] and exclaims: "Leave me, Lord; I am a sinful man." His recognition of his sinfulness perhaps has less to do with moral guilt than with the realisation that he is in the presence of the holy and an awareness of his own inadequacy, a response not unlike that of the prophets of old (Exod 3:5–6; Isa 6:5–8).[8] He books an early place among those who in the later Gospel narrative recognise their need for forgiveness and salvation, and who respond positively to Jesus (5:30, 32; 7:34, 39; 15:1–2, 7, 10; 18:13; 19:7).[9] Rather than joining his townsfolk in possessively wishing Jesus to stay with them or seeking to use Jesus for his own benefit, Simon tries to create a distance between sinfulness and the holy. The evangelist then observes that Simon's companions share his awe, his wonder tinged with fear (*thambos*), and he mentions for the first time the two sons of Zebedee, who are his partners. Their role in Luke's version of the events is somewhat muted in comparison with the Markan story.

Jesus responds: "Do not be afraid; from now on it is people you will be catching." The injunction not to fear is already familiar to the reader from the Infancy Narrative (1:13, 30; 2:10). Jesus ignores the fisherman's plea for distance, his recognition of his inadequacy, and instead of departing, he offers him a new life, drawing him "from now on" into discipleship and mission. His prophetic word, couched in metaphorical language, has the effect of a command.[10] The verb here translated "catch" (*zōgrein*) means to "take alive". In the LXX, it is used for saving someone from danger (Num 31:15, 18; Deut 20:16).[11] It is interesting that Jesus, who has come for the release of captives, should himself be engaged in the "capture" of people for the Kingdom! The success of this brief fishing expedition is also symbolic of the disciples' later mission.

The story concludes: "Then, bringing their boats back to land they left everything and followed him." In Mark's narrative, first Peter and Andrew, and then James and John, respond to the simple command to follow. There is no such explicit command here. Luke creates a context and motivation for a response. Simon is central to the narrative. Somewhat awkwardly, the partners are included in his following; there is no mention at all of Andrew.[12] As Johnson says, "his following Jesus on a path unknown is a logical progression for one who had already 'put out into the deep' on the basis of a word only."[13] This response seems more radical in Luke, for they leave, not just their nets (Mk 1:18) or their father with his hired men (Mk 1:20), their kinship group and source of security, but "everything".[14] For Luke, the surrender of everything is an indication of surrender to Jesus (see 5:28; 14:33; 18:22–23); discipleship is a costly business. They now join Jesus in his journey and begin to share his destiny. "Leaving all that has been of value, they will now find their fundamental sense of belonging and being in relationship to Jesus, the community being built around him, and the redemptive purpose he serves."[15]

The Call of Levi (5:27–28)

After the call of Peter, Luke continues the Markan sequence, relating the cure of the leper and the man suffering from paralysis, and then the call of Levi. The brief storyline, part of a broader unit, reads:

> Jesus went out and saw a tax collector named Levi, sitting at the tax booth; and he said to him, "Follow me." And he got up, left everything, and followed him.

As is so often the case, the initiative lies with Jesus. The choice he makes is quite unexpected, shocking in fact. Because of his occupation, Levi is a man despised, a sinner in the popular estimation, outside the community of Judaism.[16] Technically, Levi was a customs officer in the service of Herod, a Jewish client king (or, more accurately, tetrarch) appointed by Rome. He collected taxes or tolls at customs booths for the transporting of goods.[17] These people had a reputation for dishonesty and extortion; they also mixed with prostitutes and with non-Jewish merchants, and so were considered ritually impure.[18] In any society, tax collectors are not popular, but in Jesus' day they would be understood as serving Herod, who was feared and hated in Galilee, and also as supporting the pagan Roman domination system centred in the Jerusalem temple; they could therefore be suspect as collaborators. They therefore contributed to the severe hardship endured by the peasants. Their profession made them religious and social outcasts, barred from the synagogue.

The freedom, originality, "provocative inclusiveness"[19] and gracious generosity of Jesus are startling, as he cuts through conventional barriers and reaches out to those on the margins of religion, an outreach which upsets the religious elite. It was scandalous that he should include such a person in his circle;[20] it was a challenging gesture, which powerfully conveys a message about the inclusive and surprising nature of the Kingdom. "The new praxis of God's reign does not mix well with conventional ways of ordering the community's life."[21]

Levi accepts the invitation of Jesus; he stands and leaves his desk and his wealth and the possibilities of his job in order to follow him. His life now has a different orientation and meaning. Whereas the other disciples were self-employed fishermen and could return to their boats if things didn't work out, Levi, having opted out of Herod's administration, probably would not have been able to resume his former employment, had he later wished to do so.[22] Levi does, however, provide a banquet for Jesus; continuing connection to household and further expressions of generosity are not totally ruled out.[23]

The Fox, The Funeral and The Furrow (9:57–62)

The ministry of Jesus moves on and expands.[24] There are controversies with the religious leaders, the Sermon on the Plain, with its beatitudes and woes, several miracle stories and parables. Large crowds are often in attendance, wishing to listen to him or be healed of their infirmities. The Twelve are sent on mission, Jesus feeds the five thousand and raises the issue of his identity. When Peter acknowledges that he is the Messiah of God, Jesus responds by speaking for the first time about his coming passion, which leads into the transfiguration event.[25] Shortly afterwards, the narrative takes a fresh and decisive twist: "When the days drew near for him to be taken up, he set his face to go to Jerusalem" (9:51). For the next ten chapters, the theme of the journey to Jerusalem forms the structural spine of Luke's story of Jesus.[26]

After commencing the journey, Jesus sends messengers ahead of him, but they are not welcomed by a Samaritan village community. James and John suggest calling down fire from heaven to burn up the inhabitants, but Jesus rebukes them, for this is not his way (9:51–56). As the journey continues, Luke includes three short episodes that illustrate the radical and stringent nature of discipleship. As well as being linked thematically, these episodes form a unit structurally. The first and third follow the same pattern: a person makes an offer to follow Jesus and Jesus replies, using images from the outdoor world (from nature and from farming). The dialogue thus consists in one statement by each and the flow of thought is follow, go and then a parabolic illustration of the high cost involved. In the second episode, it is Jesus who takes the initiative; the person responds to him; and Jesus speaks again. There are therefore three "speeches" here, and the imagery this time is drawn from village society. The flow follows the pattern of inverted parallelism: follow, go, cost; cost, go, follow/proclaim.[27] Nothing is said of the identity of those involved, nor of the final outcome of their encounter with Jesus. The reader's attention is centred on the utter commitment required for discipleship and the immediacy of its demand. The first two episodes are also found with almost identical wording in Matthew (8:18–22), as Jesus is about to cross the lake from Capernaum to Decapolis. The people involved there are a scribe and a disciple.

The Lukan text reads as follows:

> As they were going along the road, someone said to him, "I will follow you wherever you go." And Jesus said to him, "Foxes have holes, and birds of the air have nests; but the Son of Man has nowhere to lay his head." To another he said, "Follow me." But he said, "Lord, first let me go and bury my father." But Jesus said to him, "Let the dead bury their own dead; but as for you, go and proclaim the kingdom of God." Another said, "I will follow you, Lord; but let me first say farewell to those at my home." Jesus said to him, "No one who puts a hand to the plough and looks back is fit for the kingdom of God."

The Fox (57–58)

As Jesus and the disciples travel along, an unnamed man whom they have met on the road says to Jesus: "I will follow you wherever you go." Jesus replies in parabolic language: "Foxes have holes and the birds of the air have nests, but the Son of Man has nowhere to lay his head."

This first encounter, in which an individual volunteers to join the group of Jesus' close disciples, contrasts favourably with the preceding incident in inhospitable Samaria. The man generously offers to follow Jesus "wherever" he goes, evincing a remarkable level of openness for discipleship. However, the destination towards which Jesus is travelling is Jerusalem, where he is to suffer, as the reader has twice been informed (9:22, 44). The would-be disciple is unaware of the implications of his offer.

So, Jesus spells out the cost involved. Foxes have the security and safety of their holes; birds have places to roost. Jesus, on the other hand, referring to himself as the "Son of Man",[28] has nowhere to lay his head. He is a homeless itinerant; in his culture, the household was the primary source of identity. It is true that Jesus was frequently offered hospitality while on his travels, but it seems that he was, in fact, dependent on it. The basic point is that he knew rejection, as recently happened in Samaria, and that this was his destiny in Jerusalem.

Some scholars have suggested that there may be another dimension to the parabolic imagery used by Jesus, a political symbolism. The "birds of the air" in apocalyptic literature were the gentile nations. The "fox" was a symbol for the Ammonites, who were political enemies of Israel. Herod's family was racially mixed and looked upon as foreign. Jesus calls Herod "that fox" (13:32). Manson writes:

> Everybody is at home in Israel's land except the true Israel. The birds of the air—the Roman overlords, the foxes—the Edomite interlopers, have made their position secure. The true Israel is disinherited by them: and if you cast your lot with me and mine you join the ranks of the dispossessed and you must be prepared to serve God under those conditions.[29]

Oppressed people are obliged to talk in symbols. "The terrors of the Herodian era, with its torture and murder, were fresh in the minds of all. No one dared criticise Rome. The Romans and their Herodian supporters were the powerful of the land and their spies were everywhere."[30] So perhaps Jesus was suggesting in a veiled fashion that if the man wants power and influence, he should look elsewhere unless he is really serious about following a rejected Son of Man. Other scholars, on the contrary, question these identifications. For in the book of Enoch, the Edomites are represented by boars; it is not certain that "birds", without more specific reference, referred to gentiles; all Israel was, in fact, disinherited, not just the "true Israel".[31]

The outcome of the dialogue is not revealed. The reader is left unsure whether the man joined Jesus and his band, or was so taken aback by Jesus' reply that he remained at the roadside as Jesus and his entourage journeyed on. The emphasis therefore falls on Jesus' description of his own way of living, without the safety, security and claims of a personal household.[32] His close disciples must have taken note of his words.

The Funeral (59–60)

In the second episode, Jesus himself takes the initiative and invites someone, who probably belongs to the wider group of disciples, to follow him more closely, using the same phrasing as earlier in the call of Levi.[33] The man replies: "Let me go and bury my father first." To this Jesus responds: "Leave the dead to bury their dead; your duty is to go and spread the news of the kingdom of God."

The man's reply to Jesus' call is positive but conditional. It is usually taken literally to mean that his father was dead. The burial of deceased relatives, especially parents, was a sacred duty, a religious obligation of the utmost importance (Tobit 4:3–4; 6:13–14; 14:11–13). It took precedence over all else, even the study of the Law.[34] It was considered an aspect of the commandment to respect one's parents (Exod 20:12). Failure to make the request would have been a scandal, neglect to carry it out a "gross impiety".[35] Bailey, however, strongly maintains that in its cultural context the man's request does not imply that his father is dead, but means that he wants to go and serve his father as long as he is alive, thus postponing his following of Jesus until after his death and burial. The phrase is a traditional idiom, which refers specifically to a son's duty to remain at home and care for his parents until their death. The recruit is pleading the demands made upon him by the expectations of his community and culture, which is a strong kind of peer pressure.[36]

Whichever position is taken, Jesus brooks no delay. His reply is demanding and radical in the extreme. Discipleship requires a willingness to break with normal social patterns in favour of commitment to the promotion of the Kingdom. Jesus' statement, "Leave the dead to bury their dead", is sometimes taken metaphorically to refer to the spiritually dead burying the physically dead.[37] The idea is that followers of Jesus are spiritually alive, and their responsibility is to concern themselves with the demands of the Gospel,[38] whereas those who have not accepted Jesus are viewed as spiritually dead in that they have failed to embrace the new life of the Kingdom. They are the ones who must attend to the responsibilities of their community.

The second part of Jesus' statement, "your duty is to go and spread the good news of the kingdom of God", in which the "your" is emphatic, underlines the importance and urgency of announcing the presence of the Kingdom, of preaching of the Good News.[39] This has priority over every other claim, even sacred duties.

The Furrow (61–62)

In the third episode, another individual approaches Jesus and says: "I will follow you, sir, but first let me go and say goodbye to my people at home." To this Jesus replies: "Once the hand is laid on the plough, no one who looks back is fit for the kingdom of God." Like the man in the first episode, the protagonist here is a volunteer; like the man in the second episode, he offers a precondition for his following. At face value, the request simply reflects the desire respectfully to take leave of his family. Elisha made a similar request of Elijah, and it was granted (1 Kings 19:20). In itself, the request does not seem unreasonable. However, the verb means more than simply saying farewell, it means "take leave", which implies asking those remaining for permission to go (Mark 6:46; Acts 18:18, 21; 2 Cor 2:13). In reality, then, the man is asking Jesus to allow him to go home and ask permission of his father to leave home, a permission which his father would probably refuse. He wishes to submit to parental authority his desire to follow Jesus, which implies that parental authority is higher than that of Jesus. In that culture, such a procedure would be normal and expected.[40]

Jesus' reply is much more radical than the lenient response of Elijah. He employs a parabolic saying, taken from the world of agriculture. Ploughing was a very precise and demanding operation, requiring dexterity to manage the instrument (keep it upright and regulate its depth) and to drive the oxen, calling for intense concentration and singleness of purpose. Distraction or lack of close attention could damage the plough, destroy work already done or make future work more difficult. "The image is strong and clear. The tension illustrated is between loyalty to Jesus as the inaugurator of the Kingdom of God and its all-consuming demands, and loyalty to the authority of the family."[41]

To become a disciple in that culture was to enter a deep relationship with one's teacher. Jesus clearly believes his authority and the urgent demands of the Kingdom take precedence over all other relationships and responsibilities.[42] Anyone struggling to resolve the tension of conflicting loyalties and, as we would put it today, repeatedly looking into the rear-view mirror, is in Kingdom terms quite useless, something of a liability. Discipleship requires "single-minded detachment from the life and social systems one has known."[43] Again, we are given no further information as to the decision that the volunteer takes when faced with this unexpected conflict of loyalties. But Jesus is not asking of others anything different from what he himself has embraced and is living.

Reflections

These three episodes illustrate very powerfully the costly nature of discipleship. It demands a willingness to give absolute priority to Jesus and the Kingdom; loyalty to Jesus takes precedence over other loyalties. Family ties, cultural demands, sacred responsibilities and personal security take second place. The Kingdom not only relativises allegiances, conventions, normal commitments and sacred customs, it turns them upside-down. The awareness of Jesus about the urgency and uniqueness of his mission is apparent, as is his total commitment to his mission. To be caught up in his mission, to share his values, entails the sharing of his cross.

Among the Synoptic Gospels, Luke offers the most radical critique of conventional family ties. Family ties are part of the structures and securities of this life that are broken, set aside, to follow Jesus. The old family structure is no longer the place of identity and social relations for the Christian; instead, a new spiritual family based on the hearing and obeying of the word of God replaces conventional family ties. But brokenness is never an end in itself; it is always "for the sake of the Kingdom".[44]

The Call of The Rich Aristocrat (18:18–23)

The final episode in this chapter, which we are devoting to the 'call' theme, concerns a rich aristocrat. The incident is found also in Mark and Matthew; the latter refers to him as a "rich young man", an epithet which has stuck in popular understanding. In Luke's narrative structure, the journey of Jesus to Jerusalem is nearing its end. Jesus will shortly enter Jericho, where he will encounter and heal a blind man, and then, as he leaves the city, he will transform the life of the wealthy Zacchaeus. Luke follows Mark in adding to his account of Jesus' meeting with the rich ruler a number of sayings of Jesus about wealth.[45]

The narrative, which continues the radicality theme of the previous section of this chapter with its emphasis on detachment from possessions and loyalty to Jesus, reads as follows:

> A certain ruler asked him, "Good Teacher, what must I do to inherit eternal life?" Jesus said to him, "Why do you call me good? No one is good but God alone.

You know the commandments: 'You shall not commit adultery; You shall not murder; You shall not steal; You shall not bear false witness; Honour your father and mother.' " He replied, "I have kept all these since my youth." When Jesus heard this, he said to him, "There is still one thing lacking. Sell all that you own and distribute the money to the poor, and you will have treasure in heaven; then come, follow me." But when he heard this, he became sad; for he was very rich. Jesus looked at him and said, "How hard it is for those who have wealth to enter the kingdom of God! Indeed, it is easier for a camel to go through the eye of a needle than for someone who is rich to enter the kingdom of God."

In its immediate context, this episode stands in contrast with the previous event, in which infants were brought to Jesus for his blessing.[46] When the disciples sought to intervene, scolding the mothers[47] and seeking to prevent this happening, Jesus exclaimed: "Let the little children come to me, and do not stop them, for it is to such as these that the kingdom of God belongs. Truly I tell you, whoever does not receive the kingdom of God as a little child will never enter it." Jesus does not openly upbraid the disciples, but his words are an implicit rebuke. It is true that infants and children can be self-centred and difficult at times, and Jesus would know this from village experience, but his point is that they cannot earn what they need; they are passive and powerless; they receive everything as gift, and delight in it; they can only give trust and affection in response. It is the same with God's free gift of the Kingdom, which calls for a loving response.[48] There is no place for pretensions of greatness and achievement. Status, self-sufficiency, independence and power are not Kingdom values.[49] Jesus continues to turn the world upside-down, to deconstruct systems and values that are contrary to God's plan.[50] This presents a profound challenge for the disciples both in outlook and practice. Now, as the story continues, with no change of setting, it is a mature man, wealthy and with influence, a member of the social elite, who approaches Jesus. But the fundamental issue is the same, that of entry into the Kingdom.[51]

Luke presents this man as a "ruler". This suggests he is a religious authority, perhaps involved in synagogue leadership or could even be a member of the Sanhedrin;[52] usually "rulers" are opponents of Jesus (14:1; 23:13, 35; 24:20). Without introduction, probably motivated by what he has just heard Jesus say,[53] he respectfully asks him: "Good Master, what shall I do to inherit eternal life?" The form of address, "Good Master", is very rare in Jewish literature; the term "good" was usually reserved for God. Rabbis were generally thought highly of and treated with respect, but perhaps there is element of flattery here, or maybe the man is trying too hard, attempting to impress with a compliment, which would merit one in return.[54] The question is the same as that of the lawyer in

10:25, which was intended as a way of testing Jesus. Some wonder whether this is the case here rather than a sincere request;[55] others do not sense a dubious motive.[56] The mentality of achieving entry into the Kingdom by dint of personal effort or earning a future reward by performing well now, in the present, is the same in both cases.

Jesus responds first with a question, then follows with an affirmation (as in Mark): "Why do you call me good? No one is good but God alone." This response has created interpretive problems for a very long time (as far back as Matthew!).[57] The statement about God's goodness probably stems from the piety of the psalms, where one frequently finds the affirmation that God is good (Pss 53:6; 72:1; 134:3; 135:1; 117:1ff).[58] It is a recognised truth. Jesus considers it as appropriate only for God. Jesus is not disclaiming goodness, or confessing sinfulness, but acknowledging his devotion to God. His response is "the reflex deflection of human praise in favour of God as the source of all being and goodness."[59] It seems that Jesus is challenging the man for his rather glib and casual use of a term that Jesus considers appropriate only for God,[60] and questioning the sincerity and seriousness of his intentions.[61]

Jesus then reminds the ruler of the traditional way to the obtaining of eternal life, the keeping of the commandments, a way he knows well. In the list that Jesus provides, the first part of the Decalogue, which concerns God directly, is omitted. The prescriptions mentioned concern relationships with others, and the order in which they occur is unusual. Whereas some suggest that in early catechetical teaching there was considerable freedom and variety in listing the last six commandments,[62] Bailey maintains that the order is a deliberate rearrangement so as to give emphasis to the subjects of loyalty to family and attitudes towards wealth.[63] In fact, this defines the community of Jesus' followers, those who will "inherit eternal life".[64]

The man responds by claiming to have observed all these commandments from his youth; he is a good member of the Jewish people. This can be understood as a sincere avowal, which is in no way boastful, not untypical of Pharisee claims. The ruler's remark can also be taken as an expression of uncertainty as to whether, since he has kept the commandments, something additional might be required, or as a complacent statement of achievement which needed to be punctured by a further radical demand.[65] Jesus neither praises nor condemns the ruler's claim. He simply tells him that he is lacking one thing and invites him to move further and become a disciple. "There is still one thing lacking. Sell everything you own and distribute the money to the poor, and you will have treasure in heaven; then come, follow me."

There are two elements to Jesus' response: the man is to sell his possessions and to follow Jesus. Again, Jesus' demands are both radical and all-embracing. While the emphasis seems to be on selling what he owns, in that culture the issue of possessions is closely linked with that of personal identity and family loyalty. The family home and estate is very important. So, the fundamental challenge is once again that of placing loyalty to Jesus over loyalty to his family and property. This implies placing his security in God rather than his wealth and social status.[66]

The ruler, on hearing this, becomes deeply distressed and sad, "for he was very rich". The invitation to discipleship that Jesus extends to him comes at a price he is unable to pay. His wealth and the status and security it brings hold him bound, fatally hindering any possibility of growth.[67]

Luke omits the comment in Mark and Matthew that the man then went away. The result is that the subsequent severe words of Jesus about the danger of riches are addressed not only to the disciples, but also to him. As he stands there silently in distress, disappointment and confusion, Jesus looks at him and states: "How hard it is for those who have wealth to enter the kingdom of God." He illustrates this with a parable: "Indeed, it is easier for a camel to go through the eye of a needle than for someone who is rich to enter the kingdom of God." A common characteristic of parables is a tendency for poetic exaggeration,[68] but even so Jesus' imagery can take one's breath away. A camel is the largest animal in Palestine; the eye of a needle is minuscule.[69] Impossible means impossible. The audience, clearly in shock, ask, "Who can be saved, then?" Jesus looks straight at them, and declares: "What is impossible for mortals is possible for God."[70] God is able to achieve what human beings cannot do.

It was the commonly accepted view that wealthy people were in a better position to obtain salvation. Wealth and privilege were considered a sign of God's approval and favour (see Prov 3:16; 22:4; Ecclus 11:21). Jesus' view is therefore extremely disturbing and challenging, and demands a completely different way of thinking. But he is a realist and is well aware that wealth, the freedom and self-reliance it can bring, the drive to achieve, the difficulties in relinquishing it, can be insurmountable barriers to openness to God. Salvation is not a human achievement; it is not earned or won; it is a gift of God, an expression of his graciousness and merciful compassion.[71]

A puzzled and pondering Peter, his worldview threatened, intervenes, speaking for himself and his companions: "Look, we have left our homes and followed you." Implicitly he is seeking clarification and assurance about where they stand in all this.[72] The word here translated as "homes" is in Greek *ta idia*, which literally means "what is ours", and so applies both to property and people, wealth and family ties: house, wife, children, job and the kinship and security that they imply. For the disciples, too, the cultural pressures concerning property and family, kinship and status applied, but, for all their weaknesses and limitations, they have been able to break free and "follow" Jesus, placing him before everything and everyone else.[73] They are experiencing the possibility of the impossible when God is involved.

Jesus replies with a solemn tone: "Truly I tell you, there is no one who has left house, or wife or brothers or parents or children for the sake of the kingdom of God, who will not get back very much more in this age, and in the age to come eternal life." Peter's question takes us back to the episode at the beginning of this chapter, and the mention of eternal life takes us back to the rich ruler's original question.[74] There is an irony in God's abundant generosity, security in Jesus' promise and wonder in the present experience of the Kingdom. Disciples receive far more than they sacrificed, now in the present, and they have the assurance of enduring life beyond the grave. This is the corollary and fruit of responding positively to the invitation of Jesus to "follow me", not a reward. In the next episode of Luke's narrative, Jesus will for a third time speak about his coming passion, which will, of course, have repercussions for their ongoing discipleship.[75]

Reflections

The theme of discipleship runs through the whole of Luke's narrative. In fact, in our earlier reflections, we have sought to identify and understand the implications for discipleship that arise from the narratives, and we will continue to do so throughout this book. From the episodes that we have considered in this chapter, several aspects merit some pondering. Luke's story of the call of Simon Peter is sensitively told. Jesus, presumably already acquainted with Simon, having cured his mother-in-law, confidently hijacks Simon's boat as a floating pulpit. Simon is prepared to abandon the cleaning of his nets and obliges, pushing off a little from the shore. After finishing his sermon, Jesus pushes Simon a little further, inviting him to move out into deeper water and start fishing all over again. An experienced and successful fisherman with an intimate knowledge of the waters and ways of the lake, he goes along with Jesus' suggestion, obviously not convinced that it is a good idea. A level of openness, respect and trust can be detected.

The result is dramatic. Having sorted out the immediate danger of sinking because of the size of the catch, and trying to cope with the shock and amazement at what has occurred, Simon humbly acknowledges that he is personally out of his depth here. This healer, preacher, prophetic Jesus is too big for him. Something is happening that is way outside his comfort zone, that he cannot take on board. Aware of his limitations, he asks Jesus to move off, to go elsewhere, and let him get on with his normal life. But Jesus has other plans. He encourages Simon not to be afraid. He has a use for his business management and teamwork skills and his basic generosity and energy; he invites him to use his gifts and his life in a very different way, directing his efforts to drawing people into the ambit of the dawning Kingdom of God. Simon Peter and his friends beach their boats, leave them there and walk off with Jesus into an uncertain future.

To some extent we can identify with Simon Peter in his awe and wonder at becoming involved with Jesus and his Kingdom dream. Maybe we prefer that Jesus should leave us be and choose others to share his life and his task. We are well aware of our weaknesses and limitations, the danger of failure and embarrassment. For Jesus, that kind of humble, realistic awareness is a good starting point. He is also aware of our qualities, gifts and potential. He knows, too, that deep down we do want him to be our friend and guide and support, and in some way to be of service to his life project in our day. He tells us, too, not to fear and to launch out into deep waters; he is with us in the boat if we take that risk.

In his calling of Levi, we see a different side of the Master, for unlike Simon, who has some standing in the village community, Levi is a rank outsider. As well as initiative, there is a remarkable streak of originality about Jesus. Clearly, his way of assessing people, his level of respect and openness, his sense of inclusion, is quite extraordinary. He is genuinely happy to share life with someone despised, marginalised, labelled a sinner. Jesus' action must have caused a stir among the onlookers and really upset them. It must have been something of a shock for Levi; here was someone who treated him as a person, who didn't argue with him and use abusive language, who invited him into a very different way of living. And he grasped the opportunity as he had previously grasped bags of coins. The later meal that he hosted for Jesus was an expression of his appreciation, joy and gratitude, and his liberation too.

This aspect of Jesus, which caused him problems with the religious elite, can cause us problems too. To be so outrageously inclusive presents a challenge to our discipleship. We all have our comfort zones, our reasonable parameters, our particular groups and boundaries. With many of us, Levi would never have had a look in. Who are the Levi types in our local world, our church and beyond? Is genuine inclusion part of our mindset and value system? Are we selective in the aspects of Jesus' style and mindset that we embrace?

With the later threesome and the rich aristocrat, we encounter a frank and demanding Jesus, a Jesus with a strong sense of being sent by God with a clear mission to fulfil. The depth of his personal commitment, his awareness of what is at stake, means that he doesn't beat about the bush. He does not hesitate to make demands of people who show interest in joining his band. Two particularly stringent areas clearly emerge. For any disciple, Jesus must come first before any other relationship, even the most sacred. A casual bystander may have wondered who on earth he thought he was. This, of course, is a crucially important question. And then, being involved with him relativises everything else: property, money, status, security, family ties, even life itself. It's the establishment of the Kingdom, God's reign in love, which is paramount.

This is a challenge for us today. For some of our brothers and sisters in recent years, following Jesus has indeed cost their lives. It is still a serious business. For some of us, discipleship may entail deeply upsetting or alienating members of our family and friends. That is very painful. The story of the rich aristocrat always leaves me wondering what it is in my life at present that may in some way be an obstacle to my following of Jesus. It certainly isn't my bank balance or large estate, but there are other things in which I can invest my security and status, and which restrict the freedom and generosity of my response. "Costing not less than everything" can be scary for most of us. Jesus does set high ideals because he wants the best for us and wishes our potential to be realised. But, as he tells Peter in the story, with God's help, for whom "nothing is impossible", we can probably go much further than we can imagine. I often find myself taking heart from the incident at Bethany during Jesus' final week, when, in Mark's account (14:3–9), a woman comes into the room during a meal and anoints Jesus' head with expensive perfume. She is roughly upbraided by the disciples for wasting money on ointment (and on him!), money that could have been given to the poor. Springing to her defence, Jesus says: "she has done what she could". We are back with Peter in the boat, heading for deeper water. We know that we are sinful men and women; we do fail, as do the disciples in the rest of Luke's narrative.

But we still keep trying to do what we can, and Jesus is still with us in the boat, and his invitation to discipleship still stands.

Notes

1   This fishing aspect contains elements that are similar to the post-resurrection narrative of John 21, and other elements which are quite different. Some scholars (like Byrne, *Hospitality*, 58, n.7) maintain that Luke has retrojected a post-resurrection incident; others (like Dodd in Marshall, *Luke*, 200) are of the opinion that essential features of the post-resurrection narrative form are lacking, which suggests that the story comes from the ministry period. Caird, *Luke*, 91, suspects some interaction between two independent stories in the course of oral transmission. Evans, *Luke*, 288, considers it plausible that Luke and John are variant versions of the appearance of the risen Lord to Peter. Tannehill, *Luke*, 100, dubs the story an extended pronouncement story containing a wondrous provision (of fish).

2   The other evangelists refer to the Sea of Galilee or Tiberias.

3   In Mark 4:1 Jesus preaches to the crowds from a boat on the lake. Wright, *Luke*, 53, notes how the inlets of the shoreline form natural amphitheatres, enabling people to hear clearly. Evans, *Luke*, 289, points out that the expression "the word of God", for the message of Jesus, is confined to Luke among the evangelists. He uses it in Acts for the apostolic message.

4   Marshall, *Luke*, 203. See 8:24; 8:45; 9:33; 9:49; 17:13.

5   Carroll, *Luke*, 125. Green, *Luke*, 232, notes that Peter's response echoes that of Mary in 1:34, 38: "incredulity leading to service". E. Earle Ellis, *The Gospel of Luke* (London: Oliphants, 1974), interprets this reply as an indication of sceptical obedience rather than expectant faith.

6   Luke is probably intending to bring out the prophetic insight of Jesus, his knowledge of what is going to happen, rather than his control over nature. Johnson, *Luke*, 88, notes that by using terms suggesting a pooling of interests and possessions, Luke also prepares the reader for the Galilean community in Jerusalem in Acts (2:41–47; 4:32–37).

7   See 22:41; Acts 7:60; 9:40. "Lord" is equivalent to "Master", but contains a resurrection resonance.

8   Marshall, *Luke*, 205. Caird, *Luke*, 90, writes of "humbling and exhilarating awe." Tannehill, *Luke*, 101, notes how the manifestation of the holy can be threatening and repel. Green, *Luke*, 233, mentions the parallels between 5:1–11 and Isa 6:1–10.

9   Green, *Luke*, 231, writes that Jesus' commission to Peter, a sinner, lays the groundwork for Jesus' ministry of forgiveness and the growing reputation of Jesus as the "friend of sinners". Evans, *Luke*, 291, devotes considerable space to a discussion of

128

the meaning of *hamartōlos* here.

10   Marshall, *Luke*, 205.

11   Byrne, *Hospitality*, 57, observes that Luke moves from the everyday sense of fishing, in which the fish inevitably die, to a symbolic sense in which fish are caught for keeping in a protected way, like an aquarium or fishpond. People will be caught in order to live more fully. Similarly, Green, *Luke*, 235.

12   He is named for the first time in the list of The Twelve in 6:14. This episode, in which Jesus, after prayer, calls The Twelve and names them "apostles", will be considered later.

13   Johnson, *Luke*, 91.

14   Tannehill, *Luke*, 101, notes the group-oriented culture of the Mediterranean world and the importance of the family unit, which was the source of identity and economic security.

15   Green, *Luke*, 235.

16   Moloney, *Mark*, 63–64. McBride, *Luke*, 77, refers to tax collectors as "professional outsiders." Some approach the Baptist (3:12–13), and are told to treat people fairly. Levi is not mentioned again. In Matthew, Levi is called Matthew (9:9).

17   Donahue & Harrington, *Mark*, 101.

18   Dennis E. Nineham, *Saint Mark* (London: Penguin, 1963), 99; Byrne, *Hospitality*, 60; Boring, *Mark*, 81; Caird, *Luke*, 95.

19   Byrne, *Hospitality*, 60.

20   Morna D. Hooker, *The Gospel according to St Mark* (London: A&C Black, 1991), 94.

21   Carroll, *Luke*, 132.

22   A point made by George Martin, *The Gospel according to Mark: Meaning and Message* (Chicago: Loyola Press, 2005), 44. Marshall, *Luke*, 219, acknowledges that Levi would have needed to formally settle his business; Luke is stressing his decisive break with his old life.

23   Carroll, *Luke*, 133. Green, *Luke*, 246, comments that for Luke, the ownership and disposition of possessions were embedded in a larger network of social relations and personal commitments.

24   The title for this section is taken from Kenneth E. Bailey, *Poet & Peasant and Through Peasant Eyes* (Grand Rapids: Eerdmans, 1983), 2:22. He considers this trilogy under the umbrella of Jesus' parabolic speech.

25   Many of these episodes will be treated in other chapters of this book.

26   The journey provides the context for a great deal of Jesus' teaching; this is derived from the 'Q' source and also from Luke's special tradition. Caird, *Luke*, 139, comments that it is impossible to plot a route, given the topographical inconsistencies.

27   Bailey, *Through Peasant Eyes*, 23.

28   Green, *Luke*, 407, calls "Son of Man" a "self-referent designed to intimate what was unique about his person."

29   Thomas W. Manson, *The Sayings of Jesus*, (London: SCM, 1937), 721.

30   Bailey, *Through Peasant Eyes*, 25.

31   Evans, *Luke*, 440.

32 Carroll, *Luke*, 230.

33 In Matthew's version of the incident, the man himself, who is a disciple, takes the initiative, and Jesus replies in two stages.

34 Marshall, *Luke*, 411.

35 Evans, *Luke*, 441.

36 Bailey, *Through Peasant Eyes*, 26–27.

37 Marshall, *Luke*, 411; McBride, *Luke*, 131; Fitzmyer, *Luke*, 1:836.

38 McBride, *Luke*, 131.

39 Marshall, *Luke*, 412, considers this a Lukan addition.

40 Bailey, *Through Peasant Eyes*, 27–28.

41 Bailey, *Through Peasant Eyes*, 30; Johnson, *Luke*, 163, sees a parallel with the demand to "hate father and mother" of 14:26.

42 Bailey, *Through Peasant Eyes*, 30.

43 Carroll, *Luke*, 232.

44 Resseguie, *Spiritual Landscape*, 60. See 12:52–53; 14:26; 18:29–30: 17:26–30.

45 This episode follows soon after the two parables about prayer which we will consider later.

46 Here Luke rejoins the Markan sequence of events that he left at 9.51. For this episode, see Mark 10:13–15. The word Luke uses is *brephos*, which means a babe in arms or infant, rather than Mark's *paidion*, which can refer to a child up to twelve years old.

47 Tannehill, *Luke*, 268, maintains that children were part of the women's world.

48 Byrne, *Hospitality*, 145. Children have appeared in the narrative already in 9:46–48. Carroll, *Luke*, 362, comments: "God's realm belongs not to the wealthy, powerful or high in status—or those who are preoccupied with enhancing their status and honour—but precisely to those whose honour is conferred by God alone." Green, *Luke*, 650–651, reminds us that children "might be valued for their present or future contribution to family business, but otherwise they possessed little if any intrinsic value as human beings." This explains the response of the disciples, especially when an important adult was waiting in the wings. Resseguie, *Spiritual Landscape*, 54, notes that children, like slaves, are at the margins of society—dependent, vulnerable waifs ... The modern tendency to dote on children is alien to ancient culture. Evans, *Luke*, 646, suggests that the disciples' view is probably that rabbis are teachers of adults, and have better things to do than concern themselves with babes in arms.

49 Evans, *Luke*, 648. Resseguie, *Spiritual Landscape*, 55, takes the meaning to be that the Kingdom is received as though one were the same status as a little child. It comes as a gift.

50 Green, *Luke*, 651. On p. 653 he refers to "status transposition" or reversal.

51 Mark's version begins: "As he was setting out on a journey" (10:17), but in Luke, Jesus has been journeying for some time already. Luke omits Mark's comment that the man ran up and knelt before him.

52 Marshall, *Luke*, 684.

53 Green, *Luke*, 654. He believes that he has been present while Jesus was speaking earlier.

54 Bailey, *Through Peasant Eyes*, 162; Green, *Luke*, 655, suggests that in the way

in which the ruler addresses Jesus, he signifies his commitment to a particular set of conventions, his identity within a particular social group and his understanding of the speech event he has initiated. Evans, *Luke*, 650, questions the validity of the view that "fulsome flattery" is involved; Marshall, *Luke*, 684, believes it could be regarded as flattery, cheapening a word usually applied only to God.

55   Johnson, *Luke*, 280.

56   Carroll, *Luke*, 363, is one of the latter. Marshall, *Luke*, 684, believes Luke presents the man sympathetically.

57   In Matthew (19:17) Jesus says: "Why do you ask me about what is good? There is only one who is good."

58   Johnson, *Luke*, 276.

59   Johnson, *Luke*, 276; Carroll, *Luke*, 363.

60   Some put the emphasis on "me", raising the issue of Jesus' identity: if God is good, and you call *me* good … Evans, *Luke*, 650, rules this out as introducing later doctrinal considerations, as does Marshall, *Luke*, 684.

61   Bailey, *Through Peasant Eyes*, 162.

62   Marshall, *Luke*, 685.

63   Bailey, *Through Peasant Eyes*, 159, suggests a cyclic structure (ABCBA): no adultery (loyalty to family); no murder (physical destruction of another); no stealing (respect for property); no false witness (verbal destruction of another); honour parents (loyalty to family). Green, *Luke*, 655–656, notes that the middle commandment, about stealing, also has to do with human relationships, for it is an affirmation of the priority of the community of God's people.

64   Green, *Luke*, 656.

65   Evans, *Luke*, 650; Carroll, *Luke*, 364, suggests the former option, Bailey, *Through Peasant Eyes*, the second.

66   Carroll, *Luke*, 364, n. 131; Johnson, *Luke*, 277; Caird, *Luke*, 205. Green, *Luke*, 656, makes the point that Jesus is not primarily advocating an ascetic of renunciation; the disposition of property is for the sake of the poor, thus following a biblical concern, participating in Jesus' ministry to the poor, rejecting concerns of status honour, and denoting identification with Jesus himself.

67   Byrne, *Hospitality*, 146; Resseguie, *Spiritual Landscape*, 109, speaks of "the consuming power of plenty."

68   Byrne, *Hospitality*, 146, notes the lack of evidence that Jesus was referring to a small gate in Jerusalem at the time. Carroll, *Luke*, 365, refers to "humorous hyperbole", which does not mask the seriousness of Jesus' words. The man asked about "eternal life"; Jesus speaks about "treasure in heaven", and later refers to the "kingdom of God"; the issue of "being saved" is then raised. These are virtually synonymous. He sees these as images of the blessed life that God purposes for human beings, which they in turn desire and seek.

69   Bailey, *Through Peasant Eyes*, 165–166, notes various attempts at mitigating the imagery, which are to be rejected. The words are to be taken literally (also Ellis, *Luke*, 219).

70   See also 1:37; Gen 18:14 LXX. The later story of Zacchaeus (19:1–10) illustrates

this in practice. Bailey, *Through Peasant Eyes*, 169, writes that Jesus is fully aware of the radical rupture of the fabric of cultural loyalties which his words create. Marshall, *Luke*, 686, notes that God can work the miracle of conversion in the hearts even of the rich.

71   Johnson, *Luke*, 281, comments that the kingdom proclaimed by Jesus is entirely about the power of God at work to heal and liberate and empower, not about humans accomplishing things for themselves.

72   Matthew (19:27) adds: "What then will we have?" In 5:11 and 5:28 (and Mark 10:28) *panta* (everything) is used.

73   Bailey, *Through Peasant Eyes*, 169, writes: "The two unassailable loyalties that any Middle Easterner is almost required to consider more important than life itself are family and the village home. When Jesus puts both of these in one list, and then demands a loyalty that supersedes them both, he is requiring that which is truly impossible to the Middle Easterner, given the pressures of his culture ... Jesus is fully aware of the radical rupture of the fabric of cultural loyalties that his words create."

74   Comparison with Mark (10:28–30) is interesting. Mark, in the first part of Jesus' answer, includes sisters and fields, and mentions father and mother separately, but omits wife. He spells out in detail point by point the "very much more" of Luke, calling it a "hundredfold": houses, brothers and sisters, mothers and children, and fields, adding persecutions.

75   Resseguie, *Spiritual Landscape*, 62, notes that brokenness results in gain. On p. 68 he writes that family ties are rendered relative in relation to the fulsome expectations of contemporary discipleship. Family ties are part of the securities of this world that must be broken to follow Jesus. The primary allegiance is Jesus. But a new family is taking shape; it is all-inclusive and based on hearing and doing God's word (8:21).

Chapter Five
Jesus and Prayer

One of the most beautiful themes in the Gospel of Luke is that of prayer. It is introduced in the Infancy Narrative with the three canticles and the presence of several obviously prayerful individuals. It reaches a climax in the Calvary scene with the prayers of Jesus from the cross. It flows through the Gospel narrative like a stream in the hills, with many references to the prayer of Jesus himself, and with episodes in which he teaches his disciples and the crowds, directly and through his parables. In this chapter, I propose to concentrate on the prayer of Jesus, which includes some of his teaching about prayer; in the next chapter, I will examine three of his parables on the theme.

The Prayer of Jesus

Luke refers explicitly to the prayer of Jesus several times: at his baptism in the Jordan river (3:21); after he has spent the day preaching to the people (5:16); when about to choose The Twelve (6:12); prior to Peter's confession of faith (9:18); at the time of the transfiguration (9:28); before the disciples' request that he should teach them to pray (11:1); in the hillside olive grove (22:41) and when on the cross (23:34, 46). He prays on mountains and hills (6:12; 9:28, 37; 22:39), in the wilderness (5:16) and in other unspecified locations (3:21; 9:18; 11:1).[1] These references span the various stages of his ministry. Luke tends to refer to the prayer of Jesus at crucial moments in his mission.

The Baptism of Jesus

The first reference to Jesus praying is found in connection with his baptism by John:

> Now when all the people were baptized, and when Jesus also had been baptized and was praying, the heaven was opened, and the Holy Spirit descended upon him in bodily form like a dove. And a voice came from heaven, "You are my Son, the Beloved; with you I am well pleased." (3:21–22)

We have reflected on this passage in Chapter Three. There we noted that, of the four evangelists who refer to the baptism of Jesus, only Luke mentions that it was after the actual baptism, while Jesus was at prayer, that the Spirit came and the voice from heaven addressed him as Son.

Early in The Ministry

The Spirit, who has come down upon Jesus at the time of his baptism, leads Jesus into the wilderness where he is tempted by the devil (4:1–13). This episode, too, we have already seen. Then, Jesus, "filled with the power of the Spirit" returns to his native Galilee and sets about preaching in the synagogues (4:14–15). He then reaches Nazareth, the place where he had been brought up. Going to synagogue, as was his wont, he is invited to read from the scroll of the prophet Isaiah. He chooses a passage that amounts to his mission statement. His subsequent words of commentary initially find favour with his audience but then things turn nasty; his words deeply upset his townsfolk and they drive him out of town, wishing to throw him off the cliff on which the town stood. He eludes them and returns to Capernaum, where he preaches, exorcises and heals people. By the lakeside he chooses his first four disciples, fishermen who then accompany him as his ministry continues:[2]

> But now more than ever the word about Jesus spread abroad; many crowds would gather to hear him and to be cured of their diseases. But he would withdraw to deserted places and pray. (5:15–16)

The tense of the verb suggests that such withdrawal to quiet, deserted spots for personal prayer was a frequent occurrence, a constant in his ministry.[3] People are coming to him in large numbers, making demands on his time, energy and compassion, pressurising him to preach to them and bring them healing. There is perhaps a danger that his rising popularity could sidetrack him from his mission.[4] And so, "Repeatedly, Jesus seeks prayerful communion with God, from time to time separating himself from the people to whom he has been sent to bring deliverance."[5] Prayer is the source of his strength and discernment of God's will for him, an expression of his dependence on God.[6] The undulating rhythm of prayer and action seems to be characteristic of his lifestyle.

Jesus Calls The Twelve (6:12–16)

The next time that Luke mentions the prayer of Jesus is in connection with his calling of The Twelve. This follows a period in which Jesus in his liberating ministry has healed a leper, a paralysed man and many other people, and has also been involved with the Pharisees in controversy. He has been criticised by the religious elite for dining with tax gatherers and sinners, for not fasting, for allowing his disciples to pluck grain on the Sabbath and for his synagogue healing of a man with a withered hand on the Sabbath.

> Now during those days, he went out to the mountain to pray; and he spent the night in prayer to God. And when day came, he called his disciples and chose twelve of them, whom he also named apostles: Simon, whom he named Peter, and his brother Andrew, and James, and John, and Philip, and Bartholomew, and Matthew, and Thomas, and James son of Alphaeus, and Simon, who was called the Zealot, and Judas son of James, and Judas Iscariot, who became a traitor.

This is clearly a crucial moment in the development of Jesus' mission.[7] In preparing for it, Jesus heads for the hills in order to pray. This time, rather than a wilderness location, he chooses a mountain. In the biblical tradition mountains are symbolic places "where the eternal and transcendent break into this world with clarity."[8] Mountains are places of revelation and of openness to God.[9] Jesus spends the whole night in prayer before selecting his special inner circle from the wider group of his followers. It is a time of discernment. "He emerged from solitude with his path clear and his resolution strong."[10] They are to be called apostles, and are symbols of the new Israel, the new covenanted people of God, and its future leadership. We are familiar with the names and with the jarring note with which it concludes. "Not even decisions guided by prayer come with the guarantee of a happy outcome."[11] After making his choice, Jesus and the group descend to the plain again, where he delivers his famous discourse which spells out the implications of discipleship, the blueprint for life in God's Kingdom (6:20–49).[12]

The Question of The Identity of Jesus (9:18–22)

Luke's story of Jesus moves on. Jesus has performed many acts of healing and exorcism, and has spoken to the people in parables.[13] He has sent The Twelve out on mission to bring the Good News to a wider audience and to cure those in need. After their return, he has provided a banquet for the large crowd of people who had spent a day with him, listening to him and seeking cures (9:1–17).[14] The issue of Jesus' identity is raised by Luke's telling of Herod's perplexity about him (9:7–9). It is in this context that the narrative continues:

> Once when Jesus was praying alone, with only the disciples near him, he asked them, "Who do the crowds say that I am?" They answered, "John the Baptist;

but others, Elijah; and still others, that one of the ancient prophets has arisen." He said to them, "But who do you say that I am?" Peter answered, "The Messiah of God." He sternly ordered and commanded them not to tell anyone, saying, "The Son of Man must undergo great suffering, and be rejected by the elders, chief priests and scribes, and be killed, and on the third day be raised."

In the overall structure of the Gospel, this episode and the subsequent event of the transfiguration are extremely significant for the clarification of Jesus' identity.[15] In both, Jesus is at prayer in the company of disciples.[16] The transfiguration will be considered in Chapter Seven. Here, after a time in personal prayer with the disciples nearby, Jesus questions them about the opinion of the crowds concerning who he is. Perhaps their recent missionary outreach has enlightened them about the popular view. The responses that they list are not unlike those mentioned earlier amid the perplexed pondering of Herod; reference is made to the Baptist, to Elijah, and to the prophets of old. Clearly the people see Jesus as a prophet, and there is truth in this perception, but it does not go far enough. Jesus then challenges the disciples about their own perception and understanding after all that they have heard and seen: "But who do you say that I am?" It is Peter who offers an answer, probably voicing the view of the group: "The Messiah of God." This assessment is correct, and is a sign of progress on their part, but it too is incomplete, as we readers know.[17]

The response of Jesus is surprising. With some sternness, he orders the disciples to be silent about his messiahship, and then explicitly spells out for the first time what his messiahship entails. For, he asserts, he will be comprehensively rejected by the constituent bodies of Jewish religion, elders, priests and scribes, and will meet his end before being vindicated by God.[18] The use of "must" indicates the will of God for him. There is an ominous ring about his words, disconcerting for his listening disciples, and very different from what the ordinary folk were expecting and hoping for.[19] The issue will dominate the rest of the story, as the disciples are challenged to integrate suffering, rejection and death into their understanding of messiahship. But for the present it is better that they keep silent.[20] The audience widens, as Jesus delineates some of the implications of following him in radical terms of self-denial and daily cross-bearing, saving one's life by losing it (14:25–27).[21] His words extend to future generations of disciples too.

Early Journey Narrative (10:21–24)

After Jesus has spoken to his disciples about the nature of his messiahship and the demands of discipleship, Luke records the incident when he is transfigured, placing it in a context of prayer. Here, mention is made of his "exodus" in Jerusalem. Soon afterwards, Luke begins a lengthy section of his story of Jesus, which is usually referred to as the journey to Jerusalem or the travel narrative. It is introduced solemnly: "When the days drew near for him to be taken up, he set his face to go to Jerusalem." There is a sense of strong determination in Jesus, for he is conscious of God's purpose. The evangelist uses this journey motif from 9:51–19:27 as a kind of framework within which he can explore salient aspects of discipleship: the way of Jesus.[22] Throughout this major block of material, mainly devoted to the teaching of Jesus, there are many clear reminders of the journey theme.[23]

As the journey gets under way, Jesus sends messengers ahead of him. They go to a Samaritan village to prepare for his coming, but the villagers are not interested in welcoming him because he is going up to Jerusalem. This reflects the prejudice and animosity that existed between Samaritans and Jews. James and John, Elijah-like, wish to respond in kind, and ask Jesus whether they should call down fire from heaven to burn them up, a suggestion which incurs a rebuke from the Master.[24] Retaliation in the face of rejection is not his style. As they journey on, there are three brief encounters that highlight the radical demands of discipleship.[25] After this, the Lord appoints seventy[26] disciples and sends them on mission to the places he is to visit on his journey. Jesus speaks with some sadness and in tones of warning about the lakeside towns for their lack of response. The seventy then return from their mission. They are delighted with what they have been able to do in Jesus' name. He states that they should rejoice rather that their names are written in heaven.

This joyful note introduces the next section in which the theme of prayer occurs. An interesting concentric or chiastic structure has been proposed: Jesus prays to the Father (10:21–22); Jesus is alone with his disciples (10:23–24); the lawyer's question, and the twofold parabolic illustration of love for God and neighbour: the compassionate Samaritan, Martha and Mary (10:25–42); Jesus is alone with his disciples (11:1); Jesus prays and teaches his disciples to pray (11:2–4).[27] The text for the first two items reads as follows:

> At that same hour Jesus rejoiced in the Holy Spirit and said, "I thank you, Father, Lord of heaven and earth, because you have hidden these things from the wise and the intelligent and have revealed them to infants; yes, Father, for such was your

gracious will. All things have been handed over to me by my Father, and no one knows who the Son is except the Father, or who the Father is except the Son and anyone to whom the Son chooses to reveal him."

Then turning to the disciples, Jesus said to them privately, "Blessed are the eyes that see what you see! For I tell you that many prophets and kings desired to see what you see, but did not see it, and to hear what you hear, but did not hear it."

The joy from the previous episode concerning mission, to which this section is closely tied, spills over, as Jesus immediately bursts into joyful prayer, like Elizabeth and Mary earlier in the story. He does so under the inspiration or influence of the Spirit, whose anointing had been such a significant aspect of his baptism, and in whose name he had launched his mission in the Nazareth synagogue.[28] In the episodes we have considered previously, Luke has simply stated that Jesus prays. Now he provides his readership with the content of his prayer.[29]

The language is poetic, has a strong Semitic ring and follows the pattern of synagogue prayers of praise and thanksgiving.[30] Jesus addresses God both as "Father" and "Lord of heaven and earth", a form of address that at the same time acknowledges God's transcendence and otherness, and also his closeness, care and intimacy.[31] "Father" occurs here five times, "Son", three. Jesus thanks this God for choosing both to conceal and to reveal.[32] The message of the Kingdom's presence, revealed by the words and works of Jesus, has been hidden from the wise and intelligent religious specialists[33] but has been made known to ordinary people, the "little ones". Jesus recognises that this is God's sovereign good pleasure, God's way, which subverts traditional Jewish religious thinking. God's predilection for the poor and lowly and needy, God's paradoxical tendency to overturn normal human values, expectations and priorities, is a theme that Luke highlights throughout his Gospel. Mary celebrates this reversal motif in the *Magnificat*, and from the outset of his ministry, Jesus has set out to bring the Good News to the poor and outsiders.[34]

Jesus moves on to reveal the relationship that stands at the basis of his prayer. Speaking in language that has a distinctly Johannine ring,[35] he shares his awareness of his unique identity and his role, his intimate relationship with the Father as Son. The sovereign Father has gifted him with authority.[36] He is uniquely known in the depth of his being by the Father, and he knows the Father as no other does. The relationship is reciprocal. And so, he alone is able to reveal the Father and does so to those whom he chooses. Recalling Jesus' words in the temple at the age of twelve (2:49) and the divine assurances in the baptism and transfiguration scenes, it would seem that "primary in Luke's presentation of Jesus is also a sense of a unique relationship with God into which he wishes to draw human beings."[37]

Jesus next addresses the chosen disciples privately, proclaiming them blessed and happy because of what they can hear and see.[38] For they, ordinary and lowly as they are, are privileged to be living in a special time, the time of revelation, the time longed for over centuries by the prophets and kings of old, the most religious and powerful people of Israel's history. They have seen God's works in Jesus' healing ministry, and heard God's words in his preaching. They are witnessing now the fulfilment of Israel's dreams in the presence and ministry of Jesus; God's Kingdom is manifest wherever Jesus is present.[39] They have been able to recognise and appreciate this also through their recent participation in his mission.

Jesus Teaches The Disciples How to Pray (11:1–4)

After Jesus has recounted the parable of the compassionate Samaritan and has visited the home of Martha and Mary, Luke again picks up the prayer theme. The structural pattern is that Jesus is alone at prayer and then teaches his disciples how to pray. The text reads:

> He was praying in a certain place, and after he had finished, one of his disciples said to him, "Lord, teach us to pray, as John taught his disciples." He said to them, "When you pray, say Father, hallowed be your name. Your kingdom come. Give us each day our daily bread. And forgive us our sins, for we ourselves forgive everyone indebted to us. And do not bring us to the time of trial."

Once again, Jesus is said to be at prayer. The location is not specified ("in a certain place"). Presumably Jesus has moved on from the village of the two sisters. The disciples are in the vicinity, aware that Jesus is again praying, aware too, no doubt, of its importance in his life. When Jesus has drawn his prayer to a close, one of them approaches him and, addressing him as "Lord", asks him to teach them how to pray. In support of his request he cites the example of the Baptist, who had done so for his disciples. Since, as good Jews, the disciples were well-versed in prayer, perhaps he intended a prayer that would become characteristic of their group, reflect something of their identity and differentiate them from other groups. The disciples are keen to learn from the Master.

In reply, Jesus provides them with a model prayer, which we know as the Lord's Prayer. A version of this prayer is found also in Matthew's Sermon on the Mount and in an early Christian document known as the *Didache* (8:2); it is Matthew's form that we are more familiar with because of our liturgy. The form in Luke is shorter and less elaborate, consisting of an opening address and five requests; of these, the first two refer to the fulfilment of God's plan for the world, the other three to the needs of the disciples.[40]

Jesus begins by addressing God as "Father", as in his earlier prayer (10:21). Although Israel understood God as "father", they rarely addressed him in prayer in this way.[41] Jesus probably used the term "Abba", more familiar than that of traditional Jewish piety. It is best rendered as "Dad", and is Jesus' characteristic way of addressing God.[42] "Jesus transformed the Fatherhood of God from a theological doctrine into an intense and intimate experience; and he taught his disciples to pray with the same family intimacy."[43] In fact, they have been drawn into the close relationship that Jesus has with God.[44]

The first two petitions or imperatives concern the Father.[45] Jesus prays that the Father's name be held holy, which means that God be recognised and acknowledged as God, the utterly Other. A name tells us something about the very being of someone; it is the extension of his person.[46] This is typical of the tradition of Jewish prayer.[47] Jesus then prays that God's Kingdom may come, that God would establish God's kingly rule in the world. This petition moves from the divine world to the human world, from reverence for God to the shaping of life in the world.[48] This coincides with the dream of Jesus, the thrust of his preaching and ministry, the heart of his mission. Jesus believed that the reign of God was already being established through him in a firm but small way, and he longed for it to be spread ever more widely and completely.[49] Discipleship has to do with participating in God's project. In fact, the disciples have only recently had a taste of what this may entail.

The rest of the petitions focus more on the needs of the community of disciples, and Jesus prays in the plural. Luke's version reads "give us each day our daily bread"; the verb implies repeated giving.[50] There is considerable scholarly discussion about the meaning of the Greek word used here (*epiousios*), which is not found elsewhere in Greek literature. Three options are commonly put forward: what is necessary, essential for existence; for the present day, today; for the next day, tomorrow.[51] The request for food probably extends beyond the strictly material realm. The main point is that Jesus' followers rely on God to provide what is needed.

This request is followed by a prayer for forgiveness of sin, a major theme in Luke's story of Jesus, and a key element of Jesus' ministry of mercy and liberation. Jesus here "grounds the disciples' request for forgiveness in their own practices of extending forgiveness."[52] The emphasis is on similarity rather than condition.[53] We can receive the gift of God's forgiveness only if we are open to forgive; being unforgiving closes one's heart and can block God's forgiveness.[54] While the term 'debt' can have a metaphorical range of meaning, it is important not to overlook the pervasive cultural reality of debts and repayment, with the personal and community problems it engenders.[55]

The final petition is couched in negative terms: "do not put us to the test." The idea is not that God authors the testing but that God would use God's power so that the disciple does not succumb to temptation.[56] Such testing may embrace inward temptations but, more so, the testing of faith, the suffering, struggles and forms of conflict that will inevitably arise for the followers of Jesus; these are often understood as foreshadowing the troubles linked with the coming of the end time. For Jesus, the phrase probably had an eschatological flavour. As it stands, the phraseology seems to suggest that it is God who does the testing, whereas in fact he allows such trials to occur. Later, Jesus acknowledges his own time of trial (22:28) and encourages his disciples to pray to avoid it (22:46).

This prayer, I believe, expresses the concerns of Jesus evident in his ministry. The link between prayer and life is so strong. It reflects his intimate and reverential love for the Father, his commitment to the Kingdom dream, his awareness of our human needs, his concern for forgiveness and the issue of faithfulness.

As The End Approaches (22:31–32)

After Jesus has responded to the request of the disciples for a special prayer by teaching them the Lord's Prayer, he continues the petitionary aspect of prayer with a parable. This, along with two other parables from later in the journey narrative, we shall consider in the next chapter. The context for Luke's next reference to the prayer of Jesus is the city of Jerusalem. The journey to Jerusalem is now completed, and Jesus has descended the Mount of Olives in triumph. At the sight of the city, Jesus weeps because it will not accept the salvation that he brings; he foretells its coming destruction. He then proceeds to the precincts of the temple, which will be the theatre of his teaching in subsequent days.[57] In a dramatic protest, he drives out from the temple (probably the court of the gentiles) the merchants selling there.[58] He accompanies his symbolic prophetic action with words:

It is written, "My house shall be a house of prayer", but you have made it a den of robbers. (19:45)[59]

The words and actions of Jesus challenge the temple institution and the priestly elite responsible for it.[60] Jesus is claiming the temple for its legitimate use, for prayer and revelatory teaching concerning God's purpose. To do so "is to brand as illegitimate its utilization by the temple hierarchy, and thus to attract opposition."[61]

From that point, while Jesus teaches in the temple, which is his Father's business (2:49), the chief priests, scribes and leaders, now his main opponents, are bent on his destruction but hesitate because of his popularity with the people. The division foretold by Simeon in the temple (2:34–35) materialises in spectacular manner. Several controversies follow as the week unfolds, before Jesus speaks, in what is often referred to as a Final Discourse, about the destruction of the temple and city, and foretells wars and earthquakes and famines, plagues and dreadful portents, events which will occur prior to the world's end. He includes the persecution of his followers, before the Son of Man finally comes in power and glory. He concludes by exhorting his followers to "Be alert at all times, praying that you might have the strength to escape all these things which will take place, and to stand before the Son of Man" (21:36). Without prayer, survival and freedom are impossible. But whatever the "ambiguities and unfulfilled promises of human history, God's purposes—God's reign—will be accomplished, with humanity flourishing as God intends."[62]

While Jesus teaches and the people listen eagerly, Judas confers with the religious leaders about how he can betray Jesus into their hands in the absence of the crowds. This forms the backdrop for the final meal, which Jesus takes with his disciples.[63] As that meal draws to a close and the power of darkness intensifies and threatens to overtake them, Jesus addresses Simon Peter:

Simon, Simon, listen! Satan has demanded to sift all of you like wheat, but I have prayed for you that your own faith may not fail; and you, when once you have turned back, strengthen your brothers. (22:31–32)[64]

There is an echo of Job (1:12) in these words, as Satan, who has already involved Judas in treachery (22:3), wishes to test the faithfulness of Jesus' group and inspire their failure and apostasy. Aware of this danger, Jesus assures Simon Peter of his prayer for him, that whatever happens, his faith will ultimately survive his initial failure, and, repentant and changed, he will have the role of restoring the confidence of the others. Peter responds by asserting his loyalty, his readiness to go to prison and even to death, but Jesus predicts that before long, despite this bravado, he will three times deny he ever knew him. This will not, however, be the end of Peter's story, for the risen Jesus will appear to him,[65] forgiving and rehabilitating him.

The Garden Prayer (22:39–46)

In the final scene before the story of Jesus' passion, prayer occupies a central place. After the final meal, Jesus, with his disciples following behind, crosses the gorge-like Kedron valley, and ascends to the Mount of Olives, a venue he frequently visited as a place for prayer.[66] Luke does not refer to the place as a garden, nor does he name it Gethsemane.[67]

> He came out and went, as was his custom, to the Mount of Olives; and the disciples followed him. When he reached the place, he said to them, "Pray that you may not come into the time of trial." Then he withdrew from them about a stone's throw, knelt down, and prayed, "Father, if you are willing, remove this cup from me; yet, not my will but yours be done." Then an angel from heaven appeared to him and gave him strength. In his anguish he prayed more earnestly, and his sweat became like great drops of blood falling down on the ground. When he got up from prayer, he came to the disciples and found them sleeping because of grief, and he said to them, "Why are you sleeping? Get up and pray that you may not come into the time of trial."

Luke reshapes and simplifies the Markan tradition with great artistic skill. He omits the reference to Jesus being sorrowful, presenting Jesus as in command of the situation.[68] As Jesus faces his time of ultimate trial, he twice exhorts all the disciples (not just Mark's chosen three) to pray that they may avoid the time of testing, echoing the final petition of the prayer he had taught them earlier.[69] These two injunctions to pray frame the central feature of the episode, the prayer of Jesus himself.[70] In Mark, Jesus, in deep anguish and distress, leaves his prayer three times and approaches the three disciples he has chosen to be close to him. Luke's version is simpler: Jesus goes off to pray and returns to the group of his friends only when his prayer is finished; the focus of the whole episode is firmly on him and on his prayer. The disciples, however, are overwhelmed with grief-induced sleep, which can only have deepened Jesus' distress.[71] They will shortly be overcome by the tragic challenge of the occasion, and take the escape route.

The struggle with the power of evil in the earlier desert temptation scene closed with the note that Satan departed until an "opportune time". That time has come with a vengeance; this is a time of cosmic conflict with the power of evil at its most venomous. In his profound anguish,[72] Jesus kneels in prayer; this posture "draws special attention to submissiveness in prayer as well as to the urgency or intensity of the prayer itself."[73] Jesus' own prayer is, typically, addressed to his "Abba, Father."[74] It is a heartfelt and honest request to be spared the cup of suffering awaiting him as his "exodus" begins, which is his destiny. This request is flanked by two references to the Father's will. The first reference reads: "if you desire". "The Lukan Jesus is first of all concerned with the direction of the divine planning before he asks whether in the execution of that plan the cup can be taken from him."[75] And it is the Father's will, not his own, that must prevail. The basic orientation of Jesus' life has always been his commitment to fulfilling God's design and purpose, whatever this might demand of him.[76] Nothing can change that.[77] "Abba" entails the "yes" of acceptance, generous surrender and self-gift. After praying Jesus stands, an indication that the contest (*agōn*) is over, Jesus' discernment is clear, his resolve and determination are strengthened. He again addresses his disciples, telling them to get up and to pray; "both physically and spiritually they must be ready."[78] At that point the arresting party, led by Judas, arrives.[79]

Reflections

The way in which Luke traces this theme of Jesus' prayer offers such richness for our reflection. Jesus is presented as a deeply prayerful person. Luke is also interested in outlining how Jesus' followers should pray; Jesus is our model. As a good Jew, Jesus would have prayed daily. He also frequented the synagogue and would have prayed in the traditional manner with the others present. What Luke seeks to highlight is his personal prayer in different places and situations, for it is his way of life. One important aspect is his prayer prior to important decisions in the unfolding of his mission; this occurs on numerous occasions. Clearly there is a strong element of discernment in his praying. Jesus is extremely active in his ministry of preaching and healing, but he frequently moves away in order to be alone in prayer. There is a rhythm of prayer and action. I have heard the prayer of Jesus on these occasions described as "listening to the Father's love", the Father's love for him and for the world. There is much here for us to imitate.

Luke gives us three glimpses of the content of Jesus' prayer. In his prayer after the return of the seventy disciples from their foray into mission, Jesus addresses God as "Father" and as "Lord of heaven and earth". In Jesus' approach, there is great familiarity and deep reverence. He acknowledges God's closeness; God is "Abba", "Dad"'; the relationship is intimate and unique. At the same time, there is a recognition of God's otherness and transcendence. As disciples of

Jesus through the Spirit's outpouring in baptism, we too can adopt this way of speaking to God as his beloved sons and daughters. There is a wonderful familiarity about our prayer. Likewise, we must approach the Other with respect and reverence, we must not lose our sense of God's transcendence, forgetting that we are on "holy ground" and need to discard our sandals, Moses-like (Exod 3:5). Familiarity and reverence are the two wings of our relationship with our God, two ongoing aspects of our prayer.

When asked by one of his disciples to teach them to pray, Jesus, I believe, shares with them his way of praying in what we call the Lord's Prayer. "Abba, may your name be held holy" reiterates the familiarity and reverence aspects that we highlighted above. "Abba, your kingdom come" encapsulates Jesus' relationship with the Father and his mission dream, the twin aspects of his identity highlighted in the baptism narrative. The request for bread reflects Jesus' concern for human needs, his awareness of our human situation. The request for forgiveness is in tune with one of the main concerns of his ministry. The prayer that he taught his disciples was not a sudden inspiration; it flowed from his own way of praying. His own prayer is now our prayer. In praying in this way, we are close to his mind and heart. In Jesus, prayer and life flowed into each other; that is a challenge held out to us.

The final petition of the Lord's Prayer opens the third window into his way of praying: his prayer in the garden. He invites his disciples to pray that they should be spared the time of trial. On that final evening, he is faced with the spectre of suffering, failure and death, and is tested indeed. Often in our lives we are faced with testing situations: sickness and pain, anxiety and fear, conflict and broken relationships, stress and failure—the list continues. We turn to God in prayer. The prayer of Jesus indicates the form that prayer should take. He addresses his Father with love and trust, asking that the cup be removed, if God wants it that way. But if God's will does not coincide with his, then it is God's will that is paramount. For us this can be such a challenge. Sometimes God does respond to our prayers in the way we would like. Sometimes the response of the Father, who loves us deeply, is not what we were hoping for. This is indeed a testing time, and we are called to say "OK, I accept your way, your will, trusting that you have my best interests at heart." We seek to unite ourselves with Jesus in his surrender.

In his presentation of the prayer of Jesus, Luke gives us valuable insight into the kind of person Jesus was. He also provides a rich spirituality for us to seek to embrace and live by.

Notes

1   L. Daniel Chrupcala, *Everyone will see the Salvation of God: Studies in Lukan Theology* (Milan: Edizioni Terra Santa, 2015), 202, notes that the two official places of Jewish prayer were the temple and synagogue. Jesus went to temple and frequented synagogue; in both his main focus was teaching; there is no mention of his corporate prayer. When the prayer of Jesus is mentioned, "it treats of the personal and almost always solitary activity."

2   This we reflected upon in Chapter Three.

3   Luke has intimated that the Baptist lived in the wilderness, and that it was there that God's word came to him at the beginning of his ministry (3:2). It is intriguing and surprising that in 4:42–44, although following Mark (1:35–39), where Jesus goes early in the morning to a deserted place to pray and the disciples seek him out, interrupt his prayer and seek to take him back to the town, Luke omits the reference to Jesus' prayer. Marshall, *Luke*, 198, suggests that this may be because Luke does not wish to say that Jesus was interrupted at prayer, or wishes to focus on the single point that Jesus' mission must embrace other towns. Chrupcala, *The Salvation of God*, 209, suggests that for Luke this episode was not a turning point in Jesus' ministry.

4   Green, *Luke*, 238; Marshall, *Luke*, 210.

5   Carroll, *Luke*, 128; see Johnson, *Luke*, 93.

6   In Mark (1:38), where Jesus is disturbed in his prayer by the disciples, Jesus' response is to refuse their request that he stay in that place; his moving on elsewhere is a divine "must": "for that is what I came out to do."

7   Johnson, *Luke*, 104, observes that Luke sets the appointment of The Twelve as a response to the Pharisees' rejection of Jesus and their desire to be rid of him. It is an aspect of the evangelist's narrative plot.

8   Resseguie, *Spiritual Landscape*, 20.

9   In the Old Testament, this is particularly true of Sinai. Luke is less interested in mountains than Matthew; he omits the "high mountain" in the temptation scene (4:5); he transfers the Sermon on the Mount to a plain (6:17); he omits the second account of the multiplication of the loaves (Matt 15:29), and the Galilean resurrection appearance (Matt 28:16). However, he quotes the Isaian text in 3:5; he mentions the location of Nazareth, and occasionally links mountains with the prayer of Jesus. (See Chrupcala, *The Salvation of God*, 204–205).

10   Caird, *Luke*, 100. Chrupcala, *The Salvation of God*, 214, explores the rich biblical tradition of praying at night, especially in the psalms.

11   Carroll, *Luke*, 141.

12   In Matthew, this is the Sermon on the Mount (5:1–7:29); Luke's version, "on a level place", is shorter (6:17–49).

13   After the sermon on the plain he heals the centurion's servant (7:1–10), raises to life the son of the widow of Nain (7:11–17), assures the sinful woman of forgiveness (7:36–50), speaks in parables (8:4–18), calms a storm (8:22–25), cures the Gerasene demoniac (8:26–39), restores a girl to life and heals a woman of her gynaecological problem (8:40–56).

14   Mark 6:45–8:26 does not appear in Luke; this is called the "Great Omission"; perhaps he considered the episodes unnecessary or unhelpful.

15   In Mark and Matthew this episode is located at Caesarea Philippi. Luke, in his presentation, does not name the place. For Chrupcala, *The Salvation of God*, 210, by leaving the location indefinite, Luke transfers all the attention to Jesus' prayer. Green, *Luke*, 368, suggests that the report of Peter's confession is more closely related to the material that follows than to the material that precedes it.

16   Green, *Luke*, 368, notes that it is in prayer that Jesus solidifies his relationship with God and receives guidance and empowerment from God. Marshall, *Luke*, 366, speculates that apparently the prayer of Jesus is for divine guidance before making the decisive revelation that is to follow.

17   Green, *Luke*, 368, maintains that Luke associates Peter's confession with Jesus' praying, as if to declare that access to Jesus' identity is supernaturally mediated.

18   See also 9:44; 18:31–33; he refers to his being rejected also in 17:25 and 20:17; rejection exacerbates the suffering. Green, *Luke*, 371, refers to these hostile groups as a kind of triumvirate in Luke's ongoing narrative.

19   Luke omits Mark's description of Peter's response, when the disciple seeks to deter Jesus from such a course, and Jesus takes this as a satanic temptation. Clearly the disciples are deeply unhappy with what Jesus predicts, neither understanding nor accepting this kind of messianic path. Caird, *Luke*, 129, observes that in Jesus' mind there is a fusion of three Old Testament figures: the Messiah, the Son of Man, and the Servant of the Lord.

20   Marshall, *Luke*, 367, suggests that the reason for the injunction to silence (a feature also of Mark's Gospel) could be the danger of it being misunderstood in nationalistic terms. Another reason could be the disciples' failure to fully understand its nature.

21   Johnson, *Luke*, 155, notes that this is the essential pattern for Christian identity and spirituality. Green, *Luke*, 366, points out the inseparability of Christology and discipleship.

22   "Now it happened that as the time drew near for him to be taken up, he resolutely turned his face towards Jerusalem ..." (9:51). Some scholars (like Tannehill, *Luke*, 167), maintain that the motif continues as far as 19:44/45, when Jesus enters the temple; Green, *Luke*,394, as far as 19:48, the conclusion of the temple incident. While the "way" theme is present in Mark, the material in this major Lukan section is from 'Q' or Luke's own sources. At 18:15, Luke rejoins Mark. As Caird, *Luke*, 139, puts it: this is "a somewhat artificial structure, full of topographical inconsistencies."

23   At 9:57, "As they travelled along"; 10:38, "In the course of their journey he came to a village"; 13:22, "Through towns and villages he went"; 17:11, "Now on the way to Jerusalem he travelled along the border between Samaria and Galilee"; 18:31, "Now we are going up to Jerusalem"; 19:11, "He was near Jerusalem"; 19:28, "He went on ahead, going up to Jerusalem"; 19:37, "And now, as he was approaching the downward slope of the Mount of Olives"; 19:41, "As he drew near and came in sight of the city"; 19:45, "Then he went into the Temple.*"* There are a few healing stories (11:14; 13:10–17; 14:1–6; 17:11–19; 18:35–43). Green, *Luke*, 394–399, suggests five narrative needs in this

journey section: the coming of salvation in all its fullness to all people; the expectation that Mary's son would be the cause of division in Israel; the developing portrait of Jesus as one who, in order to fulfil God's purpose, must suffer rejection and be killed; the obduracy of the disciples; Jesus' "exodus" in Jerusalem.

24   2 Kgs 1:10, 12; on this see Caird, *Luke*, 140; Green, *Luke*, 405.

25   These we considered in the last chapter.

26   The NRSV reads seventy, following most manuscripts; some manuscripts have seventy-two, and some scholars (e.g. Carroll, *Luke*, 233, n.a.) believe it more likely that this is the original.

27   John R. Donahue, *The Gospel in Parable* (Philadelphia: Fortress, 1988), 138. The parable and parabolic narrative are treated in Chapter Eight.

28   1:47; Acts 2:26; 16:34.

29   Green, *Luke*, 421, refers to a "christological peak in the Gospel of Luke as well as a high point in the characterisation of Jesus' disciples."

30   Many psalms contain the words "I thank you that ..." followed by the reason (Ps 75:1; 78:1; 138:1); this is the pattern also of the *Magnificat* and *Benedictus* earlier in the Gospel; see Johnson, *Luke*, 169. Marshall, *Luke*, 432, detects in this section a background of Jewish wisdom literature.

31   Marshall, *Luke*, 433, holds that Jesus uses the "Abba" address to the Father, as do children to their dad.

32   Marshall, *Luke*, 434, suggests that the concealing is perhaps not to be stressed: "what was happening remained obscure in its significance to one group of people, but to the disciples it constituted a revelation of God's saving action."

33   The religious elite of Jesus' day, despite their learning, have failed to recognise what is happening in Jesus. Carroll, *Luke*, 240, observes that they are wise and knowledgeable but not discerning about the ways of God.

34   1:51–53; 4:18–19; see also 1 Cor 1:18–31.

35   See especially chapter 17, the prayer of Jesus at the Supper. Byrne, *Hospitality*, 96, n. 12, maintains that there are no firm grounds for excluding its provenance from the lips of Jesus himself. Caird, *Luke*, 146, is of the view that it cannot be a product of the Greek-speaking Church; it contains little that is not implicit in the baptism and temptation scenes. Carroll, *Luke*, 241, n. 7, observes that the theological claims of the passage cohere with earlier developments in the narrative.

36   The verb "handed over" can be used of the handing down of knowledge or the transfer of power and authority. Marshall, *Luke*, 436, believes that probably both authority and knowledge are meant here.

37   Byrne, *Hospitality*, 97.

38   In Matthew, the next verses are presented in a different context after the parable of the sower (13:16–17). This is the seventh *macarism* or beatitude of the Gospel. Green, *Luke*, 400, notes that the knowledge shared by Peter, James and John in the transfiguration scene has now been made available to the larger group of his followers. He understands the words of Jesus as addressed to the seventy, who share Jesus' mission.

39   Green, *Luke*, 423–424. Carroll, *Luke*, 242, notes that this emphasis on hearing and acting is seen in the next two stories.

40 There is some discussion as to which version is the more original. Caird, *Luke*, 151, suggests that in some points it seems to be Luke's, in others that of Matthew. Matthew's form, with seven petitions, probably reflects the liturgical prayer of his community, with stronger Jewish ties. McBride, *Luke*, 144, maintains that Luke's context seems more original than that of Matthew. Evans, *Luke*, 476, opines that the original may not be recoverable if both versions have had behind them a history of liturgical use.

41 Green, *Luke*, 441, cites, for example, Deut 32:6; Isa 63:16; Deut 14:1; 2 Sam 7:14; Ps 2:7; Jer 31:9; Hos 11:1–4. The prayer is grounded in the covenant and eschatological promise.

42 Byrne, *Hospitality*, 104. Green, *Luke*, 441, n. 18, considers it virtually certain that "Abba" is used here, and that this form of address is without exact parallel in contemporary Palestinian Judaism. Raymond E. Brown, *The Death of the Messiah*, 2 vols (London, Geoffrey Chapman, 1994), 1:173, n. 15, also. He discusses this issue in 1:172–175, considering it most plausible that addressing God in Aramaic as "Abba" was a historical and memorable (because unusual) practice of Jesus himself. Luke's "Father" is more original than Matthew's "Our Father in heaven". John P. Meier, in Raymond E. Brown, Joseph A. Fitzmyer and Roland E. Murphy (eds) *The New Jerome Biblical Commentary* [*NJBC*] (Upper Saddle River, NJ: Prentice-Hall), 78:31, writes that "one is justified in claiming that Jesus' striking use of 'Abba' did express his intimate experience of God as his own father and that this usage did make lasting impression on his disciples." Evans, *Luke*, 479, too opts for "Abba"; he observes that although Father is not used of God in Jewish prayer, the idea of God as Father of Israel and individual Israelites was well established in Judaism. In Jewish piety "father" conveyed a sense of authority and lordship rather than love and care.

43 Caird, *Luke*, 152.

44 Marshall, *Luke*, 456, states that the use of the intimate form was the amazing new thing that Jesus wished to teach his disciples, initiating them into the same close relationship with the Father that he enjoyed, and it is improbable that the early Christian usage can be explained apart from a definite command from Jesus himself.

45 Byrne, *Hospitality*, 104, points out that in the Aramaic of Jesus the verbs would be stronger.

46 Evans, *Luke*, 480.

47 Caird, *Luke*, 152, states that the first petition is a prayer that God will act to display his holiness and love (Ezek 36:23); Evans, *Luke*, 480, "to act decisively in such a way that this acknowledgement may come about." For indications of Jewish prayer see Green, *Luke*, 439; Evans, *Luke*, 478.

48 Carroll, *Luke*, 250.

49 Here Matthew adds: "your will be done on earth as in heaven", which amounts to the same thing. The coming of God's reign implies liberation from Satan's control.

50 Matthew has "this day", and the tense of the verb suggests one gift.

51 Byrne, *Hospitality*, 104, prefers "bread necessary for survival"; also, Johnson, *Luke*, 178 ("the bread we need"). Carroll, *Luke*, 250, suggests: "give us day by day our bread for the coming day or age, the bread of tomorrow." Green too, *Luke*, 442, opts for "the bread pertaining to the coming day."

52   Green, *Luke*, 444.

53   Evans, *Luke*, 483.

54   Byrne, *Hospitality*, 104. Matthew uses debts for both parts of the petition. The use of debt for sin is unusual in the Old Testament, but common in contemporary Judaism; the words are the same in Aramaic (also Evans, *Luke*, 483).

55   Carroll, *Luke*, 250.

56   McBride, *Luke*, 146; Marshall, *Luke*, 462.

57   The Gospel begins in the temple (1:8); Jesus last visited the temple in 2:41–51: "Did you not know that I must be in my Father's house?" Marshall, *Luke*, 719, sees the current incident as a prelude and preparation for Jesus' ministry of teaching in the temple.

58   The temple inevitably had a financial aspect, as pilgrims brought money for taxes and bought animals for sacrifice; currency required an exchange mechanism. Carroll, *Luke*, 389, suggests that there was some "exploitative business activity", as also Tannehill, *Luke*, 286. The verb used for Jesus' action (*ekballein*) has been used by Luke for the casting out of devils (9:40, 49; 11:14–20; 13:32). Luke's description omits details of violence, and focuses more on Jesus' words.

59   The quotation is from Isa 56:7; the phrase "den of robbers" derives from Jer 7:11. Surprisingly, Luke omits the phrase "for all the nations". Johnson, *Luke*, 298, suggests that for Luke the temple did not have an enduring role for gentiles. Green, *Luke*, 694, comments that in Luke's vision the gentiles would not come to the temple to find God; rather, the Lord goes out to the gentiles though his witnesses; similarly, Evans, *Luke*, 688; Tannehill, *Luke*, 286.

60   Carroll, *Luke*, 389.

61   Green, *Luke*, 692. Marshall, *Luke*, 719, notes that the episode serves to provide part of the motive for the action taken against Jesus by the religious authorities.

62   Carroll, *Luke*, 420. Green, *Luke*, 743, n. 60, suggests that prayer here would seem to involve both discernment of the divine aim and orientation of oneself around that purpose.

63   The Last Supper is part of Chapter Twelve.

64   The literary model that Luke is using in this final section of the Supper is the Farewell Discourse (Green, *Luke*, 771). Luke here reverts to Peter's former name; Green, *Luke*, 772, suggests that this may signal to the reader that his identity and vocation as an apostle are at stake in the coming conflict.

65   Both in Paul's list (1 Cor 15:5) and in Luke 24:34.

66   Since this was Jesus' custom or habit, Judas would know where to find him. The phrase "as was his wont" might also suggest that Jesus made more than one visit to Jerusalem, as in John's Gospel. Chrupcala, *The Salvation of God*, 206, takes "as was his wont" to refer to his prayer. The tradition of Jesus' struggle with his destiny is found in John 12:27 and Heb 5:7–8, as well as the three Synoptic Gospels. Byrne, *Hospitality*, 175, asserts that we are dealing with something firmly rooted and highly valued in the early tradition; similarly, Marshall, *Luke*, 829.

67   Brown, *Death*, 1:124, notes that Luke's use of *poreuesthai* here forges a link with the overall journey motif (9:51, 53; 13:33; 17:11; 22:22). The Mount of Olives has

eschatological significance; Zech 14:4 reads: "On that day his feet shall stand on the Mount of Olives." Brown, *Death*, 1:125, reminds us that after Absalom's revolt, David went up the Ascent of Olives, wept there and prayed to God (2 Sam 15:30).

68   Brown, *Death*, 1:157, suggests that Luke presents Jesus as a model for Christian sufferers and martyrs, and is partly influenced by Greco-Roman ideas. Similarly, Paul in Acts 20:36–37. For Johnson, *Luke*, 354, Luke, sensitive to his Hellenistic audience, removes from Jesus his need for companionship and the elements of fear and sorrow found in Mark. Jerome Neyrey, *The Passion according to Luke: A Redaction Study of Luke's Soteriology* (New York: Paulist Press, 1985), 50–54, discusses the background to the term "grief" in Greek and Roman philosophy and in the Old Testament; it is considered as a vice, a punishment for sin and an indication of guilt. Aware of this, Luke omits Mark's phrasing. He simplifies Mark's threefold prayer to one prayer which focuses on God's will.

69   Chrupcala, *The Salvation of God*, 217, n. 54, links *peirasmos* with apostasy. Brown, *Death*, 1:160–162, sees *peirasmos* as a crucial moment in the great final trial with Satan. 1:218: His "reluctance and anguish were not caused simply by facing suffering and death but also by the knowledge that he was entering a great struggle with Evil, the great trial that preceded the coming of the Kingdom."

70   Carroll, *Luke*, 445, detects a chiastic structure here; Jesus' prayer is framed by two exhortations to the disciples that they should pray; also, Frank J. Matera, *Passion Narratives and Gospel Theologies* (New York: Paulist Press, 1986), 167. Green, *Luke*, 777, terms it an *inclusio*. As it stands the text refers to the prayer of Jesus three times.

71   Luke softens their failure to keep awake by asserting that they were overcome with grief! His account is briefer than Mark's, and less graphic and dramatic. Brown, *Death*, 1:193, suggests that Luke changes Jesus' grief (in Mark) to that of the disciples, making them less blameworthy for not having prayed; their sleepfulness is forgivable. Matera too, *Passion Narratives*, 168, notes that Luke typically has a benign attitude to the disciples. Johnson, *Luke*, 352, notes that it is not the case that Jesus sweats blood as a physiological reaction to stress, but that his sweat resembles globules of blood. Green, *Luke*, 780, observes that Jesus sweats profusely like an athlete in a contest; he was not sweating blood. Marshall's view, *Luke*, 833, is that the implication is that the sweat was like the shedding of blood.

72   Caird, *Luke*, 243, refers to Jesus facing rejection by his own people, the shame and guilt of national sin, the doom of Jerusalem.

73   Green, *Luke*, 779; McBride, *Luke*, 291. The normal posture for prayer was to stand. In Mark (14:35) Jesus "threw himself to the ground"; in Matthew (26:39) "he fell on his face". In Luke Jesus is more dignified.

74   Unlike Mark, Luke does not explicitly use the term "Abba" here; (see earlier comments on the "Our Father").

75   Brown, *Death*, 1:171. On 1:177, he comments that in Jesus' prayer about his impending suffering and death there are parallels drawn from early Christian prayer patterns known to us in the Lord's prayer; also, the reference to "testing". Christians knew how Jesus prayed because some of their prayers were traditionally his prayers, reflecting his style and values. For Luke's readers, there is a consistent pattern between

what Jesus taught in the ministry and how he prayed as he approached death. Neyrey, *Passion*, 60, notes that the first petition is that God remove the cup; the second prayer presupposes that God may not wish to remove the cup, and prays that God's will may be done.

76   Green, *Luke*, 778, notes points of contact here with Isaian Servant texts referring to suffering as an outworking of the divine will, submissive obedience, the offering of aid through a divine messenger (Isa 41:10; 42:1, 6; 49:5; 50:4–9; 52:13–53:12). Marshall, *Luke*, 828, refers to alignment with God's will rather than submission to it.

77   Some scholars take the reference to the angel and blood as a later interpolation and not original (Fitzmyer, *Luke*, 2:1443–1444; Carroll, *Luke*, 446, who notes the absence of angels in the temptation scene, and the tension here with Luke's picture of a composed Jesus facing martyrdom; Matera, *Passion Narratives*, 167; Evans, *Luke*, 813, maintains that on balance the verses should probably be deleted; Byrne, *Hospitality*, 175; Johnson, *Luke*, 351; Neyrey, *Passion*, 57, do not agree.) Green, *Luke*, 780, understands that the angel empowers Jesus to engage in even more ardent prayer. God's response to the prayer of Jesus is to provide strength for the ordeal, not to remove the cup. Marshall, *Luke*, 832, accepts the verses as original, "but with very considerable hesitation." Brown, *Death*, 1:185, favours Lukan authorship. He thinks Luke has transferred Mark's desert temptation angels to this point (also Neyrey, *Passion*, 63). He actualises the angelic assistance that is potential or misunderstood in the accounts of Matthew and John. Brown, *Death*, 1:187–190, notes the angel tradition in 1 Kgs 19:5–8 (Elijah) and Dan 3:20, 28. The angel strengthens Jesus in entering the *peirasmos*; he prays with an intensity which induces sweat. *Agōnia* means the tension which an athlete experienced before a contest, and he breaks into a sweat; there is trepidation before the unpredictable elements in the contest. The angel is like a trainer who readies the athlete; Jesus' resumed prayer is last-minute preparation for entering into the *peirasmos*. Jesus is aware that his baptism must be completed (12:50). Neyrey, *Passion*, 64, notes that vivid physical descriptions are characteristic of Luke's narrative style. It emphasises the gravity and importance of the contest.

78   Brown, *Death*, 1:193.

79   Evans, *Luke*, 808, observes that the account must have been, at least in part, a construct given that the disciples were at a distance and asleep. The content will presumably have been inferred from a particular theology of Jesus as Son of God in a relationship of obedience to God as Father, and of his death as a consequence of that obedience. Brown, *Death*, 1:192, refers to the "composed and masterful Jesus". Brown, *Death*, 1:225–226, maintains that "early Christians had a tradition that before he died Jesus struggled in prayer about his fate. I do not know whether they retained or claimed to retain accurate memories of the wording he used; more probably they did not. But they understood his prayer in terms like the hour and the cup, which in the tradition of his sayings he had used to describe his destiny in God's plan. They fleshed out the prayer tradition in light of the psalms and their own prayers, both of which they associated with Jesus' way of praying. Each evangelist (and the tradition before him) knew different forms of that tradition, and each developed it differently both before and in the course of fitting it into his narrative."

Chapter Six
Parables about Prayer

In addition to presenting Jesus as a man of prayer, Luke provides the reader/ listener with three of Jesus' parables on the subject: the friend at midnight, the widow and the judge, and the Pharisee and the publican. Before we examine these stories in detail in an effort to understand their original meaning, their significance for Luke and their implications for ourselves today, it would be useful to reflect a little about parables in general.

Parables

We all appreciate a good story. Jesus of Nazareth was a consummate storyteller, a creator of interesting and thought provoking short stories. We usually refer to these as his parables. Telling stories seems to have been a characteristic way of his preaching to the people.[1] He was not original in opting for this method of addressing folk. There are some classic parables in the Old Testament, like the trees wishing to anoint a king to rule them (Judg 9:8–15) or Nathan's parable about the ewe lamb, which he addressed to David (2 Sam 12:1–7) or the wonderful story of Jonah, the reluctant prophet. Other rabbis over the years adopted a similar approach, for storytelling and parables were part of Jewish culture.[2] But Jesus seems to have excelled in this art form, as he sought to communicate his message and draw people into his worldview, forcing them to reconsider their values and lives.[3] Jesus probably did not use a story on one single occasion only. It is likely that he retold it to different village audiences, maybe with slight adaptations and variations depending on the situation.[4] Parables draw the hearer/ reader in; of their nature they are challenging, stimulating thought, inviting to decision. The classic definition is: "the parable is a metaphor or simile drawn from nature or common life, arresting the hearer by its vividness or strangeness, and leaving the mind in sufficient doubt about its precise application to tease it into active thought."[5]

After his death and resurrection, the followers of Jesus repeated his stories in their preaching and teaching, and no doubt they, too, added their own nuance and flavour, adapting them to the interests and needs of their audience, while the key elements remained consistent.[6] It was quite a while before the parables were committed to writing. In the process, the original context in which Jesus used his stories was lost. This entailed that the original meaning and thrust of the story in Jesus' mind were at times to some extent obscured. Inevitably some filtering went on.[7] Of their nature, parables are open to many interpretations; there is not just a single meaning; they are open-ended.[8] They are intended to evoke a response.

The location of a parable in the Gospel story as we now have it is therefore largely the decision of the evangelists, using it as part of their overall literary structure and theological message. In doing this, they reshaped it and inevitably also provided an interpretation of the parable's meaning and an application to the situation of their own listeners and readership.[9] This process has been repeated over the centuries and happens regularly in books and sermons today. And this is fine; the word of God is alive; the Spirit of God is around and active. The texts must speak to each of us anew. However, perhaps we can lose sight of the original impact such stories would have had on their Galilean and Judean hearers. It is important to attempt to recover this, if possible, and to do so we seek to discover the possible original contexts and to understand the people of Jesus' day, their lives and views and ways. Theirs was a very different world from ours.[10] It is also helpful to be sensitive to echoes of the Old Testament.[11] So, we need to ask two main questions: how do we hear the parables through an imagined set of first-century Jewish ears, and then how do we translate them so that they can be heard still speaking?[12] There is a danger that we import historical and anachronistic readings, which deform the message of Jesus.[13]

Levine makes the point that "the parables often express concerns that appear elsewhere in the Jesus tradition; they echo themes heard in his teaching and debates."[14] He is concerned about economics and wealth management; he is concerned about relationships, emphasising caring for others, service and humility. He is concerned about priorities. He is concerned about the reign of God. He is keen on celebrating and on table fellowship.[15] What Jesus spoke in his parables, he lived.[16] A key characteristic of Gospel parables is their realism; generally, they are rooted in everyday life, the world of human experience. "The parables claim that the arena in which God summons human beings to the risk of decision is the world of everyday existence, that same world in which the life of Jesus unfolded in dialogue with the mystery of God."[17] At the same time, parables contain exaggerations and hyperbole, incompatibilities and paradoxes; they can be puzzling and enigmatic; it is often here that the religious challenge lies.

With all this in mind, we can pursue our study of the three parables of prayer.

The Friend at Midnight (11:5–13)

The first of the Lukan prayer parables is found early in the journey narrative. After the parable of the compassionate Samaritan and the story of Jesus' visit to the house of Martha and Mary, which we will consider later in Chapter Eight, Luke provides a section about prayer. This we have just reflected upon. After Jesus has taught his disciples to pray the "Lord's Prayer", he presents this parable, which is found only in Luke's Gospel (11:5–8). This is followed by some sayings of Jesus about prayer (11:9–13), which are also found in Matthew (7:7–11).

The text of the parable reads as follows:

> And he said to them, "Suppose one of you has a friend, and you go to him at midnight and say to him, 'Friend, lend me three loaves of bread; for a friend of mine has arrived, and I have nothing to set before him.' And he answers from within, 'Do not bother me; the door has already been locked, and my children are with me in bed; I cannot get up and give you anything.' I tell you, even though he will not get up and give him anything because he is his friend, at least because of his persistence he will get up and give him whatever he needs."

Jesus immediately engages his audience, encouraging them to use their imagination and see themselves in the story he is about to relate: "suppose one of you", or "which of you?"[18] The main protagonist is a person who has been thrust suddenly into the position of host by the unexpected arrival late at night of a friend of his[19] needing food and shelter.[20] Having a larder that is bare, he is plunged into crisis in a community for which hospitality is a paramount law: "I have nothing to offer him." The only course of action is to go to a neighbour, who is also a friend, and disturb him in the middle of the night with a request for three loaves of bread, which would facilitate the fulfilment of the solemn obligation of hospitality.[21] In that culture, hospitality is the concern not only of the individual, but also of the whole community. It is important that the guest leaves with positive feelings about the whole village community.[22] The phrase: "I have nothing to offer him" is a frequent idiom that means nothing adequate to uphold the honour and reputation of the village. Although one unbroken loaf would be sufficient for a guest, hospitality demands that more than is strictly necessary be placed before him. The host would be aware who in the village had baked recently. He is therefore asking the sleeper to fulfil his duty to the guest of the village; his request is modest and reasonable. He would probably go elsewhere for the other things required.[23] A refusal is unthinkable.

The friend in question has locked up for the night and is asleep with his family on a mat placed on the floor in the one room of the house. He does not wish to be disturbed, nor to disturb the other members of the family by moving around and opening the door. However, the iron bolt in the door would not be heavy or difficult to manipulate. The children, if disturbed, would soon go back to sleep. The excuses are flimsy, absurd and something of a joke.[24]

At this point, the storyline is interrupted as Jesus answers his own question, assuring his audience that in the end the man inside the house will get up from his bed and give his friend "whatever he needs".[25] It is at this point that issues of interpretation arise. Does the householder get up and respond generously because of the other's "persistence", or is he "shamed" into responding? The Greek word (*aneidia*) can mean both.[26] Is the main character the man making the request, whose shameless, impudent persistence wins out, or the man in bed, who is eventually shamed into responding in a positive and generous manner?

One interpretation argues that in its present context, the context provided by Luke, the emphasis in the parable falls on the persistence of the man seeking bread to provide a meal for his guest.[27] The parable is situated between the prayer given by Jesus to the disciples, which is largely petitionary (and which includes a request for bread), and a series of sayings taken from the 'Q' source, which stress the need to knock and to ask. This the petitioner does in the parable. The series of sayings concludes with the assurance that the Father will grant the gift of the Spirit to those who ask.

The alternative view sees this interpretation as alien to the original thrust of the parable on the lips of Jesus, and as a Lukan imposition, favoured by the prayer sayings and the later parable of the unjust judge (18:1–8). The subject of the verbs in the second stanza of the parable is the sleeping householder. The correct rendering of *aneidia* is not persistence but shamelessness, and it applies to the man in bed.[28] The demands associated with hospitality and maintenance of honour (or avoidance of shame, the diminishing of public reputation) move the sleeper to get up and assist.[29] This he does in the end, with great generosity towards his friend. The argument, like that of the later parable of the unjust judge, goes from the lesser to the greater (or *a fortiori*). If an awkward person[30] such as the sleeper will answer the request despite the inconvenience, how much more certainly will God, who is Abba and more generous and gracious than his children can imagine? God is not hard of hearing nor barricaded in; God will not send us away empty handed; God will respond to our needs with gifts in abundance.[31]

As the parable stands, perhaps there is truth in both interpretations: God will graciously answer our prayers; but it is important to keep on praying, despite a seeming delay.

Added Sayings (11:9–13)

So I say to you, Ask, and it will be given to you; search, and you will find; knock, and the door will be opened for you. For everyone who asks receives, and everyone who searches finds, and for everyone who knocks, the door will be opened. Is there anyone among you who, if your child asks for a fish, will give a snake instead of a fish? Or if the child asks for an egg, will give a scorpion? If you then, who are evil, know how to give good gifts to your children, how much more will the heavenly Father give the Holy Spirit to those who ask him!

This small block of material is carefully structured: an introductory statement; three recommendations (ask, search and knock), with a threefold assurance of success; a parabolic statement (introduced in a way similar to the earlier parable) based on the relationship of father and son, comprising a twofold asking and giving; a comparison between a human father and the heavenly Father.[32] In the Sermon on the Mount, Matthew includes a very similar section (7:7–11; see Jas 1:5–8); this suggests that the source is 'Q', and that the sayings were not originally attached to the parable.[33]

The opening statement "So I say to you" forms a link with the preceding parable. The recommendation is to keep on asking (present imperative in Greek), seeking and knocking, which are actions linked with the preceding parable and are fairly synonymous expressions for prayer; the stress falls on the importance of unwearied effort in prayer, even if results are not immediate.[34] Each is followed by an assurance of a positive outcome (receive, find, open door). The use of the passive voice in "will be given to you" and "will be opened for you" indicates God's action in responding. The certainty of a positive outcome is further emphasised for "everyone" who asks, searches or knocks, not just for an elitist few.[35]

A short parable follows, in which the imagery switches from the friendship relationship of the earlier parable to the relationship of father and son. The introduction is couched in the typical style of Jesus, as he engages the listener: "Which of you?" If a child asks for a fish or an egg, no father would offer a serpent or a scorpion.[36] The images probably refer to a barbut fish (a sea snake) and a folded-up scorpion, which resembles an egg. A human father would not play a bad joke on his son, deceiving him into thinking that he was getting what he asked for, nor would he give him something harmful instead of the gift he was seeking. If a human father, with all his faults and weaknesses, responds lovingly to his children, avoiding any form of harm, how much more can the heavenly Father be trusted to respond with love and care. Again, the argument moves from lesser to greater (step parallelism).

Whereas Matthew's version concludes with the assurance that God will give good things to those who ask, Luke's Jesus speaks of the Father giving the Holy Spirit, a significant editorial change.[37] This is God's most precious gift, the best gift of all, offered to the followers of Jesus, far beyond what an earthly father could bestow. There is a strong emphasis on God's abundant generosity. Luke is here anticipating the later event of the Spirit's coming upon the disciples after the resurrection and ascension of Jesus (Acts 2:1–13).[38] That gift "is the constant assurance of the presence of God working at the heart of reality."[39]

Reflections

The two key words used in both the parable and the additional section are "ask" and "give". Those listening to Jesus, then and now, are recommended to ask God for what they need and to keep on doing so with persistence and perseverance, boldness even. It is difficult to stick at it when a response seems slow in arriving. We quickly become downhearted, discouraged, disconcerted; our confidence takes a knock. It is easy to throw in the towel and give up, faith eroded. It is at times like this that we need to remember with trust the words of Jesus.

The ground for such persistent prayer is the certainty of God's abundant graciousness; God will give us far beyond our expectations.[40] God is essentially a giving God; that is the essence of God's being. "All I have is yours" says the father of the two sons in another parable. Jesus seeks to inculcate an understanding of God's love and care that will lead us to approach him with confidence, trusting that God will respond in the end.

The Widow and The Judge (18:1–8)

There are two parables about prayer at the beginning of chapter 18; both are found only in Luke's Gospel. The first of these has much in common with the parable occurring earlier in Luke's story, which we have just considered; the two are in parallel. In context, the parable of the widow and the judge is linked with the material in 17:20–37, in which, prompted by a question from some Pharisees, Jesus speaks about the time of the coming of the Kingdom, or the day of the coming of the Son of Man.[41] The parable is addressed to Jesus' disciples, and "is brilliantly placed after the discourse in which Jesus makes it clear that the Kingdom he proclaims is not yet the end time, that there must be a period when the disciples will 'long to see one of the days of the Son of Man and will not see it'" (17:22).[42] It is appropriate at this point in Luke's narrative sequence to have a parable with the point that one must pray constantly and not give up.[43]

The text reads as follows:

> Then Jesus told them a parable about their need to pray always and not to lose heart. He said, "In a certain city there was a judge who neither feared God nor had respect for people. In that city, there was a widow who kept coming to him and saying, 'Grant me justice against my opponent.' For a while he refused; but later he said to himself, 'Though I have no fear of God and no respect for anyone, yet because this widow keeps bothering me, I will grant her justice, so that she may not wear me out by continually coming'." And the Lord said, "Listen to what the unjust judge says. And will not God grant justice to his chosen ones who cry to him day and night? Will he delay long in helping them? I tell you, he will quickly grant justice to them. And yet, when the Son of Man comes, will he find faith on earth?"

The structure is quite straightforward: an introduction (18:1), the parable (2–5), the applications (6–8).[44] It is generally agreed that the introductory verse and the applications come from Luke's editorial hand; he has created a frame for the parable.[45]

As in the previous episode, the audience consists of the disciples. In the introductory verse Luke explicitly informs the reader at the outset what he considers the parable to be about: "he told them a parable about their need to pray always and not to lose heart."[46] The verb translated here as "lose heart" means to become discouraged, to despair at the failure to obtain what is prayed for.[47] The opening that Luke has included not only highlights the topic of prayer but, in the wider context, gives the parable an orientation towards the delayed coming of the parousia. Luke wishes to offer "a paradigm of prayer which should mark the life of the community during its pilgrimage."[48] However, the parable as originally told by Jesus may have referred simply to the need for perseverance and courageous action in the face of difficulties, or persistence in prayer in a general sense. On the other hand, "the generalised introduction could be authentic to the specific situation which Jesus himself faced, as well as an appropriate introduction to the parable at a later stage in the life of the Church." The topic of prayer and the delay of the second coming are woven together.[49]

The parable begins with the introduction of one of the protagonists, an unnamed judge in an unidentified town, clearly a stock character and not a nice man. In those days perhaps there was no uniformly organised justice system; prominent individuals in the locality were appointed to act when required.[50] Maybe monetary cases could be handled by a single judge or local magistrate; recourse to a tribunal was not necessary.[51] The judge, who would have political influence and economic security,[52] is described at the outset as "one who neither feared God nor had respect for people", the antithesis of what a judge should be (see the description of an ideal in 2 Chron 19:4–7, where a judge is said to judge on God's behalf).[53] The frequency with which perversion of justice is mentioned in the Old Testament suggests that it was a common occurrence. Judges apparently had a reputation for corruption, despite strong recommendations to impartiality, especially with regard to the helpless (Deut 10:18; 14:29; 16:11, 14; 24:17–21; 26:12–13), whose rights were to be protected (Exod 22:21–24; Deut 10:18; Ps 68:5; Isa 1:17; Jer 22:3; Job 22:9; 24:3, 21).[54] Among the prophets, their activities are heavily criticised (Amos 2:6–7; 5:10–13), whereas doing justice for widows becomes shorthand for covenantal loyalty (Mal 3:5; Isa 1:17, 23; 10:2; Jer 5:28 LXX; 7:6; 22:3; Ezek 22:7; Ps 93:6).[55] There is evidence to suggest that the judges in Jerusalem in New Testament times were known for their corruption.[56] In a shame/honour culture, being impervious to shame is a devastating criticism.

The other protagonist is then introduced in a parallel manner, and is a widow.[57] Throughout the Old and New Testament, the widow is a symbol of powerlessness. Widows were in fact victims of exploitation, oppression and injustice (see Isa 1:16–17; Ps 94:1–7; Job 22:9–11; Luke 20:46–47). They were "endemically vulnerable" in any patriarchal, agriculturally based economy; they had no standing in the community.[58] So this choice of character heightens pressure on the judge.[59] In that culture women married young, and so we should not automatically think of the woman as aged and infirm. In fact, as the parable progresses, she seems quite energetic, feisty even.[60] She repeatedly approaches the judge and, in language appropriate to official court proceedings, says: "I want justice from you against my enemy!" The term "justice" or "vindication" occurs four times and links the parable with its applications. It can apply to the punishment of an offender or to the securing of a person's rights, which is the case here.[61] In that cultural context, a widow would not normally claim her rights by appearing constantly and alone in a public court and raising an outcry. This is the shock element of the story.[62] She probably lacked male members of the extended family or influential friends to plead for her and protect her; she was unwilling to resort to bribery, which was a frequent occurrence.[63] She can rely only on herself. The story assumes that she is in the right. As readers, we tend to think the same!

The Greek suggests that the adversary is a male, possibly an in-law, or her son or stepson by her husband's previous marriage. In all probability, the issue is a dispute over an inheritance or dowry—the portion that remained to her after her husband's death, or the withholding of a debt or pledge. The harsh reality is that a life of hardship and poverty would await her if she fails in her quest for justice.[64]

The judge is unmoved by her pleading and for some considerable time refuses to act.[65] Perhaps, through laziness or lack of care he is simply unwilling to help. Perhaps he prefers to favour her adversary because he is more influential or has had recourse to bribery.[66] In the end, however, he does decide to accede to her request. He provides the reason for the change of heart in his brief soliloquy (a typically Lukan feature). He acknowledges the description of himself with which the story commenced: "Though I have no fear of God and no respect for anyone." Nevertheless, he is now willing to give the widow her just rights. His reason is twofold and humorous. The woman is a nuisance; she keeps pestering or bothering him.[67] And secondly, "so that she may not wear me out by continually coming." Actually, the verb here is more graphic than this translation, and more amusing. It is taken from the boxing world, and means "strike a blow below the eye" or "give a black eye." Some commentators doubt whether the judge really fears physical violence; that would not be countenanced in that cultural milieu, and any such attempt would result in her exclusion from the court, never to return.[68] A metaphorical interpretation is sometimes suggested: blacken his character, give him a bad name. But this hardly accords with his self-confessed disregard for the views of others! Johnson refers to delicious ambiguity—a literal sock in the eye, or damaged reputation.[69] "A complacent and fearless judge is pummelled like a faltering boxer by a woman fighting for her rights."[70] The notion of violence is introduced by the judge; the widow has not acted violently. Perhaps he is just wearying of her nagging and fuss and wants peace, and also feels threatened.

There is both humour and shock in this situation.[71] Normal expectations are turned upside-down, as happens so often in the parables of Jesus, for such reversal is the nature of the Kingdom. Contrary to popular expectation, the widow proves to be anything but powerless and vulnerable. Rather, she shatters stereotype by persistently confronting the judge, even in a manner appropriate to the boxing ring, and finally gets her way. He opts for expediency, not justice.[72]

Many scholars hold that the original parable ends at this point.[73] It could be understood as a call to persevering effort or even boldness, not least in the face of difficult and seemingly hopeless situations. It serves as an exhortation to overcome discouragement and disillusionment when results are slow in materialising. This could also apply to prayer, and the introductory verse indicates this as Luke's view. Again, *a fortiori* logic obtains: "If persistence prevails with one who cares only for his own peace and comfort, how much more will it prevail with One who has compassion on his elect."[74] Unlike the reluctant judge, God is willing to help, and quickly.

An alternative approach suggests that the view that the judge is like God (the *a fortiori* argument) is flawed. "It is the widow who is cast in the image of God and who is presented to the disciples as a figure to emulate."[75] It is God-like to resist, name, denounce injustice until right is achieved. God's power is shown in weakness.[76]

Applications (6–8)

The indication of a switch from parable to application is clear: "And the Lord said ..." Whereas the introductory verse laid emphasis on the widow's role ("to pray always and not lose heart"), now attention is focused on the words of the judge ("listen to what the unjust judge says"). Only here is the judge explicitly called unjust.

The application then takes the form of two questions (v. 7) and an answer (v. 8a):

> And will not God grant justice to his chosen ones who cry to him day and night? Will he delay long in helping them? I tell you, he will quickly grant justice to them.

This verse is difficult to translate. Carroll uses a different form but still with two questions. The first expects a strongly affirmative answer, the second a negative reply. "But God *will* effect justice for his chosen ones who are crying out to him day and night, won't he? And is he delaying [in doing so] for them? I tell you he will swiftly effect justice for them."[77]

Both protagonists of the parable feature in this interpretation, which is allegorical: now the judge clearly represents God, and the widow becomes the figure of God's elect, or the Christian community. The situation envisaged is the delay in the coming of the parousia, the injustices perpetrated against the elect, and their eschatological vindication. The elect, a term used only here by Luke, "are those who are specially called to serve God through suffering for the faith at the hands of an ungodly world. Their loyalty to God makes them pray day and night to him for that deliverance which only he can bring." [78] Jesus' word is reassuring; their prayers will certainly be answered. God can be trusted and relied upon. His saving intervention will not be long delayed.[79]

The final sentence (v. 8b) raises the issue whether the Son of Man will find faith on earth when he comes. The switch is rather abrupt, and many commentators hold that this question, with its "tentative, troubled character",[80] is an addition from a different context, probably made by Luke, who realises that the expected parousia is delayed and adapts the parable to the situation of his community, which is undergoing tribulation. It is his reinterpretation of eschatology.[81] The emphasis moves from God's vindication to believers and the challenge to their faith, which can occur when God seems to delay in responding to their requests and needs. The question perhaps reflects anxiety about the quality of faith within the community of believers.[82] Carroll captures the intensity of the human drama: in moments "when history deals unrelenting, unjust suffering and when God has seemed distant and silent, why go on believing in God? This is the challenge to persevering faith that Jesus' parable invites readers to consider."[83]

Reflections

The text that we have been considering is difficult. Taking the parable as Jesus told it, without the Lukan framework, its meaning is not self-evident. There are, however, some lessons for us to reflect on. It is difficult to like the judge. Someone who is so self-contained, and who doesn't care what God or human beings think about him, displays a level of arrogance, independence and self-centredness that is deeply disturbing. In many areas of our contemporary human experience, we come across this kind of thing, perhaps not so blatant, but no less real—in politics, business, the media, academia, even the Church. There can be hardness, intolerance, lack of compassion, abuse of power. In finally acceding to the widow's request, the judge is concerned with his own well-being, not hers. That can be the case, too, in many areas of our life experience, where expediency and self-interest prove to be key factors in decision making. Perhaps we may detect traces of this in ourselves and, at times, in our dealing with others, especially if they are the pestering type. Another point may be to avoid putting off necessary encounters, running away from real listening, hesitating long before eventually responding. In most cases this simply exacerbates the situation.

It is probably true that we feel sympathy for the widow in the story. She certainly baulks the stereotype. We can admire her courage, determination, sticking power, and can learn from this as we face difficult or seemingly hopeless situations in our own lives. In a world where we expect instant coffee, same-day delivery, immediate response, on the spot electronic access, we find it hard to cope with delays. Being obliged to wait causes us discomfort, impatience, even anger, and we can easily give up.[84] The parable challenges this and urges us to persevere, whatever the odds. Levine's suggestion that the widow is looking for vengeance rather than justice, I find disturbing.[85] Perhaps there is a very thin line between justice and punishment or vengeance. Perhaps our passion for justice can sometimes turn sour. The claims culture has introduced a new area of conflict, potential dishonesty and bad feeling. Jesus speaks of turning the other cheek, of forgiveness and reconciliation. That is certainly something to pray for without ceasing, since it is very countercultural and against the grain.

Given that we are considering Luke's presentation of the theme of prayer, we need to take on board his message, as he reminds us of the need to "pray always and not lose heart." We have all prayed, and prayed earnestly, when faced with difficult situations, whether they be personal, family, social, work-related, be they concerned with health, job, relationships … Sometimes we can acknowledge that our prayers have been answered. At other times, we may feel that God is not listening. One factor to bear in mind is that we may be praying for the wrong thing; perhaps there is selfishness or ambition or pride in our prayers. Also, it is necessary that, like Jesus, we remain open to the possibility that what we want may not be in keeping with God's will. It could be that God, in care and love, knows that the outcome we long for may be detrimental to our well-being in the long run. God's ways are not always our ways; God's time is not always our time. It remains true, however, that delay can cause us to question God's love, and it is then that we need to ask ourselves about our trust and confidence in the God of Jesus.

On a different level, and on a wider stage, Luke's message raises another challenge. Each day we pray sincerely to the Father for the coming of the Kingdom. We genuinely long for a heart, a family, a community, a country, a world which reflects the values of Jesus, a "place" where the love of God reigns. Yet, as we reflect on our own condition and experience, or as we watch the TV and read the newspapers each day, we encounter selfishness, ambition, greed, compromise. There are tales of brutality and oppression, war and violence on a massive scale, terrorism, racism, genocide, real hatred and prejudice, crushing injustice. The presence of the Kingdom of God is far from evident. The widow in the parable invites us to resist these evils, though without the violence she may seem to threaten! We are called to action.[86] And Luke, as he and his community struggled to come to terms with the delay in the expected parousia, exhorts us to pray day and night without ceasing for justice, change and transformation. The danger is that we give up hope and give up prayer. And Jesus' question "Will you persist in faith?" is addressed to us.

The Parable of The Pharisee and The Publican (18:9–14)

The prayer theme continues with a further parable, again found only in Luke. Once more there are two protagonists, but this time both are male. The immediate context remains the travel narrative, but the parable forms part of Luke's wider interest in exploring the issue of fitness for entry into the Kingdom.[87] It reads as follows:

> He also told this parable to some who trusted in themselves that they were righteous and regarded others with contempt: "Two men went up to the temple to pray, one a Pharisee and the other a tax-collector. The Pharisee, standing by himself, was praying thus, 'God, I thank you that I am not like other people: thieves, rogues, adulterers, or even like this tax-collector. I fast twice a week; I give a tenth of all my income.' But the tax-collector, standing far off, would not even look up to heaven, but was beating his breast and saying, 'God, be merciful to me, a sinner!' I tell you, this man went down to his home justified rather than the other; for all who exalt themselves will be humbled, but all who humble themselves will be exalted."

Again, the basic structure of the parable is straightforward: there is an opening verse, the parable proper and a brief application. The introduction and the concluding application form a Lukan frame for the parable itself.[88]

The connective *de kai,* translated here as "also", links the parable with the theme of prayer in the previous parable; it is a familiar Lukan introduction (5:36; 12:16; 14:7). This introductory verse was probably added by Luke himself, or taken over from his source.[89] The topic of the parable is not stated directly, as in the previous story (18:1); it is indicated indirectly through the naming of those who are addressed: "some people who prided themselves on being righteous, and despised everyone else." The meaning of righteousness is explored through a description of two men at prayer. Righteousness is an aspect of other parables too.[90] In the Old Testament, righteousness is shown through faithfulness to the covenant; in the New it stems from faith in Christ, which is a gift from God (Rom 3:1–26).

Some scholars take the view that the parable is addressed to the Pharisees and lawyers (or scribes).[91] Others consider this identification too facile, and maintain that the disciples, who are the audience of the previous story, may well be included.[92] There are two issues: these people were self-confident, convinced of their uprightness, their "living in accordance with the requirements of the covenant";[93] and they despised and dismissed others, the rest of humankind. This topic is paired with that of acceptable prayer. "Jesus uses prayer to speak to the issue of what sort of people, with what sort of character and commitments as well as behaviours, are fit for the kingdom of God."[94] There are instances in the Gospel story where the Pharisees behave like this, but the disciples, too, manifest this proclivity.[95] Luke does not wish to condemn a particular group; he wishes to highlight dispositions, views, attitudes that are not in keeping with the values and style of the Kingdom.[96] The issue is relying on oneself for salvation rather than on the mercy of God.[97]

Once again, Jesus exploits the potential of contrast or polarisation in order to make his point; he also employs a touch of exaggeration and caricature. The two men, a Pharisee and a tax collector, come from the opposite ends of the religious spectrum; they are contrasted also in position and body posture, in the content of their prayers, in their basic attitudes and in their dramatically different way of life.[98] The story unfolds in the temple, a favourite Lukan setting, where both have "gone up" in order to pray.[99] The temple is a significant aspect of the story.[100] Public prayer took place there twice a day, in the morning at dawn and at 3 in the afternoon; private prayer could take place at any time. It is highly probable that they go for corporate worship; they offer their private prayer at the appropriate time within the context of the public daily atonement ritual.[101]

Pharisees were known to keep the commandments and follow meticulously the observances of ritual purity; they paid tithes and they were pillars of the temple. They were admired and respected for their exemplary piety, their religious fervour.[102] Mention of a tax collector present in the temple would come as a shock for the original hearers of the story. Tax gathering was a proscribed occupation. Its exponents lived on the verge of excommunication, for they were deemed to be ritually impure because of their contact with gentiles; they were considered to be dishonest, swindlers and extortioners, and, naturally, they were unpopular in a country that was suffering oppression and economic exploitation through widespread taxation, and were thought to be traitors to the nation.[103] The *telōnes* did not collect land taxes for the empire; they were a lower class employee who worked at the gates of cities like Capernaum and in collection booths along the commercial highways, charging tolls and taxes for the importing and exporting of merchandise. They were judged to be unredeemable.[104]

So far in the narrative, Pharisees and tax collectors have featured several times. The former have shown opposition to Jesus, resisting his acceptance of sinners, criticising him for his interpretations of the Law and have been inclined to justify themselves.[105] Luke's depiction of them tends to be rather negative and uncomplimentary.[106] The tax collectors, on the other hand, have been portrayed as being open to Jesus and have responded to him quite positively. Inevitably, as readers we are somewhat conditioned by this in our expectations of the parable, whereas for the original Jewish hearers of the story this would not have been the case.

The Pharisee adopts a standing posture for prayer and prays aloud, as was the custom. He chooses to stand by himself, away from the others present for prayer.[107] In the context of public worship, he steps apart from the other worshippers, probably to avoid incurring uncleanness. This is a gesture of superiority.[108] He utters a prayer which can be heard by all, almost giving a sermon during the liturgical pause.

Formal prayer usually consisted in thanksgiving to God for his gifts and petition for one's needs.[109] The Pharisee's prayer has, indeed, a twofold thrust: it is a prayer of thanksgiving to God for his having been preserved from sin, and an account of his piety. He thanks God first for what he is not: he is not into extortion and swindling nor adulterous, like everyone else.[110] The first two words are probably chosen with the tax collector in mind, whom he then explicitly, publicly and disparagingly singles out from among this despised mass of wrongdoers for special attention as an apposite illustration.[111]

This type of prayer would not have shocked the original hearers of the parable, for such boasting is not entirely out of the ordinary. "It is an extension of the thanksgiving of Israel for its election by God from among the nations (Deut 26:18f), to cover the distinction within Israel between those who cared supremely for the divine law in its greatest possible application, and those who cared little or not at all."[112] Paul boasts of his piety and observance, and contrasts himself with others (Phil 3:4–6; Gal 1:14; 2:15), and there are similar examples in the Talmud and Qumran. "To thank God for election and to speak of one's devotion do not of themselves make a prayer hypocritical or self-congratulatory."[113]

The Pharisee then moves on to give an account of his fidelity, listing what he does positively, focusing on his own performance.[114] Structurally, this forms the centrepiece of the parable. He claims to fast twice a week. The only obligatory fast was for the Day of Atonement (*Yom Kippur*). There are references in the Old Testament to fasting on other occasions.[115] The Essenes and disciples of the Baptist used to fast (5:33–39). As well as observing the public fasts, some pious Jews and Pharisee circles also undertook private fasting twice a week (Monday and Thursday) on a voluntary basis (see 2:27; 5:33; Acts 13:2–3; 14:23). This Pharisee goes beyond what is legally required of him; his asceticism would have been considered admirable.[116]

Another important aspect of Jewish piety was the payment of tithes. The Pharisee states that he pays tithes not only on the grain, wine, oil and the firstborn of herd and flock, as prescribed in the Torah (Deut 14:22f; Luke 11:42 adds some herbs), but on everything that he gets. This meant that he avoided the danger of using materials which had not been properly tithed by others. Again, he exceeds the norm and would seem to be an exemplary model of faithfulness.[117]

In his praying, however, the focus is not on God but on himself and what he has achieved. All the verbs are in the first person, the "I"; he is at the centre, not God.[118] The other questionable aspect of his prayer is the gap that he arrogantly creates between himself and the rest of humankind, who are dubbed as adulterers, rapacious, unjust. He is so negative, judgemental and uncompassionate.

The spotlight now falls on the tax collector, whom we encounter as he really is rather than through the eyes of the Pharisee.[119] His approach to God is dramatically different and exhibits four features.[120] First, he too stands apart, at a distance from the Pharisee and the other pious worshippers. "He stands apart because he knows such is his proper place as an outsider."[121] He does not consider himself worthy to take his place alongside the other worshippers and be in God's presence. Perhaps he is afraid of the reaction of others to his presence.[122] Secondly, he does not dare to raise his eyes to heaven, let alone his hands in a posture of prayer.[123] Thirdly, he beats his breast. This is a gesture normally denoting extreme anguish and sorrow, and not usually made by men in that culture; here it is a sign of profound contrition (as in 23:48 after the death of Jesus). And fourthly, a further contrast, he offers a short, simple prayer: "God, be merciful to me, a sinner." He does not list his sins, nor compare himself with others. He does not promise God that he will change his way of life or make restitution for what he has stolen.[124] With great humility and trust, he acknowledges his sinfulness, his deep need for God's graciousness. "He shelters his 'me' in the mercy of God."[125] The verb used in his prayer (*hilasthēti moi*) is not that usually employed in requests for mercy (like that of the blind man later or the lepers in 17:13). It is the language of atonement[126] and fits the context of the atoning sacrifice well, as he longs for reconciliation.[127] Jesus' original hearers would not expect God to accept his prayer.

The parable concludes with a solemn and authoritative statement by Jesus, which would have shocked his audience and seemed outrageous:[128] "this man went home again justified; the other did not." Once again, a dramatic reversal has occurred. The two men "go down" from the temple together at the end of the service, but this time, in contrast with the opening of the parable, it is the tax collector who is mentioned first, ahead of the Pharisee. The verb "justified" is in the perfect passive, implying that it is God who justifies. This is the only use in the Gospels of the term "justified" applied to an individual. It becomes clear that justification is not the result of one's own activity, a reward for one's observance of the Law; it is the free gift of a merciful God.[129] God approves the prayer of the tax collector but not that of the Pharisee, indicating that what is required when approaching God is acknowledgement of our sinfulness and trust in God's compassion.[130]

Jesus would have surprised and shocked his self-righteous audience. The Kingdom that he speaks about, and which he is introducing, is a very different world. The God whom Jesus reveals is a different kind of God. Jesus' stance, with its emphasis on mercy rather than Law, threatens to undermine the religious system and spirituality of the temple.[131] "The social map of the time is being abandoned and the kingdom of God is no longer found in the temple. The holy is outside and the unholy inside."[132] What Jesus says in his parable is fully in keeping with the way we have seen him act as the Gospel story has unfolded, as people on the religious periphery are included at his table and in his new family.

Application (14b)

Luke adds a comment to the parable: "For everyone who raises himself up will be humbled, but anyone who humbles himself will be raised up." This statement is found *verbatim* in 14:11 after Jesus has been discussing places at table;

it appears also in Matthew 23:12. It is a kind of proverb or wisdom comment, an independent saying of Jesus, which was free-floating, used by the evangelists in different contexts to highlight the theme of divine reversal.[133] Structurally, this conclusion, which highlights the meaning of righteousness, balances the introduction to the parable, and underlines the saving action of God, the God of surprises.[134] On the other hand, Luke's appended saying can lead the reader to be judgemental about the Pharisee. Jesus is opposed to such judgementalism; the parable is aimed precisely at those with this propensity. The original hearers were aware that the tax collector could be justified, but would not have been happy with it.[135]

Reflections

As it stands, the opening of the passage invites us to examine ourselves and see if in some ways or on some occasions, we are numbered among those who are self-righteous. This is frequently a danger for religious people. Similarly, we need to ask whether we look down on others. Comparison and competition are always dangerous. It is so easy to find ourselves noting people's faults and weaknesses and commenting critically about them with subtle arrogance. It is easy to become adept at putting others down, which is often a way of coping with our own inadequacies. All this reflects the religious culture of achievement, the idea that we must win God's love and approval, we must gain salvation.

As the parable unfolds, we are invited to share the Pharisee's prayer of thanksgiving to God for God's many blessings. We are who we are, we have achieved in life what we have achieved through the gift of God, through the inspiration and support of other people, through fortunate and providential circumstances. We are called to compassion for those less fortunate, those who in different ways may have made a mess of their lives.

While we may not be cheats and swindlers and adulterers and traitors, as the tax collector was thought to be, there are probably areas of our living and relationships that leave something to be desired. We are sinful people; we are in need of forgiveness and reconciliation; we are in need of God's mercy. The parable invites us to take a leaf from the taxman's book and throw ourselves humbly and with deep trust on the mercy of God.

Although Jesus does not introduce this parable with the phrase "The Kingdom of God is like ...", as in other parables, Jesus is in fact describing the God of the

Kingdom and the attitudes required by those who wish to be part of his new family, Kingdom people. This God is a God of generous mercy, freely offered, a God who is accessible and inclusive. This God is not a God who rigidly keeps a tick list of our successes and failures, or who can be controlled by systems. The basic attitudes recommended in this new world are gratitude, recognition of our need or poverty of spirit, compassion towards others and humble trust in God. These attitudes will fashion our approach to prayer.

Notes

1   Mark 4:33–34: "With many such parables he spoke the word to them, as they were able to hear it; he did not speak to them except in parables, but he explained everything in private to his disciples." Charles H. Dodd, *The Parables of the Kingdom* (London: Collins, 1961 [1935]), 13, writes: "The parables are perhaps the most characteristic element in the teaching of Jesus Christ as recorded in the Gospels. They have upon them, taken as a whole, the stamp of a highly individual mind, in spite of the re-handling they have inevitably suffered in the course of transmission. Their appeal to the imagination fixed them in the memory, and gave them a secure place in the tradition. Certainly, there is no part of the Gospel record which has for the reader a clearer ring of authenticity. But the interpretation of the parables is another matter..." As Meier, *A Marginal Jew*, 5:49, points out, however, though parables were an important and major part of his teaching, they were not the only type of teaching method and discourse which Jesus used. Donahue, *Gospel*, 1–2, notes the rich imagery of biblical literature, a tradition to which Jesus is heir. His speech reveals the characteristic devices of Hebrew poetry; this is particularly true of his parables.

2   Levine, *Stories*, 5–7; Meier, *A Marginal Jew*, 5:48. Levine notes that rabbinic parables usually began: "I will tell you a parable. To what can the thing be compared." Jesus, of course, often began: "The kingdom of heaven is like ..."

3   Meier, *A Marginal Jew*, 5:33. Denis McBride, *The Parables of Jesus* (Chawton: Redemptorist Publications, 1999), 22–28, stresses that Parables are challenges to change, ways of indirectly confronting people, invitations to think differently. Sometimes they are subversive.

4   Meier, *A Marginal Jew*, 5:81, n. 68, agrees with this view; also, p. 34.

5   Dodd, *Parables*, 16. Meier, *A Marginal Jew*, 5:35–40, notes that there is a lack of consensus among scholars concerning the number of Jesus' parables and what constitutes a parable. Part of the problem stems from the unclear etymology of the Hebrew term (*māshāl*) normally translated as parable, and the wide range of meanings it can have. The parables of Jesus are not aphorisms or proverbs, but mini narratives ("stretched out" similes or metaphors) with at least an implicit plotline. See also Donahue, *Gospel*, 5.

Meier, *A Marginal Jew,* 5:41 states: "Developing the narrative *māshāl* out of the traditions seen in the Former and Latter Prophets, Jesus the prophet told striking short stories that employed figurative language meant to be puzzling enough to tease the mind into active thought and personal decision—all within the larger context of prophetic conflict with the ruling class at a critical moment in Israel's history."

6   Levine, *Stories,* 17.

7   Donahue, *Gospel,* 3. Situation, tone, bodily expressions are lost to us. Jesus originally spoke Aramaic and probably some Hebrew and some business Greek (see Lohfink, *Jesus of Nazareth,* 100; Meier, *A Marginal Jew,* 1: 255–268); the parables come down to us in a Greek text and then in an English translation. Altered in transmission, the text we have is a reconstructed one.

8   Levine, *Stories,* 2, comments: "This surplus of meaning is how poetry and storytelling work." Also p. 7. Meier, *A Marginal Jew,* 5:32–33, and Donahue, *Gospel,* 12, 17, highlight the openness of parables to multiple meanings and a wide variety of interpretations.

9   Sometimes their interpretations are not in keeping with the thrust of the parable (e.g., Luke's addition about repentance to the shepherd parable), but are a distortion. Given that the Gospel parables are two stages removed from Jesus' original words, we want to find out how Jesus' original hearers understood them. Jan Lambrecht, *Once More Astonished: The Parables of Jesus* (New York: Crossroad, 1981), 12–14, detects four stages: Jesus; the oral preaching (sometimes in another language and spoken to another culture); then written down and fairly standardised; incorporation into the Gospels.

10   Levine, *Stories,* 9, writes that "when the historical context goes missing or we get it wrong, the parables become open to problematic and sometimes abusive readings." On p. 20 she refers to "millennia of domestication".

11   It is the view of Meier, *A Marginal Jew,* 5: 40–41, that the analogue for the narrative parables of Jesus is not to be found in the Old Testament wisdom literature but the prophetic books, the "Former prophets" in Samuel-Kings, and the later writing prophets. Jesus should be described in terms of the prophet rather than the sage. This does not mean that Jesus did not engage in debates over the Law or make wisdom statements. His use of narrative parables fits in with his being an eschatological prophet.

12   Levine, *Stories,* 19. Barbara E. Reid, *Parables for Preachers: Year C* (Collegeville, MN: The Liturgical Press, 2000), 13, describes this as retrieving what the story means in its original telling, and then re-effecting such a dynamic in the contemporary context.

13   Levine, *Stories,* 21–25, suggests several reasons for this: parables function as children's stories; clergy don't take the time to develop the challenge of the parable, preferring to play safe; folk see the sermon as entertainment; clergy present anti-Jewish stereotypes, contrasting Jesus and "the Jews" in an ill-informed manner; sacrificing Jesus' context and voice to our own; the allure of newer approaches that don't respect historical considerations. Detached from their original setting, parables can become more anti-Jewish.

14   Levine, *Stories,* 12.

15   Levine, *Stories,* 4–15, writes: "What is infectiously appealing about Jesus is that he likes to celebrate. He is consistently meeting people not at the altar but at table ... He

is indiscriminate in his dining companions ... In his dining, Jesus is providing a foretaste of the messianic age."

16   Donahue, *Gospel*, 11. Reid, *Parables*, 11, states that the power of Jesus' preaching came from his very life being a parable.

17   Donahue, *Gospel*, 14. Meier, *a Marginal Jew*, 5:42, warns that some parables go beyond "everyday events".

18   This is characteristic of Luke and 'Q' (11:11; 12:25; 14:28; 15:4; 17:7). Marshall, *Luke*, 463–464, maintains that there are no contemporary parallels to this formula, which suggests that it originates with Jesus. Johnson, *Luke*, 179, refers to Luke's capacity vividly to evoke with a minimum of words the circumstances of real life and social relationships; and Evans, *Luke*, 484, calls it a "vignette of Palestinian village life." Bailey, *Through Peasant Eyes*, 119, notes that the opening question demands an emphatic negative answer. No one could imagine a person refusing such a request.

19   Carroll, *Luke*, 447, n. 40, supports the would-be host interpretation; also, Marshall, *Luke*, 464; Bailey, *Through Peasant Eyes*, 125.

20   Marshall, *Luke*, 464, maintains that such a late arrival was not uncommon because people tended to travel late to avoid the heat. However, Bailey, *Through Peasant Eyes*, 121, disputes this with regard to Palestine and Lebanon because the altitude is higher and there is often a breeze; a midnight arrival would, in his view, be unusual.

21   As Byrne, *Hospitality*, 105, points out, there are three friends in the story. For him, the host is the main character (the "you"). McBride, *Luke*, 148, refers to "letter-box diplomacy". Green, *Luke*, 447, notes that bread is baked and consumed daily, so its dearth is not unusual; three is the appropriate number of loaves for an evening meal. Bailey, *Through Peasant Eyes*, 122, maintains that Middle Eastern peasants do not bake each day; a supply could last a week. Since the women helped one another, it would be known who had baked that day. A guest had to be offered an unbroken loaf. This was probably more than he could eat.

22   Bailey, *Through Peasant Eyes*, 122. Carroll, *Luke*, 251, refers to "pivotal values and practices" of the social world of Jesus (friendship, hospitality, honour and shame).

23   Bailey, *Through Peasant Eyes*, 123, notes the custom of doing the rounds of the village to provide other items necessary for the meal.

24   See Caird, *Luke*, 152; Bailey, *Through Peasant Eyes*, 124.

25   Green, *Luke*, 448, notes that for Jesus the demands of friendship would normally be enough to evoke a response; the threat of dishonour would lead to the same outcome.

26   For a thorough discussion of this, see Bailey, *Through Peasant Eyes*, 125–129, who highlights the history of the spread of the "persistence" translation. He maintains that "persistence" is the message of the parable in chapter 18, but not here. There is no "persistence" element in the story; it is found in the poem that follows.

27   This is the view of the translators of the text used here. Johnson, *Luke*, 178, refers to the *aneideia* shown by the effrontery of making a demand in the middle of the night, and refusing to take "no" for an answer. Byrne, *Hospitality*, 106, n. 14, notes that there is no word connoting "persistence" in the text; the persistence idea is imported from a parallel parable, the unjust judge and the widow (18:1–8). He prefers to stay

with the application of "shame" to the householder. On the other hand, the "his" in the text more naturally refers to the one who knocks. So, there are problems with either interpretation. Green, *Luke*, 445, n. 37, emphasises the absence of the concept of "persistence" in the actions of the would-be host. Rather than persistence, the issue is honour and shame in the community.

28   Bailey, *Through Peasant Eyes*, 128.

29   Carroll, *Luke*, 252; he refers to the primary importance of hospitality; the desire to maintain honour by being generous to a neighbour, despite the inconvenience.

30   Byrne, *Hospitality*, 106, sees him as the typical "rogue", forced to do the right thing against his personal interest.

31   McBride, *Luke*, 147. See also Byrne, *Hospitality*, 106; Marshall, *Luke*, 465. Bailey, *Through Peasant Eyes*, 119, 133, holds that the parable teaches that God is a God of honour and that man can have complete assurance that his prayer will be heard. Chrupcala, *The Salvation of God*, 220, suggests that the petitioner's perseverance would be unfounded, if it had not been accompanied by trust in the friendship and paternity of God who is always ready to grant the requests of his children.

32   Marshall, *Luke*, 466, sees it as composed of two units. Bailey, *Through Peasant Eyes*, 134–135, calls it a parable/poem; a poem on the Father's gifts, consisting of three stanzas, the first and third in step parallelism (a pattern of three items, with a movement from second to third person), the centre stanza being a parable with three double images.

33   Bailey, *Through Peasant Eyes*, 119, n. 2, notes that the parable is followed by a related yet distinct piece of tradition which may have had no original relationship to it; it was not part of the earlier parable. Nor was it intended as a commentary on the first. The imagery and emphasis are different.

34   Carroll, *Luke*, 252, refers to "assertive petition". Evans, *Luke*, 485, links seeking with Rom 10:20 (Isa 65:1), and sees the door as a figure of entry into the Kingdom.

35   Bailey, *Through Peasant Eyes*, 135, sees "everyone" as an appeal to outcasts who have not prayed, and a defence of the universality of the Gospel (challenging the Pharisees).

36   This sequence is found earlier in 10:19: "I have given you power to tread down serpents and scorpions and the whole strength of the enemy; nothing shall ever hurt you." Matthew has requests for bread and fish, with offers of a stone and a snake (7:9–10). Some Lukan manuscripts include the bread/stone image, which would make a triple form, as in the previous verses. Bailey, *Through Peasant Eyes*, 136–137, discusses this, and believes that originally there were indeed three elements.

37   Evans, *Luke*, 487. Johnson, *Luke*, 178, prefers the translation "your Father will give you the Holy Spirit from heaven"; similarly, Evans, *Luke*, 487, who comments that this would stress the heavenly origin of the gifts of the divine Father compared with the earthly gifts of earthly fathers.

38   Green, *Luke*, 450, observes that this promise carries Luke's audience beyond the Gospel into Acts. Evans, *Luke*, 487, notes that in Acts this gift is the characteristic possession of the Christian, and is given in answer to prayer.

39   McBride, *Luke*, 149.

40   Evans, *Luke*, 484; Carroll, *Luke*, 252.

41   Bailey, *Through Peasant Eyes*, 129. Green, *Luke*, 627, sees 17:20–18:8 as one unit, entitled "Faithfulness at the Coming of the Son of Man."

42   Johnson, *Luke*, 273. Caird too, *Luke*, 201, believes that the two parables contribute to our understanding of the final paragraph of 'Q'. Byrne, *Hospitality*, 142, sees the two parables and the next episode (Jesus blessing the children) as referring to the appropriate way disciples should pray during this time of waiting for the full arrival of the Kingdom. Similarly, Green, *Luke*, 638. Reid, *Parables*, 227, refers to 17:11–19:44 as the eschatological section of Luke's Gospel; McBride, *Parables*, 169, sees the eschatological discourse as running from 17:20–18:34. Carroll, *Luke*, 637, comments that its narrative location provides this unit with decidedly eschatological edge, an emphasis which comes explicitly to the fore in vv 7–8.

43   Bailey, *Through Peasant Eyes*, 127, notes that the deceptively simple story hides a complex series of theological themes and interpretive problems.

44   Donahue, *Gospel*, 180; Fitzmyer, *Luke*, 2:1176. Green, *Luke*, 638; McBride, *Parables*, 171; and Bailey, *Through Peasant Eyes*, 127, consider Sirach 35:15–19 its prototype; some of this material is used, some transformed, some omitted; the similarities are hardly accidental. Evans too, *Luke*, 636, sees this as a possibility.

45   Donahue, *Gospel*, 181, notes how this parable offers an excellent example of a text that reflects the three levels of the Synoptic tradition: Jesus, the early church, the evangelist and the progressive reinterpretation of tradition. Reid, *Parables*, 228, refers to "layers of interpretation". The original parable runs from 2–5. Verses 1 and 6–8 are secondary additions reflecting early Christian attempts to understand the story. See Levine, *Stories*, 244–245: "Whether we take the verses surrounding Luke 18:2–5 as from Jesus, the early tradition, Luke's special source, or the hand of the evangelist, the core text is a proper parable." Evans, *Luke*, 637, comments that the element of the "grotesque" in the parable indicates the mind and parabolic method of Jesus.

46   Reid, *Parables*, 228, Luke alone uses *legein* when introducing a parable. Prayer is a favourite theme of his. The use of "the Lord" in v. 6 is a sign of a later interpretation, being a post-resurrection insight. Verse 7 relates to the situation of the Lukan community. Marshall, *Luke*, 671, believes that v. 1 shows features of Luke's style, and has at least been edited by him. McBride, *Parables*, 170, sees this verse as Luke's own construction, relating the parable to the previous discussion.

47   See 2 Thess 3:13; Eph 3:13; Gal 6:9; 2 Cor 4:1,16.

48   Donahue, *Gospel*, 180.

49   Bailey, *Through Peasant Eyes*, 130.

50   Marshall, *Luke*, 672; Bailey, *Through Peasant Eyes*, 133.

51   McBride, *Luke*, 231; Joaquim Jeremias, *The Parables of Jesus*, trans. S. H. Hooke (London: SCM, 1963), 153.

52   McBride, *Parables*, 172.

53   Green, *Luke*, 639, notes the ambiguity: the judge may appear as he ought: unbiased, objective, neutral. Yet in the Roman and Lukan world, the phrase suggests "thorough wickedness".

54   Caird, *Luke*, 201. Deut 27:19 states: "Cursed be he who prevents the justice due to the sojourner, the fatherless, the widow." Resseguie, *Spiritual Landscape*, 58, believes

that his attitude exemplifies a corrupt judicial system that exploits rather than protects the disenfranchised.

55   Johnson, *Luke*, 269.

56   Bailey, *Through Peasant Eyes*, 131.

57   Reid, *Parables*, 232, n. 14, observes that in the New Testament, Luke has most stories about widows; this probably reflects their growing prominence in ministry in the early Church.

58   Green, *Luke*, 640. Levine, *Stories*, 239–240, lists biblical widows who "defy the convention of the poor and dependent woman." She maintains that Luke's introductory verse domesticates her; this undermines the challenge of the parable.

59   Johnson, *Luke*, 269; Donahue, *Gospel*, 182. Reid, *Parables*, 232, notes that according to Deut 27:9; Isa 10:2, anyone violating the rights of a widow was cursed.

60   Resseguie, *Spiritual Landscape*, 59, notes that her speech is confrontational, she offers no respectful title, "and refuses to coat her language in treacle." Tannehill, *Luke*, 263, refers to her as bold and brash.

61   Evans, *Luke*, 635, translates *ekdiken* as "to secure a favourable verdict at law for"; Wright, *Luke*, 212, is similar. Levine, *Stories*, 242–243, prefers the vindication/vengeance connotation. Does the widow want money, access to property, or vengeance and punishment for her opponent? Bailey, *Through Peasant Eyes*, 133, maintains that she is looking for justice and protection, not vengeance. Marshall, *Luke*, 672, what the widow wants is not the punishment of her opponent but the payment of whatever is due to her.

62   Donahue, *Gospel*, 182.

63   Green, *Luke*, 640; Bailey, *Through Peasant Eyes*, 133.

64   Donahue, *Gospel*, 182; Reid, *Parables*, 232. Levine, *Stories*, 248, while not wishing to dismiss real concern for poor widows, does question the stereotype. "Not all widows are poor, without agency, and completely dependent on the good will of others." The parable gives no indication of the widow's economic status. On p. 250, she writes: "The widow might well be destitute, oppressed and desperate. She may also be wealthy, powerful and vengeful. Or she may be somewhere in between." McBride, *Parables*, 174, maintains that the parable assumes that that either the adversary is influential or that he has paid off the judge with bribes.

65   Fitzmyer, *Luke*, 2:1179 suggests "for a long time" rather than "for a while" as the translation of *epi chronon*.

66   Levine, *Stories*, 252–253, maintains that the judge's lack of "respect" for others could indicate a refusal to defer to a person of higher status; the parable says nothing about bribery. However, first century auditors would have seen him as a negative figure, and a good match for the widow.

67   Resseguie, *Spiritual Landscape*, 59, notes that the judge's soliloquy is a reluctant tribute to her wearisome persistence. The verb translated "bother" literally means "give me work". I disagree with Reid's assertion, *Parables*, 233, n. 16, that these two verbs (bother and pester) have an overtone which is sexist. Green, *Luke*, 640, n. 92, maintains that "bother" is weak; it suggests neither the duress the judge was under nor the level of the widow's shocking behaviour had reached in the judge's view. He prefers "badgered".

68   Bailey, *Through Peasant Eyes*, 136. He prefers "lest she give me a headache." The

judge exaggerates as an indication of the extent to which her persistence has irritated him.

69   Johnson, *Luke*, 270. The verb (*hypōpiazein*) refers to a black eye, and the boxing ring. Byrne, *Hospitality*, 143, prefers the physical violence meaning to besmirching his reputation or wearing him out. Maybe a real incident was behind the story where a woman did throw punches! Tannehill, *Luke*, 264, feels it is not meant to be taken literally; he suggests "keeps battering me". Reid, *Parables*, 232, rejects a connotation which dilutes the irony which the literal meaning conveys, which is part of the intentional twist of the story. Green, *Luke*, 641, refers to a macho judge cornered and slugged by the least powerful in society.

70   Donahue, *Gospel*, 183.

71   Carroll, *Luke*, 356, notes that while this is humorous, it is the sort of serious humour that knows, and names, stark reality ... of oppression and injustice suffered by persons to whom the judicial, economic and political systems continually turn a cold, silent shoulder.

72   Levine, *Stories*, 254. She maintains that the widow wants vengeance; the judge is co-opted by and so complicit in the widow's schemes.

73   Byrne, *Hospitality*, 142, comments that the use of "Lord" does suggest that the story has come to an end, but without v.6, the point of the parable is not clear. The post-resurrection title "Lord" is a characteristic of Luke's style.

74   Caird, *Luke*, 201. Similarly, Byrne, *Hospitality*, 143: if the judge (even from base motives) grants her justice, how much more certainly and readily will God who is good; Bailey, *Through Peasant Eyes*, 137; Wright, *Luke*, 213; McBride, *Parables*, 176. Levine, *Stories*, 255, suggests that it is unlikely that the original audience would understand the widow's badgering as about prayer to God.

75   Reid, *Parables*, 234. She maintains that Luke has tamed this story of an unconventional woman and cast her in a docile and acceptable role as an example of praying always. His redaction of this parable, and the translations and interpretations of subsequent scholars have tamed and trivialised a powerful portrait of a godly widow persistently pursuing justice.

76   Levine, *Stories*, 262, considers this view anachronistic for Jesus and Luke. She maintains that this widow is not weak; widows in biblical narrative rarely are.

77   Carroll, *Luke*, 355. McBride, *Parables*, 170–171, notes that some scholars see vv. 6–8 as Jesus' interpretation, others as the interpretation of the early Church.

78   Caird, *Luke*, 201. Bailey, *Through Peasant Eyes*, 137–140, argues at length that the word translated "delay" (*makrothumeō*) really means "be slow to anger"; the phrase is a statement, not a question. God is slow to anger over his elect, who are sinners; God is long-suffering with them, willing to put off judgement. Johnson, *Luke*, 270, favours "show patience towards" the elect. Marshall, *Luke*, 674–675, rehearses all the arguments, and concludes in favour of "delay"; similarly, Carroll, *Luke*, 355; Green, *Luke*, 642, n. 99.

79   There is also discussion as to the best translation of *en tachei*. Some take it to mean "speedily" or "soon"; it will not be necessary to wait, like the widow. Others prefer "suddenly"; the idea being that God could delay for a long time, like the judge, and then act suddenly and decisively. Marshall, *Luke*, 676, prefers "soon". Donahue, *Gospel*, 181,

refers to "imminent eschatology" in vv. 7–8a; this is in tension with Luke's realisation of the delay in the parousia.

80   Johnson, *Luke*, 271.

81   Donahue, *Gospel*, 181. Reid, *Parables*, 230, sees this verse as a transplant from the discussions in chapter 17. There is no mention of faith in the parable. Similarly, Levine, *Stories*, 255. Bailey, *Through Peasant Eyes*, 137, notes that the saying could be a reflection of the evangelist or the Church or a separate saying of Jesus attached here by the evangelist or his source.

82   Bailey, *Through Peasant Eyes*, 137. On p. 140–141 he wonders whether 18:6–6, which has long been interpreted in the context of expectation of the parousia, could be understood as applying to the ministry of Jesus, as opposition intensifies on approach to Jerusalem. There is a promise that God will vindicate them; the resurrection is God's vindication of Jesus.

83   Carroll, *Luke*, 357. McBride, *Luke*, 232, notes that Jesus ends with a question: will his hearers follow the example of the persistent widow and continue in their prayer, or will they give up their life of faith as a lost cause?

84   McBride, *Parables*, 178–179.

85   Levine, *Stories*, 264–265. Carroll's translation of the text, *Luke*, 355, does not sound at all vindictive and vengeful: "Give me what is my just due from the one who has treated me unjustly."

86   Donahue, *Gospel*, 185–186: "Luke understands continual prayer not simply as passive waiting but as the active quest for justice." Green, *Luke*, 642, notes that "crying out to God must be correlated with the dogged pursuit of justice."

87   Green, *Luke*, 644: the parable is followed by the stories of Jesus and the children, the rich ruler, riches and rewards, the Passion prediction, Jesus and the blind man, and Zacchaeus. Reid, *Parables*, 237, notes that after this parable Luke returns to his Markan source for what follows; also, Evans, *Luke*, 641.

88   Reid, *Parables*, 237; Donahue, *Gospel*, 187; John D. Crossan, *In Parables: The Challenge of the Historical Jesus* (San Francisco: Harper & Row, 1973), 68–69; McBride, *Parables*, 181. Evans, *Luke*, 642, maintains that the first verse should read "because" rather than "that". Bailey, 143–144, considers it a seven-stanza parabolic ballad, using inverted parallelism.

89   Bailey, *Through Peasant Eyes*, 144. Levine, *Stories*, 186, suggests that Luke provides the literary context in which negative images of Pharisees drive the interpretation.

90   Reid, *Parables*, 238: the children in the market place (7:29–35), the good Samaritan (10:29–37), which is addressed to a scribe who seeks to justify himself, and the unjust steward (16:1–13), which is followed by a critique of the Pharisees.

91   Johnson, *Luke*, 271.

92   Green, *Luke*, 644. Carroll, *Luke*, 358, refers to "unspecified listeners assured of their own uprightness". Levine, *Stories*, 186, notes that the charge could fit any listener.

93   Byrne, *Hospitality*, 143. He notes that we should not conclude that the type of behaviour represented by the Pharisee in the story was typical of the Pharisees in general or of Judaism. It affects all religions. Levine, *Stories*, 187, notes that judging others is not particularly Jewish; it is a human trait. Jesus' disciples can be guilty in this regard.

McBride, *Parables*, 182, notes that the great Pharisee leader, Hillel, was aware of the danger of spiritual pride among his fellow Pharisees, and warned against it.

94   Green, *Luke*, 644.

95   For Pharisees, see 10:29; 11:37–44; 14:1–14; 15:1–2; 16:14–17; for disciples see 9:46–50.

96   Green, *Luke*, 646.

97   Bailey, *Through Peasant Eyes*, 144.

98   Carroll, *Luke*, 359; Green, *Luke*, 645.

99   Green, *Luke*, 646, notes that the temple is also a cultural centre, the place in Jewish society where the world is ordered through its layout of courts that segregate Jews and gentiles, men and women, priests and non-priests, clean and unclean. The social polarisation is concretised in the story. For a different appreciation of the temple and its role, see Levine, *Stories*, 194–198.

100   McBride, *Parables*, 182–185; it held a religious and cultic role, and functioned at a political level. Its construction in concentric rectangles reflected degrees of purity and access. As well as a centre of worship, the focus of God's presence, it served as a central bank and treasury, and was supported by taxes and tithes from the people. He sees the Pharisee as a dedicated supporter of the temple and its system, and the tax collector as a supporter of the Roman imperial system. See also Reid, *Parables*, 244–245.

101   Bailey, *Through Peasant Eyes*, 145; McBride, *Parables*, 187.

102   Reid, *Parables*, 239. See McBride, *Parables*, 185–189, for a full description. Evans, *Luke*, 642, quotes Josephus that they had the reputation "of excelling the rest of their nation in the observance of religion."

103   Donahue, *Gospel*, 187; Levine, *Stories*, 188, points out that tax collectors were thought to be corrupt, and unmerciful to others; they were often rich (19:2), well connected and ostentatious enough to host banquets (5:29).

104   Pagola, *Jesus*, 142; see McBride, *Parables*, 189–191.

105   Carroll, *Luke*, 360; Green, *Luke*, 647.

106   See Levine, *Stories*, 189–194; she highlights the difference between Luke's presentation and the views of most of Jesus' Jewish audience. She also points out that Pharisees were not temple based, nor did they run synagogues; they were respected teachers.

107   The Greek text (*pros heauton*) is problematic here. It could modify "pray", indicating that he prayed quietly to himself, rather than to God. (Johnson, *Luke*, 271, follows this interpretation.) Others have suggested "with himself", or "to himself". Or it could modify "stand", suggesting that he stood by himself, adopting a prominent position. For the discussion see Bailey, *Through Peasant Eyes*, 147–8; he gives seven reasons in favour of standing by himself. Green, *Luke*, 648, agrees; also, McBride, *Parables*, 187.

108   Bailey, *Through Peasant Eyes*, 149. Donahue, *Gospel*, 188, suggests that this was not uncommon among religious leaders at the time. Levine, *Stories*, 199, would see such views as an overstatement; she maintains that Pharisees were not obsessive concerning ritual purity.

109   Bailey, *Through Peasant Eyes*, 150.

110   Johnson, *Luke*, 271, notes that Pharisees have been criticised by Jesus for these

180

kinds of things (11:39, 42; 16:14–18). Green, *Luke*, 648, observes that the prayer does not thank God for God's acts, as it should, but his own acts. Bailey, *Through Peasant Eyes*, 148, points out the distinction between those who kept the details of the Law ("associates" or *haberim)* and the "people of the land", who were looked down upon.

111   Bailey, *Through Peasant Eyes*, 150–151. Evans, *Luke*, 643, comments that it is part of the artistry of the parable to bring contrasted figures together by having one refer to the other. Byrne, *Hospitality*, 144, says he moves to detach himself from the sinful mass of mankind. He bolsters his own self-image by putting down others. Life is a competition in virtue.

112   Evans, *Luke*, 643.

113   Donahue, *Gospel*, 188. Reid, *Parables*, 239–240, also gives examples of such prayers from the Talmud and the Tosephta, documents dating from after Jesus, but probably expressing values current in his day; similarly, McBride, *Parables*, 187–188. See also Ps 17:4–5 and Qumran (1 QH 7:34). Levine, *Stories*, 200–201, offers a different slant on these prayers, viewing them as expressions of genuine gratitude to God, rather than sanctimonious and hypocritical. For her, what is negative about the prayer of the Pharisee in the parable is its negative judgement of the tax collector.

114   McBride, *Luke*, 233.

115   Reid, *Parables*, 240, notes Ps 35:13; 2 Sam 1:12; 3:36; 12:13–25; 1 Kgs 21:27.

116   Evans, *Luke*, 643, quotes Tacitus and Suetonius about Jewish fasting. Levine, *Stories*, 203–204, notes that the dominant Jewish view was to enjoy the good world God provided. His fasting and tithing would be considered meritorious acts performed on behalf of and in solidarity with the rest of the covenant community.

117   Green, *Luke*, 648, says that this shows his conformity not only to Torah but also to the forms of Torah-interpretation specific to this Pharisee's community. Thomas Keating, *The Kingdom of God is like* ... (Slough: St Paul's, 1993), 22–23, maintains that the Pharisee only did what the temple map required of those who were considered insiders and members of the religious elite of the time. His conduct and prayers are typical of the devout Pharisee. Levine's take on tithing, *Stories*, 203, is that his prayer is a caricature, and would have brought a smile to Pharisee bystanders. McBride, *Parables*, 188, notes that there is no criticism of the Pharisee inside the parable, no indication that he is a hypocrite. The expectation of Jesus' hearers would be that the God of the temple would be favourable to him.

118   Caird, *Luke*, 202, notes that the verbs are all in the first person; his trust is in his righteousness and achievement; he despises those who don't reach his standard. Carroll too, *Luke*, 359, notes the five first person verbs; Donahue, *Gospel*, 189; McBride, *Luke*, 233.

119   For Bailey, *Through Peasant Eyes*, 152, this is the turning point of the ballad format.

120   Johnson, *Luke*, 272.

121   Keating, *The Kingdom of God*, 23.

122   Levine, *Stories*, 205, observes that ritual purity is not an issue here; one needed to be ritually pure to enter the Temple.

123   See 1 Enoch 13:5. On all this see Bailey, *Through Peasant Eyes*, 153.

124   McBride, *Parables*, 191. Byrne, *Hospitality*, 144, asks whether his sin is that he is trapped in an occupation he can't get out of. The parable leaves it open.

125   McBride, *Luke*, 233.

126   See Heb 2:17; as a noun Rom 3:25; Heb 9:5; 1 John 2:2; 4:10.

127   Bailey, 154. *Through Peasant Eyes*, Caird, *Luke*, 203, notes that he is focused on God; his only help can be from God.

128   McBride, *Parables*, 191.

129   Luke could well have been acquainted with Paul's teaching in some form, but the motif is also found in the Old Testament (Ps 51; 24:3–5).

130   Caird, *Luke*, 203.

131   Pagola, *Jesus*, 143; see also Carroll, *Luke*, 360. McBride, *Parables*, 192 links this with occasions in the Gospel where Jesus is critical of the temple (Mark 11:12–25).

132   Keating, *The Kingdom of God*, 23.

133   Reid, *Parables*, 238; Bailey, *Through Peasant Eyes*, 155; McBride, *Parables*, 181; Levine, *Stories*, 207. Byrne, *Hospitality*, 144, mentions reversal too. On p. 145 he comments that in many situations today God can cope with "disorder" in terms of objective morality or church discipline far better than those who guard the tradition imagine.

134   Carroll, *Luke*, 358, speaks of Jesus' assertion "of the table-upending activity of God that subverts conventional notions of status and honour". Crossan, *In Parables*, 69, speaks of the radical reversal of accepted human and religious judgement; God does not play the game by our rules.

135   Levine, *Stories*, 208. She goes on to note that *para* is usually translated as "rather than"; but it can also mean "because of" or "alongside". This could have been the original meaning, had Luke not added 14b. Possibly, by God's generosity, the tax collector has been able to tap into the collective repentance of the temple system and the good deeds of the Pharisee; both go home justified.

Chapter Seven
The Transfiguration

The story of the transfiguration of Jesus appears in each of the Synoptic Gospels and is referred to in 2 Peter. It is alluded to in the Gospel of John.[1] It is a powerful narrative, rich in symbolism, spirituality and theological meaning. And yet it is a neglected tradition in the Western Church and in modern biblical scholarship, whereas for centuries it has held a central place in the art, liturgy and theology of the Eastern Church.[2] On August 6th each year, the Catholic Church celebrates the transfiguration as a feast but not a solemnity; the Gospel reading for the second Sunday of Lent in each cycle is the story of the transfiguration.[3] Pope Saint John Paul II included it in his "luminous mysteries" of the rosary, thus giving it greater prominence in the reflection and prayer of the Church. In this chapter, I propose to examine and ponder Luke's version of the event, which reads as follows:

> Now about eight days after these sayings Jesus took with him Peter and John and James, and went up on the mountain to pray. And while he was praying, the appearance of his face changed, and his clothes became dazzling white. Suddenly they saw two men, Moses and Elijah, talking to him. They appeared in glory and were speaking of his departure, which he was about to accomplish at Jerusalem. Now Peter and his companions were weighed down with sleep; but since they had stayed awake, they saw his glory and the two men who stood with him. Just as they were leaving him, Peter said to Jesus, "Master, it is good for us to be here; let us make three dwellings, one for you, one for Moses, and one for Elijah"—not knowing what he said. While he was saying this, a cloud came and overshadowed them; and they were terrified as they entered the cloud. Then from the cloud came a voice that said, "This is my Son, my Chosen; listen to him!" When the voice had spoken, Jesus was found alone. And they kept silent and in those days told no one any of the things they had seen. (9:28–36)

Context usually provides the key for unlocking the meaning of a text. The story of the transfiguration of Jesus, as recounted by Luke, must be taken in conjunction with Peter's earlier declaration about Jesus' identity, which is followed by Jesus' prediction of his passion and vindication (9:18–22). The two episodes form a diptych. Luke's narrative is similar to that of Mark, which is probably his main source. Some scholars suggest that Luke may have had access to a second source, which would explain many of the variations.[4] Others believe that he has been creative in editing Mark to produce a version which is longer due to additional material, and which displays his own characteristic style and emphases.[5] The story has a hinge-like function, as it brings the Galilean ministry to a climax and launches the lengthy journey of Jesus to Jerusalem.

The opening sentence sets the scene, giving an indication of time and place, and the names of the participants.[6] The time reference, "about eight days after these sayings", provides a link with the preceding episode at Caesarea Philippi (though Luke neglects to name the place); the two events are closely related.[7] However, the wider context of the Gospel narrative recalls Herod's perplexity and his question, "Who is this about whom I hear such things?" and the various erroneous answers that people were putting forward (9:7–9). Jesus posed a similar question to his disciples concerning the popular view about his identity, before challenging them directly about their own opinion. To this Peter, as spokesman, responded: "You are the Christ of God" (9:18–20). This reply led to Jesus' words to his disciples about his own coming suffering and death, and their call to share that path; this he set against a background of ultimate vindication and glory.[8] These are the "sayings" referred to in the link sentence. But the issue of Jesus' identity still hangs in the air.

About a week later, Jesus takes three of the disciples, Peter, John and James, with him up the mountain; they are named in a slightly different order than usual.[9] Across the scriptures, mountains are places of prayer and of revelation, where the divine and the human meet. Elsewhere in this Gospel, mountains are oases where Jesus goes specifically to commune with the Father.[10] Luke does not name the mountain, nor does he suggest that it is particularly high; for him geographical and altitudinal concerns are not paramount.[11]

Jesus makes this trek because he wishes to pray, a purpose not rendered explicit in the Markan version and clearly a Lukan addition. In Luke's Gospel, there are a number of references to the prayer of Jesus, often prior to important events or turning points: Luke also provides us with a considerable amount of Jesus' teaching about prayer. It is a significant theme of his Gospel, as we have seen in Chapters Five and Six.

And it is while Jesus is praying on the mountain that a transformation occurs.[12] Luke, unlike Mark, does not use the term "transfiguration", which is the way this event is normally designated. The appearance of Jesus' face is changed, and his clothes become dazzling white, the hue of heavenly garments as described in apocalyptic literature.[13] It would seem that Jesus is caught up in the intimate presence and love of God, an intense mystical experience that totally transforms his being and his appearance in such a way that the three disciples catch a glimpse of a deeper dimension to his identity.[14]

At this point, Moses and Elijah appear on the scene, introduced with "behold", which suggests something extraordinary is happening.[15] As well as being great prophetic figures in Israel's past,[16] who had also experienced theophanies on mountains[17] and were thought to have been translated into heaven, both featured prominently in popular expectations connected with the coming of the Messiah and the end time.[18] Luke specifies that they are in the radiant state of heavenly glorification.[19]

Luke is also original in stating that they were speaking with Jesus about his "departure which he was to accomplish in Jerusalem."[20] The word used here in the Greek is *exodos*; its literal meaning is departure but figuratively and euphemistically it can also mean death; the Jerusalem location is made explicit. But the word obviously conjures up the Old Testament epic of the liberation of the Jewish people from Egyptian slavery under Moses, an event in which God's glory was revealed, and it suggests that the exodus of Jesus in Jerusalem, his "passing over" through death, resurrection and ascension into heaven, will be the time of the new exodus, a freeing from a different bondage and a leading into the new promised Kingdom, the new creation.[21] It thus refers to the main events in the history of salvation. The role of Moses and Elijah is probably to relate this "departure" of Jesus to what has been said about him in the Old Testament;[22] they are symbols of continuity.[23] As the narrative continues, however, they also become symbols of what has been superseded.

As in Gethsemane on a later occasion (22:39–46), the disciples are struggling to keep awake, and they fail to hear this conversation.[24] Nevertheless, they see the "glory" of Jesus, they glimpse his otherness.[25] Jesus reflects the brightness of the divine presence; this also points to the future, confirming the final part of the passion prediction at Caesarea Philippi that Jesus' suffering and death will not be the end of his story.

The focus of the narrative now switches from Jesus to the disciples. As the vision starts to fade, and Moses and Elijah begin to take their leave of Jesus, Peter gives expression to his wonder at what is happening and seeks to prolong the experience or render it permanent. Addressing Jesus as "Master" (as in 5:5; 8:45),[26] he suggests the construction of three shelters (booths or tabernacles), one for Jesus himself, one for Moses and one for Elijah. Such shelters made of plaited branches were originally erected in the fields at harvest time. Later, they came to be associated with the tents used by the people on their wandering journey through the wilderness when God was close to them. They were a key feature of the annual weeklong celebration of the great pilgrimage feast of Tabernacles, an occasion of intense joy and festivity.[27] One of the many expectations for the messianic age was that folk would again live in tents and that God would pitch tent with the people.[28] Peter may have had this in mind, or possibly the tent in the wilderness where God dwelt, or even the tents in heaven where the righteous dwell. Luke omits any reference here to Peter's fear, but gently acknowledges his drowsy confusion, which perhaps contributes to his mistake in placing the three figures on the same level, failing to recognise the uniqueness of Jesus. Peter is also grasping the glory and sidestepping the suffering. He does not really know what he is saying, nor does he understand what the whole experience is about.[29]

At this point, "a cloud came down, covering them in shadow." In scripture, the cloud is the sign of God's presence, revealed and concealed at the same time; it was associated with God's glory.[30] The disciples become fearful, filled with awe, which is the normal scriptural response to theophany. It is not clear who enters the cloud. Some maintain that Jesus, Elijah and Moses enter the cloud and the disciples remain outside; others hold that Elijah and Moses have left the stage and the disciples enter the cloud; a further possibility is that all six are overshadowed by the cloud.[31] "If the disciples do enter the cloud, as seems likely, Luke is depicting the presence of God as something that is both beyond the disciples' comprehension and at the same time embracing of them, with all their limitations."[32]

Just as God spoke to Moses out of the cloud on Sinai, so now God's voice reveals Jesus' identity, informing the now fearful disciples that Jesus is "my Son, the Chosen One", thus echoing God's words to Jesus privately at the baptism (changing "beloved" to "chosen") and Isaiah's Servant song.[33] The statement, making it clear that Jesus is Son and Servant, corrects Peter's misunderstanding and provides an answer to Herod's earlier puzzled questioning. There is no need for tents as places in which God's presence is enshrined; Jesus is revealed as the focal point of that presence and glory. The voice interprets the visual phenomena. Seeing and hearing go together.

The voice from the cloud enjoins that the three should "listen to him".[34] It is Jesus, not the figures of old, whose words are authoritative. The listening refers particularly to Jesus' words at Caesarea Philippi concerning what lies in store for him and for them as his disciples. Listening to him entails a response of obedience.[35] The phrasing recalls the words of Moses, and suggests that Jesus is the expected prophet like Moses who will speak God's words.

Suddenly it is all over; the voice is silent, the cloud disappears, and Jesus in his earthly state is alone in his uniqueness and humanity. His will be a lonely "exodus"; only at the end will his glory be manifest again.[36] Luke informs us that the three disciples kept silent about what they had witnessed, telling no one of the experience "in those days". Later, after the "exodus" is fulfilled, and its meaning has become evident, they will understand and proclaim it. For the time being, without being instructed to do so by Jesus (as in Mark), they remain silent about "what they had seen"; it has been overwhelming, ineffable.[37]

This mountain-top experience has confirmed the earlier words of Jesus to his disciples that his destiny was to suffer and die in Jerusalem,[38] but that this would be a prelude to vindication and glorification. They have caught a glimpse of the glory to come in the resurrection and later parousia, an indication of his true identity. Jesus' choice in the Nazareth synagogue early in his ministry to express his understanding of his mission in the terms of the Isaian Suffering Servant is further clarified and deepened. His prayer on the mountain, his listening as the Chosen One to the Father's love, confirms his identity as Son and steels his commitment and surrender to his costly mission. Jesus began his mission in Galilee after his baptism in which he was anointed by the Spirit and proclaimed, "my Son, the beloved". The heavenly voice has confirmed that relationship, and Jesus, with strong determination, now begins his journey to Jerusalem, the place of his "exodus" and his being "taken up".[39] "When the days drew near for him to be taken up, he set his face to go to Jerusalem" (9:51). The disciples, though perplexed, are strengthened in their accompanying Jesus on this journey.

History

Over the years, the impression has grown on me that the transfiguration is not a favourite text for preachers. I have often felt uncomfortable myself in that role. It is one thing to reflect on the story as it stands, opting for the narrative critical approach, an approach that uncovers amazing theological and spiritual depths in the narrative. Pondering what may have happened historically is a different and more difficult proposition, certainly to be avoided in a sermon. Some scholars consider the episode a retrojected resurrection appearance narrative, a view which is clearly on the wane nowadays.[40] Others suggest that it is an apocalyptic vision, given the supernatural elements and rich symbolism and its emphasis on the future.[41] A further alternative is to consider the story as an epiphany, which means that its focus would be concerned with the revelation of the heavenly origins and identity of Jesus, manifested in bodily form in the present.[42]

To regard the narrative as a straightforward report of an event in the life of Jesus is problematic.[43] It does, however, seem likely that the story has a historical core or nucleus, recalling an occasion when Jesus, probably at prayer, is caught up in the presence and love of God, which totally transforms his being so that the three disciples who are with him catch a glimpse of a deeper dimension to his identity.[44] The import of this experience only became clear to the disciples in hindsight after the death and resurrection of Jesus, when, through the appearances and the gift of the Spirit, his deepest reality as the glorified Lord was revealed. It is possible that early Christians later forged links with the stories and symbolism of the Old Testament, especially the Moses and Elijah traditions.[45] In the other direction, influenced by apocalyptic ideas, connections were made with expectations concerning the future end time.[46] Mark inherited this tradition, which was probably circulating orally, and included it in his Gospel narrative, closely associated with the episode at Caesarea Philippi and its aftermath: the issues of Jesus' identity and his suffering way, and the implications for discipleship.[47] In terms of Luke's narrative, the location of the transfiguration serves to clarify and justify Jesus' words to his disciples, with his emphasis on the need for him to suffer and die and then be vindicated. It provides an explanation and assurance for the disciples, but they are unable to understand. The event triggers the journey to Jerusalem, where the "exodus" will take place.

Reflections

Whatever the origins of Luke's transfiguration narrative, it invites us to reflection from many angles. The setting for the experience on the mountain is prayer. Jesus goes there to pray, taking his disciples with him. Luke places him before us as a model, inviting us to become people of prayer. It is true that we can pray at all times and in any situation. Clearly, Jesus did.[48] Prayer must be rooted in daily experience; it is there that God finds and encounters us. But there were times when Jesus sought silence and solitude. In our hectic and noisy world, we too need 'mountain' moments; we need to find innovative ways of getting away. I believe that Luke is also suggesting that prayer is a creative context for discernment, for Jesus is said to be at prayer before several important moments in his ministry. Through listening in prayer to the Father's love, we can reach a deeper awareness of our true identity as a child of God, beloved and chosen. We can also come to a clearer understanding of the meaning of Jesus in our lives and of the implications of discipleship.

As always, the narrative invites us to think about our own experience. Mountains have for me a powerful attraction. I'm fascinated by their shape, texture, colour, rugged beauty. And I feel the urge to reach the top, though with the passing of the years that can now be a daunting prospect! On mountain heights over the years there have been many 'wow' moments in snow, in dazzling sunshine, in bracing wind, in thick cloud, alone and with others. And in that awesome wonder I've sometimes sensed the transforming presence of God, reassuring, affirming, challenging. For other people, the 'mountain of revelation' can be music, art, poetry or water, the stars, the kitchen table, the look in a friend's eyes, the smile on a child's face ... situations and settings where somehow God's presence gently or dramatically breaks through, revealing a deeper dimension embedded in the ordinary and the normal. For yet others, the moment of revelation or epiphany may be recovery from serious illness, success after failure and disappointment, reunion after separation or estrangement, relief from tension, anxiety or depression, liberation from any form of darkness ... in short, any death situation transformed into a situation of newness, life and promise. Though such transfiguration moments may be fleeting, their effect can be tenaciously lasting. For the followers of Jesus, the ordinary is far from ordinary; it is shot through with transcendence.

But, while such 'mountain' moments are special and we may wish to linger long, we cannot stay there. Like Jesus, we must come down and continue our journey, a journey that will at times be difficult, uncomfortable, demanding, a journey made under the shadow of the cross, a journey into a future that is unknown. But these moments can sustain us when we have returned to the valley and the plain and are struggling with our everyday problems and cares.

The voice from the cloud invited the three disciples to "listen to him", to take seriously the message of Jesus, uncomfortable though it was, and to respond to it positively with openness and trust. We too, centuries later, are called to listen to the word of Jesus, to mull over his message, allowing it to penetrate mind and heart. We need to seek its meaning and its challenge. It will lead us to deepen our identity as God's beloved children. The Greek verb implies an obedient listening, which leads to action. That can be one of the reasons why we are reluctant listeners! Real listening involves the call to discern the needs of others in our fractured and disfigured, but wonderful, world and to respond in love and self-giving. It will help us to grasp what love is demanding of us. It will lead us to respond with compassion and generosity, courage and hope.

The reading also, and especially, invites us to reflect upon the person of Jesus. The transfiguration discloses his true identity, his unique being. The symbolism of dazzling light, the presence of Moses and Elijah in glory, the symbolism of the cloud, show that in Jesus, heaven and earth coalesce; he belongs to both worlds. The voice from the cloud confirms that this human being is God's Son, uniquely beloved and chosen.[49] The deeper dimension of his being, permanently present but hidden, shines through. This Sonship is expressed through trust and obedience, self-giving and service, to the point of death.[50]

The light, the transformation of face and clothing, the heavenly visitors, are aspects of apocalyptic literature, a genre that points to the future, the end time, usually described as eschatology. The transfiguration therefore points forward to Jesus' resurrection, ascension and second coming. It points to God's final triumph over evil and suffering and death, and the full establishment of God's reign. It is therefore a proclamation of hope. The journey to Jerusalem leads to the "exodus" of Jesus. But his suffering, seeming failure and shameful death, accepted in obedient trust, is not the end. The resurrection and exaltation to the Father's right hand follows. "The glory of the mountain is the glory he will receive on the other side of death, and also at the world's end."[51]

Through baptism we have become God's sons and daughters, dearly beloved, personally chosen. Through the gift of the Spirit we are made one with Christ, and are able to address God as "Abba, Father". Like Jesus' disciples, we too are called to share his Servant way in self-emptying and generous self-giving. We do so in the conviction that this way will lead to fullness of life with him beyond the grave in resurrection. Such a style of living is profoundly prophetic; it proclaims an alternative worldview. It subverts the power structures, greed and ambition so prevalent in our society and even in our Church. It is the only way to transform or transfigure our world, so that the eschatological reign of God takes hold in the present, now. His future is also our future.

Notes

1   Dorothy Lee, *Transfiguration: New Century Theology* (London: Continuum, 2004), 100, observes that the whole of John's Gospel can be viewed as a transfiguration narrative.

2   Lee, *Transfiguration*, 1–2.

3   R. Alan Culpepper, *Mark* (Macon: Smyth & Helwys Publishing, 2007), 318, observes that the feast was introduced in the Western Church in 1457.

4   The main differences between the versions of Luke and Mark are: the time setting; the prayer context; the change in Jesus' facial appearance; mention of his "glory"; the conversation about his "exodus"; the sleepfulness of the disciples; the association of fear with the coming of the cloud; the voice which names Jesus as "chosen"; the ending in silence rather than conversation during the descent. See Marshall, *Luke*, 381; Lee, *Transfiguration*, 66.

5   See Lee, *Transfiguration*, 66; Fitzmyer, *Luke*, 1:791–791. Marshall, *Luke*, 381, suggests that it may be best to assume that ongoing oral traditions lie behind Luke's reworking of Mark.

6   Lee, *Transfiguration*, 68, suggests a simple structure for the narrative: ascent (9:28), Jesus' transfiguration (9:29–31), the disciples' response (9:32–36), descent (9:37). This structure is different from that of Mark, so the story is different, even if much of the symbolism is the same. Resseguie, *Spiritual Landscape*, 21, divides the narrative into two parts: what the disciples see (9:28–34); what they hear (9:35–36).

7   As Carroll, *Luke*, 217, n. 60, observes, Luke's shift from Mark's six days to eight has no obvious motive; such a precise temporal marker is unusual in Luke outside the passion.

8   Byrne, *Hospitality* 89, notes that the location of the transfiguration episode here in the narrative is designed to help the disciples come to terms with what they have just been told.

9   See also 8:51. Lee, *Transfiguration*, 69, suggests that this may anticipate the frequent pairing of Peter and John in Acts (3:1–4:22; 8:14–17). In Luke, the three are not singled out on the Mount of Olives. In Exod 24:1, 9, Moses has three named companions as he ascends Sinai.

10   6:12; 19:29; 21:21; 22:39–46.

11   Mark and Matthew mention that the mountain was "high". Carroll, *Luke*, 217, notes that for Luke altitude is irrelevant. Marshall, *Luke*, 382, points out that Luke is not concerned about which mountain it was; he has not mentioned Caesarea Philippi in the previous incident, so he may not have had Mount Hermon in mind, as Mark probably does. Tradition names the mountain as Tabor, and a church was built there in 326; but Hermon is more majestic and is situated near Caesarea Philippi, and most scholars prefer this option; see Caird, *Luke*, 131.

12   The verb "pray" is used twice here in close proximity. Green, *Luke*, 380, notes that the reference to Jesus' prayer is parallel with the opening of the previous incident in which he questions Peter about his identity (9:18). Prayer provides the context for both events; both events are highly significant for Jesus and his mission.

13   Lee, *Transfiguration*, 71, suggests an astonishingly brilliant light flaming forth from Jesus—the radiance of his body shining through his garments in flashes of fire, like light pouring through a window. See Dan 7:9; Rev 2:17; 6:2; 7:9, 13–14; 20:11; also, Luke 24:4 at the empty tomb; Acts 1:10 at the ascension. Green, *Luke*, 380, writes that in the Old Testament and Jewish tradition, one's countenance is a mirror of one's heart and a manifestation of one's relationship with God. Jesus' inner being was made transparent to those accompanying him; it is a disclosure of his status to the disciples. The apostles are given a glimpse of Jesus' future glory in order to provide an unimpeachable endorsement of the grounding of his mission and message in the divine purpose. The glory that will be manifest upon his exaltation is proleptically unveiled. Marshall, *Luke*, 383, refers to 2 Cor 3:7, 13; Dan 12:3; 2 Bar 51. With regard to countenance and clothing, he refers to Moses typology. Resseguie, *Spiritual Landscape*, 92, notes that ordinary people did not wear white, bleached garments. Jesus' garments are not only white but gleam like lightning; this transformation "provides a glimpse of his inner character: his transcendent glory, his Otherness."

14   Caird, *Luke*, 132, notes that the intense devotions of saints and mystics are often accompanied by physical transformation and luminous glow. The account may therefore be literally true. Green, *Luke*, 377, 381, notes Luke's emphasis on sight (a seeing which is not enough); then on hearing. The whole scene is a moment of revelation. The *idou* ("behold") draws the audience in. Resseguie, *Spiritual Landscape*, 21, too notes the division into seeing and hearing: the hearing interprets the seeing; "God's clarifying word interprets the meaning of Jesus' altered appearance." Seeing alone is insufficient and is open to misunderstanding. There are five references to sight in the narrative, but a clarifying word is needed.

15   The text reads "two men", before specifying their identity; this seems awkward. Lee, *Transfiguration*, 71, suggests that Luke may be aligning this episode with the later stories of the empty tomb and the ascension, which refer to the appearance of two men (24:4; Acts 1:10). Green, *Luke*, 377–378, notes the background of the exodus theme (story or interpretation): three companions (Exod 24:1); a mountain; Moses; change of countenance (34:29); tents; the cloud (24:15–18); fear; conversation about "exodus"; and Deut 18:15—the promise of a prophet like Moses. Luke also draws on the new exodus theme in the prophets and especially Isaiah. Luke sees the mission of Jesus as a virtual, divinely ordained, re-enactment of the exodus from bondage; (also Resseguie, *Spiritual landscape*, 23). Green, *Luke*, stresses the interpretive background. The echoes are shaped by the mission statement of Jesus in 4:18–19; Jesus' mission of liberation in his ministry so far has been very effective; the transfiguration goes on to intimate the redemptive power of his upcoming journey through death to exaltation. He notes echoes from the narrative before and after the transfiguration. This scene summarises critical issues concerning Jesus' status in relation to God; proleptically alerts representative apostles to the full significance of his heavenly status; and supplies an interpretive framework for making sense of the ensuing narrative, including the fulfilment of Jesus' predicted suffering and death. (379).

16   See Deut 18:15–18; 34:10, regarding a prophet like Moses; Mal 3:1, 23; 4:4–5 concerning the return of Elijah. It is sometimes stated that they represent the Law and

the prophets; but both were prophets. (Lee, *Transfiguration*, 85, n. 36).

17   Exod 24:15–18; 1 Kings 19:8–13.

18   In 2 Kings 2:9–11 Elijah is taken up to heaven in a fiery chariot. Deut 34:5–6 tells of Moses' death, adding that no one knows where he was buried. This led to speculation that he was "assumed" into heaven. (See this tradition in the document 'The Assumption of Moses' or 'The Testament of Moses'.) Green, *Luke*, 381, notes that the presence of Elijah shows that the crowds are wrong in their speculation concerning Jesus. Luke associates Elijah with Jesus in that Jesus, like Elijah, engages in a prophetic ministry in which the power of God is active on behalf of those not normally regarded as the elect—that is, gentiles, Samaritans and the poor.

19   Carroll, *Luke*, 218, comments that their "glory" indicates that Jesus' change of appearance results from the intrusion of the heavenly into mundane space and time.

20   Johnson, *Luke*, 156, observes that Luke places the suffering element in the middle of the vision of glory, confirming Jesus' earlier prediction, and preparing for the journey narrative and passion. Carroll, *Luke*, 217, notes that Heaven endorses Jesus' declaration of the meaning and goal of his messianic mission.

21   Byrne, *Hospitality*, 89; Lee, *Transfiguration*, 73. Evans, *Luke*, 418, speaks of "departure through death to glory." Resseguie, *Spiritual Landscape*, 23, refers to Jesus leading a new Israel on a new exodus to a new promised land, the Kingdom of God. Similarly, Wright, *Luke*, 115: "Jesus will lead all God's people out of the slavery of sin and death, and home to their promised inheritance—the new creation in which the whole world will be redeemed." Carroll, *Luke*, 218, notes that later, Jerusalem will also be the departure point for the exodus on mission to the world. Caird, *Luke*, 132, regards this incident as a crisis in Jesus' religious life, the realisation of coming rejection and death.

22   Fitzmyer, *Luke*, 2:800. Johnson, *Luke*, 156, sees the presence of Moses and Elijah as confirming Jesus' identity as the Deuteronomic prophet raised up by God (see 7:16).

23   Green, *Luke*, 382, refers to the continuation and consummation of God's ancient, eschatological purpose.

24   Green, *Luke*, 383, prefers that "they were weighed down with sleep but stayed awake," barely awake. Marshall, *Luke*, 385, believes that the disciples fail to hear the conversation and the heavenly confirmation of Jesus' destiny. There were therefore no witnesses to the conversation, so its content must have been supplied later by Jesus or supplied by the narrator. Evans, *Luke*, 418, maintains that the disciples do not witness the transfiguration of Jesus nor the appearance of Moses and Elijah, but only the consequences on waking. Lee, *Transfiguration*, 74, believes that it is unclear whether they have fallen asleep and missed the conversation, waking to perceive the "glory" and the presence of the two men, or are sleepy and later roused to full wakefulness.

25   Evans, *Luke*, 417, describes "glory" as "the manifested being and presence of God" and "the nature of those belonging to the heavenly eschatological realm." Lee, *Transfiguration*, 72–73, states that light and glory are closely related concepts in the Old Testament, where "glory means the powerful and radiant reality of God in its holy otherness and engaging nearness to human life"; it can refer to the essence or manifest presence of God.

26   For Lee, *Transfiguration*, 75, "Master" is a more exalted form of address than Mark's "Rabbi" (see also 8:24; 9:49; 17:13); it "indicates Jesus' divinely given power and authority." Other scholars seem to think the title is inadequate as a designation of 'Jesus, and an aspect of Peter's lack of understanding.

27   Caird, *Luke*, 133, links the term with the tabernacle built in the wilderness to enshrine God's presence.

28   Evans, *Luke*, 419, notes the close connection between the "tent" and God's dwelling with Israel, his glory and revelation. Lee, *Transfiguration*, 75, also mentions the tradition of the dwellings of the righteous in heaven in the end time.

29   Carroll, *Luke*, 219, comments that their lack of understanding continues into the rest of the narrative; the journey narrative unfolds as an educative experience for them. Marshall, *Luke*, 386, concludes that probably Peter wishes to erect earthly counterparts to the heavenly dwelling places of the three visitors so that they would have somewhere to stay on earth, and thus the glorious experience might be prolonged.

30   See Exod 13:21–22; 24:15–18; 33:9–10; 40:29; Dan 7:13. Luke uses the term "overshadow" in 1:35 concerning Mary. Lee, *Transfiguration*, 77, links the annunciation, baptism, and transfiguration: "the cloud signifies the descent and overshadowing of the Spirit." Green, *Luke*, 383, notes that so far in Luke, God usually operates behind the scenes. The cloud is referred to three times here. Evans, *Luke*, 419, calls it the cloud of theophany.

31   Green, *Luke*, 384, thinks it refers to the disciples, as does Evans ("probably"), *Luke*, 420; Marshall, *Luke*, 387, Jesus with Moses and Elijah; Lee, *Transfiguration*, 76, on balance opts for the six.

32   Lee, *Transfiguration*, 77.

33   Isa 42:1–2. The Servant here is both beloved and chosen and anointed with God's Spirit (see Luke 4:18; the term "chosen" is also used as a form of mockery on Calvary: 23:35). Green, *Luke*, 384, says that God's word identifies Jesus in three ways: Son of God; Isaian Servant of Yahweh; and prophet, like Moses. So far, the apostles have not been privy to this information. God has identified Jesus for them; Jesus' words are therefore reliable. God has sanctioned Jesus' status and mission. Jesus is the authorised interpreter of the Law and the prophets. Lee, *Transfiguration*, 78, notes the links with the annunciation and baptism, the temptation, the saying in 10:22. Jesus is proclaimed as Son of God in Acts 9:20; 13:33. Marshall, *Luke*, 388, supports the Servant reference. Evans, *Luke*, 420, is also open to the link with Isa 41:1: "chosen one". McBride, *Luke*, 124, states that before he sets his face towards the place of his exaltation, he experiences the confirmation of his Father.

34   The words are emphatic: "to him, listen." Johnson, *Luke*, 154, sees the reference to listening as linked to Deut 18:15 LXX. Also, Evans, *Luke*, 421; the injunction establishes the ultimate authority of Jesus' words on earth for his Church.

35   Lee, *Transfiguration*, 79, notes how Mary has been portrayed as the exemplar of this kind of obedient, faithful listening (1:38, 45; see 11:27–28; 24:8). The disciples struggle with listening in 9:44, when Jesus predicts his passion again.

36   Lee, *Transfiguration*, 79–80, sees the glory of Jesus at the beginning of Luke's story, the divine visitation and birth stories and the end of the journey in resurrection

and ascension; the transfiguration occupies centre ground, looking both to past and future.

37   Lee, *Transfiguration*, 82, says that the silence, by their volition, dramatises the ineffability of the event and the impossibility of the apostles' speech until empowered from on high for mission (24:48). They are indeed "blessed for what they have a seen and heard" (10: 23–24).

38   Rejection "by the elders, chief priests and scribes" (9:22) implies the Jerusalem location.

39   The terminology of being "taken up" recalls the story of Elijah in 2 Kgs 2:1. The "exodus" and being "taken up" refer to the whole sequence of events: death, resurrection and ascension. The ascension completes Jesus' journey.

40   Boring, *Mark*, 260. McBride, *Luke*, 123, rejects the idea of a misplaced resurrection appearance; also, Byrne, *Hospitality*, 89, n. 4; Evans, *Luke*, 413; Culpepper, *Mark*, 393; Lee, *Transfiguration*, 3–4. The resurrection appearances are of a different literary genre. Donahue & Harrington, *Mark*, 273–4, believe this is not implausible, while acknowledging the absence of key elements in such stories. They consider the transfiguration as at least a preview of the glory of the risen Jesus, and so an anticipation of the resurrection.

41   Lee, *Transfiguration*, 4–5, discusses this as a possible genre for the story. This way of understanding the story "depicts Jesus as he will be at his future coming, already anticipated in his ministry and resurrection."

42   Lee, *Transfiguration*, 5.

43   Boring, *Mark*, 260.

44   See N. Tom Wright, *Mark for Everyone* (London: SPCK, 2001), 116; Marshall, *Luke*, 381. Lee, *Transfiguration*, 4, refers to "stubborn elements ... that suggest an historical kernel, even if we allow for the development of the symbolic." "Taken together with a persistent tradition in mysticism of holy people surrounded by inexplicable light, it is hard to dismiss the transfiguration historically." Caird, *Luke*, 132, notes that the intense devotions of saints and mystics are often accompanied by physical transformation and luminous glow. The account may therefore be true. Donahue & Harrington, *Mark*, 273, while acknowledging the symbolic and imaginative elements, consider it highly likely that the story reflects the disciples' experience of Jesus' brilliance. The precise details of this experience are hard to determine.

45   We suggested a similar process with the temptation narrative.

46   Evans, *Luke*, 413, believes that it could be a theological construction of Christian creation.

47   Lee, *Transfiguration*, 39, suggests that the transfiguration narrative as it stands can be read as both an apocalyptic vision and an epiphany. "It expresses, on the one hand, the revelation of Jesus' heavenly identity in the context of his ministry and, on the other hand, his role in bringing to birth God's future, where that identity will be fully and finally manifest." Donahue & Harrington, *Mark*, 274, prefer the term "Christophany", a revelation of Jesus' "true identity and the glorious goal to which his journey will lead."

48   In his village community, Jesus from childhood would have embraced the daily rhythm of prayer (the *Shema* recited first thing in the morning and last thing at night),

the weekly Sabbath observance and the service in the (makeshift) synagogue, and would have embraced the importance of the *Torah*, which was woven into every aspect of ordinary life.

49   In the Prologue of the Fourth Gospel we read that "the Word became flesh and pitched his tent in our midst, and we have seen his glory, the glory of the Father's only Son" (John 1:14). Divine glory abides in the humanity of Jesus.

50   The Fourth Evangelist expresses this through the phrase *eis telos*, which means to the end of life, and to the utmost (13:1).

51   Lee, *Transfiguration*, 125; it is the "anticipated glory of the crucified Lord, risen and ascended."

Chapter Eight
Listening and Doing

One of the great challenges that we face in life is the integrating of the active and contemplative dimensions of our response to God as disciples of Jesus. This is by no means a modern phenomenon, though the speed and 'noise' of life today does exacerbate the problem. Luke, in his Gospel, explores the importance of both listening to God's word and doing it, by placing together a parable and a parabolic narrative: the parable of the compassionate Samaritan, and the story of Jesus' visit to Martha and Mary. Generally, these two episodes are treated separately. In the mind of the evangelist, however, they hang together.[1]

The wider context for our material in the structure of Luke's Gospel is the earlier part of what is usually referred to as the journey narrative, the dynamic framework that he uses as the context for a great deal of his special material and his teaching on discipleship. The journey begins: "When the days drew near for him to be taken up, he set his face to go to Jerusalem" (9:51).[2] References to its progress punctuate the next ten chapters, until Jesus and his followers, having passed through Jericho, finally reach Jerusalem (19:29–45).

The Parable of The Compassionate Samaritan

As it stands, the parable itself (10:30–35) is introduced by an opening dialogue (10:25–29),[3] and is followed by a concluding dialogue (10:36–37).[4]

Opening Dialogue

This runs as follows:

> Just then a lawyer stood up to test Jesus. "Teacher," he said, "what must I do to inherit eternal life?" He said to him, "What is written in the law? What do you read there?" He answered, "You shall love the Lord your God with all your heart, and with all your soul, and with all your strength, and with all your mind; and your neighbour as yourself." And he said to him, "You have given the right answer; do

this, and you will live." But wanting to justify himself, he asked Jesus, "And who is my neighbour?" (10:25–29)

The lawyer seems to interrupt the conversation that Jesus is holding privately with his disciples.[5] He shows respect in standing and addressing Jesus as "teacher", and therefore as an equal.[6] In Mark's Gospel, during Jesus' final week in Jerusalem, one of the scribes, impressed by Jesus' answers to a series of challenging questions, asks him which is the first commandment. Jesus answers:

> The first is, "Hear, O Israel: the Lord our God, the Lord is one; you shall love the Lord your God with all your heart, and with all your soul, and with all your mind, and with all your strength." The second is this, "You shall love your neighbour as yourself." There is no other commandment greater than these. (Mark 12:29–31)

The scribe expresses his agreement with Jesus, and Jesus praises him, assuring him that he is not far from the Kingdom of God. In Matthew's version, the context is more tense, and the purpose of the question is to test Jesus (Matt 22:34–40). Luke moves the incident to its present location earlier in the ministry, retaining the flavour of hostility[7] but changing the terms of the question: "What must I do to inherit eternal life."[8] With its emphasis on "doing", suggesting a single action, this is the wrong question. "It presumes that eternal life is a commodity to be inherited or purchased on the basis of a particular action rather than a gift freely given."[9] Jesus responds by asking a counter-question, which forces the lawyer to answer his own question and gives him the opportunity to display his knowledge, massaging his ego a little.[10] This he does according to classical rabbinic teaching, the *Shema*, the foundation and core of Jewish life and prayer, recited twice daily (Deut 6:5), but he adds to the love command "and your neighbour as yourself" (Lev 19:18).[11] The answer is a good one; Jesus is in agreement; they are on common ground. Jesus then tells him to "Do this, and you will live." Knowledge isn't enough; it is essential to do what you know.[12] "Jesus turns the tables on him, first by showing that he already knew the answer to his own question, then by compelling him to measure his own life against the standard which he had been prepared to use as a weapon in an intellectual sparring match."[13] "The answer is given in a command for an open-ended lifestyle that requires unlimited and unqualified love for God and people."[14] Whereas in Mark there are two commandments—love of God and love of neighbour—in Luke's formulation there is a single unified love command with a twin focus.[15] The meaning of the commandment is then illustrated by the parable of the Good Samaritan and the parabolic narrative of Martha and Mary.[16]

The Parable

The lawyer in the narrative finds it hard to let go of the idea of earning eternal life with which he has begun his encounter with Jesus. He continues to press for answers, to assert himself and regain the initiative.[17] Jesus has forced him to answer his own question and challenged him to live by what he knows. So, he next attempts to clarify the meaning of the Law by seeking a definition of the term "neighbour", or a clear delineation of the limits of his responsibility.[18] Levine suggests that he was really interested in who was not his neighbour! Usually, the Jews considered fellow Jews to be resident aliens,[19] and proselytes as belonging to the category of neighbour; there were others classified as non-neighbour, and there were exceptions within the community.[20] With a clear list in mind, the lawyer would be able to tick off those loved and feel justified in being able to say: "I have done it."

The lawyer's initial question sought a definition of neighbour, a list of categories that would fall under this rubric. He hopes that by fulfilling the requirements of the list, a prescriptive law, he will be able to earn eternal life for himself. How many people have I to love in order to earn righteousness by my own efforts?

To his question: "And who is my neighbour?" Jesus replies with the famous parable. Naming this parable "the Good Samaritan" over the centuries has "dulled us to the explosive tension of the phrase in the world of Jesus; a modern-day equivalent would be a 'good drug dealer'."[21] It is a classic oxymoron. I prefer to call the story the parable of the 'compassionate Samaritan'.[22]

The Story

> Jesus replied, "A man was going down from Jerusalem to Jericho, and fell into the hands of robbers, who stripped him, beat him, and went away, leaving him half dead. Now by chance a priest was going down that road; and when he saw him, he passed by on the other side. So likewise a Levite, when he came to the place and saw him, passed by on the other side. But a Samaritan while travelling came near him; and when he saw him, he was moved with pity. He went to him and bandaged his wounds, having poured oil and wine on them. Then he put him on his own animal, brought him to an inn, and took care of him. The next day he took out two denarii, gave them to the innkeeper, and said, 'Take care of him; and when I come back, I will repay you whatever more you spend'."

A man,[23] whom we presume to be a Jew, is travelling the lonely seventeen-mile (23 km) road that descends some 3,300 feet (1 km) from Jerusalem to Jericho.[24] The terrain is rough and rocky, and provides ideal cover for robbers, organised bands or gangs of highwaymen, and it offers ready escape routes too.[25] The man is ambushed, beaten up, stripped and left half dead. The detail that he is stripped and unconscious is essential to create the tension at the heart of the drama. He cannot identify himself; nor can his identity or nationality easily be ascertained by another; conversation is impossible (and his accent or dialect would betray his origins), and any distinctive garb has been removed. He is, therefore, anonymous, belonging to no ethnic group or religious community; he is simply a human being in need.[26] But he is still alive! The audience would identify with the man in the ditch.[27]

A priest happens to pass that way.[28] Many of the priestly families resided in Jericho; the priests would go up to Jerusalem when their turn for ministry came around. Presumably this one is returning from one of his two weeks of service.[29] The structure of the parable suggests that he was probably riding; he steers his donkey to the far side of the road and passes by.[30]

Although the text is silent about motivation, several motives are frequently put forward to explain his passing by. Many scholars opt for his theological and legalistic mentality, his fear of incurring ritual defilement. Sir 12:1–7 indicates that help offered to "sinners" may go against God, who detests sinners. The priest is unable to identify the victim securely as a Jew, and he may be dead. Contact would in either case defile a priest, at least according to the Sadducee interpretation. If defiled, he would not be able to officiate at services or wear phylacteries; nor could he collect, distribute or eat tithes, and his family and servants would suffer as a consequence. To incur defilement would be a great humiliation for a priest, especially so soon after finishing his term of office. Purification would take a week, would be financially costly and would entail returning to the East Gate and standing among others who were "unclean". It is better to maintain status and righteousness within the system and the supporting community than to reach out to one in need.[31]

Many other scholars discount this idea as unconvincing. Were the man dead, there was an obligation to bury him and if injured, to care for him. Fear of a trap or an ambush could have been a factor;[32] but it seems that he just did not wish to get involved. He saw but ignored.

The next person on the scene is a Levite. The Levites, too, formed a privileged group. They were cultic officials involved in temple liturgy; they also exercised a policing role there.[33] This man would not be bound by as many regulations as the priest; he was required to observe ritual cleanness only while on duty. So, he approaches, probably takes a closer look, and decides against helping. In his case the motive would not be fear of defilement. He could be walking and is afraid to linger because of the danger of robbers. He would most probably be aware of the priest ahead, since it was possible to see a good distance; if the priest were mounted, he could have overtaken him earlier. Perhaps he argues that it isn't his duty to help, since the priest has not done so.[34] To do so could be construed as a criticism of the priest's conduct. Although professionally a religious man, there is nothing in his orientation which moves him to help. Both are caught in a moral dilemma: to observe the Torah on uncleanness or on love of neighbour.[35] Levine writes that their responsibility was to save a life, but they failed. Saving life overrides every other concern, even Sabbath. Had the man died, their responsibility was to bury him; and they failed here too.[36] Those listening to the parable would have been shocked that their religious officials acted in this way; they would not easily have excused them in the name of ritual purity.[37]

A third man reaches the scene.[38] Popular stories like threes. Perhaps Jesus' original hearers, not adverse to a little spicy anti-clericalism, expected this protagonist in the drama to be a Jewish layman (an Israelite). This would be the natural sequence; laypeople also worshipped in the temple and travelled home. To their shock and dismay, Jesus disrupts the sequence by choosing as hero a Samaritan, the traditional enemy.[39] It is difficult for us to imagine the impact that this would have had on Jesus' audience. There had been centuries of animosity between Jews and Samaritans.[40] The Samaritans had opposed the restoration of Jerusalem after the exile and had later helped the Syrians against the Jews. In 128 BCE, the Jewish high priest burned the Samaritan temple on Mount Gerizim. In Jesus' time, hostility had intensified because of an incident (6 CE) in which the Samaritans had defiled the temple and prevented the celebration of Passover by strewing dead men's bones there. They were cursed in the synagogue worship; there was a prayer that they would be refused eternal life. So, Jesus was really rocking the boat, chancing his arm, stirring and exposing the deepest hatreds and emotions and religiously institutionalised prejudices of his audience. It must have taken great courage to make a despised, mistrusted, heretical, as-bad-as-gentile Samaritan, a socio-religious outcast, appear as morally superior to religious Jews and as exemplar of the true fulfilment of the Law! Jesus raises the very basic question about the people's understanding of God and the nature of God's approval.[41] The Samaritans were hostile to Jesus' own ministry in 9:53, a detail which reflects his magnanimity.

A Samaritan was also subject to the Law and risked contamination. He, too, would be exposed to attack from robbers if he lingered, especially if carrying merchandise; and he wasn't a man of the cloth. He would doubtless be aware that the other two had ignored a man who was probably a fellow Jew, and so might wonder why he should get involved. But, "when he saw him, he was moved to compassion." The verb in Greek is strong; it comes from the same root as bowels and womb; it means moved to the depths of one's being; a gut-wrenching feeling. Compassion is the turning point of the narrative, a compassion that finds immediate, concrete, practical expression. "Compassion is the bridge between simply looking on injured and half-dead fellow human beings and entering their world with saving care."[42]

To begin with, he renders first aid.[43] He cleans and softens the wounds with oil, disinfects them with wine, and bandages them up. The word order is unusual. Perhaps it is meant to recall God's binding of wounds (Jer 30:17; Hos 6:1–10).[44] The second stage of the rescue is that he provides transport. He may have had several donkeys. It is not clear whether the two ride the same animal or whether the Samaritan puts the victim on his own mount and then leads the animal as would a servant. In Palestine, the social distinction between the rider and the one leading the animal is important. The third stage is rehabilitation. He takes him to an inn,[45] presumably in Jericho, and remains overnight ministering to his needs. This is a marvellous act of self-giving love, easy for us to overlook. In that culture, blood revenge is deeply rooted. If someone is hurt and the assailant cannot be found, anyone (even if only remotely connected) could suffer. So, in taking him to Jericho, he runs the risk of the community blaming him and attacking him (as an irrational group response, especially as he belonged to a minority group). Caution would suggest that, at the very most, he should take him to the inn and then disappear. In staying around, in offering to return later, he displays great courage. What a price he is prepared to pay to complete the act of compassion![46] Finally, to complete the balanced framework of the parable, he compensates for the robbers. They rob, leave, abandon. He pays, leaves, promises to return. Innkeepers had an unsavoury reputation for dishonesty and violence. If simply left there, the man on awaking would not be able to pay the bill since he had been robbed, and so could be arrested for debt. The Samaritan's advance payment and promise of settling further expenses with the innkeeper on his return guarantees the man's freedom and security, for someone with an unpaid debt could be enslaved until the debt was paid (Matt 18:23–35). He recognises his ongoing responsibility, almost providing a blank cheque. There is no mention of his being reimbursed.[47]

The story is an amazing delineation by Jesus of the meaning of compassion. Note the cost in time, effort, convenience, finance, personal danger—a cost completely disregarded. Utter self-forgetfulness, generous attention, service far beyond the call of duty, thoughtful concern and foresight ... , and the contrast between the action of the hated Samaritan and the inaction of the respected Jewish religious elite is quite stunning. "Jesus deliberately shocks the lawyer by forcing him to consider the possibility that a semi-pagan foreigner might know more about the love of God than a devout Jew blinded by preoccupation with pettifogging rules."[48] "The Samaritan participates in the compassion and covenantal faithfulness of God, who sees and responds with salvific care."[49]

The Concluding Dialogue

> "Which of these three, do you think, was a neighbour to the man who fell into the hands of the robbers?" He said, "The one who showed him mercy." Jesus said to him, "Go and do likewise." (10:36–37)

Concluding the parable, Jesus enters once again into dialogue. He rephrases the lawyer's question and switches the focus: "Which of these three, do you think, was a neighbour to the man who fell into the hands of the robbers?"[50] Jesus is not primarily interested in responding directly to the definition-seeking question, but in exploring the nature of neighbourliness. The commandment had been quoted as "love your neighbour". For Jesus, it is the verb that matters. The lawyer's answer, which avoids the naming of the Samaritan, is again correct, "the one who shows kindness."[51] Neighbour has become subject rather than object;[52] the one who actively ministers to the needy. "Neighbour is a way of being in the world, it is a way of relating to other people and to God."[53] But Jesus has, in fact, answered the original question; neighbour means any human being in need, beyond ethnic and religious restrictions and prejudices.

The encounter closes in parallel with the earlier question with a further challenge from Jesus: "Go, and you do likewise." This is the way to eternal life. To become neighbour to anyone in need, to reach out in costly compassion to all people (even enemies) without any limits, with no boundaries, is a demanding ideal.[54] And of course the lawyer cannot, the standard is too high. The verb means "keep on doing it", make treating everyone with compassion a way of life. Though we cannot achieve it, the standard remains. And in the end, eternal life will be God's gift. "The parable summons us to a solidarity with suffering men and women and tells us that such solidarity can come only when we can acquire hearts of flesh and a compassionate vision."[55]

Reflections

From our perspective today, we can see that the parable can serve as a kind of commentary on the life and ministry of Jesus himself and on God's actions throughout the Old Testament. Reaching out to others in compassion, serving their needs with care, being prepared to take risks, not looking for recompense—these are qualities that are characteristic of Jesus of Nazareth. There is something quite subversive in Jesus' approach, even if he is bringing out the deeper meaning of the Law. He seeks to overturn prejudices, change attitudes, adjust values, deconstruct our world and create a new world, which he calls the Kingdom. The God of Luke, as we have seen, is a God of faithful compassion. Jesus is a man of great compassion.

As disciples, we are called today to be sacraments of the compassion of Jesus. It has been said that our Western world is becoming increasingly lacking in compassion, more self-centred and exclusivist. Sadly, there is much truth in that. Given our economic system, it is probably inevitable. There are, however, many examples of amazing compassion and care, especially evident in times of crisis and disaster. There are many instances, too, which go unnoticed. As Christians, we are called to make real the dream of Jesus, to model an alternative lifestyle with compassion at the centre. We are called to reflect to our family and community in the first place, to those with whom we work and minister, to those whom we serve and to anyone in need, the compassionate presence of God. We are called to be a window into God's faithfulness and constancy, God's compassionate care, God's tender love, God's thirst that we should have life in its fullness.

This means that, like Jesus, we are called to be prophetic in our world and in our Church. Compassionate solidarity and caring action is also critique and challenge; it undermines current structures and styles in our world; it proclaims an alternative value system and way of living, a different world (called "Kingdom"). It is a sign of hope. It holds the promise of transformation. "Be compassionate as your heavenly Father is compassionate (Luke 6:36)." We need constantly to ask ourselves who are the people we pass by, often without a second glance? And, why do we develop strategies of avoidance, rationalisation, excuses for doing little or nothing? Compassion is not a single act; it is a lifestyle.[56]

Martha and Mary

One of the best known Lukan narratives, still capable of stimulating quite heated group discussions, describes the visit of Jesus to the home of Martha and Mary.[57]

The episode concerning these sisters is found only in Luke; presumably it stems from his special source.

> Now as they went on their way, he entered a certain village, where a woman named Martha welcomed him into her home. She had a sister named Mary, who sat at the Lord's feet and listened to what he was saying. But Martha was distracted by her many tasks; so she came to him and asked, "Lord, do you not care that my sister has left me to do all the work by myself? Tell her then to help me." But the Lord answered her, "Martha, Martha, you are worried and distracted by many things; there is need of only one thing. Mary has chosen the better part, which will not be taken away from her." (10:38–42)

In Luke's mind, I believe, the story of the two sisters, Martha and Mary, is to be taken in tandem with the parable of the Good Samaritan, which we have just considered. Viewed together, they illustrate the two aspects of the one commandment of love that the lawyer has articulated in reply to Jesus' question. The story is also an instance of Luke's tendency to juxtapose two narratives in which a woman and a man are in turn the principal protagonist.[58] He is a forerunner in the call for equal opportunities! In the much-loved parable, the contrast is drawn between the Samaritan and the two Jewish wayfarers who have close connections with the temple. Here, it is the sisters who are contrasted. The two sisters appear in the Fourth Gospel in connection with the raising of their brother Lazarus from death. Their home is in the village of Bethany, situated just outside Jerusalem. Such a location does not fit Luke's scheme. Already in his Gospel, Luke has noted that women are among the close followers of Jesus, and that some of them support him and the male disciples (8:1–3).

As Jesus proceeds on his journey to Jerusalem, he reaches an unnamed village. He is in need of hospitality, and a lady named Martha makes him welcome in her home.[59] Luke does not indicate whether Jesus arrives at the door by chance or by design;[60] I suspect that the latter is implied. Maybe Jesus and his disciples were frequent visitors. The disciples travelling with Jesus are sidelined; we are not told how they fared; Jesus is at the centre of the narrative. Martha appears to be the head of the household[61] and immediately gets involved unselfishly in busily preparing a rather elaborate meal. Mary, her sister, "seated herself at the Lord's feet and stayed there listening to his words." She adopts the normal posture of a disciple and is clearly keen to listen to what Jesus has to say and, student-like, to learn from him. She acknowledges his authority[62] and is attentive to his word, a key motif for this evangelist (1:41; 8:21; 11:28). Jesus, far from shrinking from this, as most rabbis would have done, encourages her interest. This is another example of his freedom with regard to social and religious convention in his treatment of women and of his advancing their status. They, too, are allowed to listen and learn and are deemed capable of doing so.[63]

It soon emerges that Martha has a problem. The pressure of hospitality, as she understands it, prevents her from listening, which she doubtless would have appreciated and enjoyed. She is "distracted by all the serving." The verb means to be pulled or dragged about, to be overburdened.[64] There is just too much to do. She probably feels rather peeved that she has been left to do everything herself, and maybe thinks her sister is being a little selfish. Perhaps she is somewhat disappointed that Jesus does not seem to notice her frustration, so she attempts to enlist his support. She assumes a slightly confrontational attitude. There is an emphasis on 'me' in her words. One might detect a touch of resentment in her voice, a tone of accusation against her sister: "Tell her to come and lend a hand." Martha really ought not to have asked her guest to become involved in a family dispute.[65]

As is generally the case in the Gospel narrative, Jesus resists the pressure to intervene.[66] He is not unsympathetic to her plight and her problem and her feelings of annoyance; but he insists on priorities. There is great affection in his voice as, with a gentle reproach, he indicates the real issue: "Martha, Martha, you are fretting and fussing about so many things." The first verb means to be anxious, to be unduly concerned. Anxiety usually has a negative connotation in scripture, implying a lack of trust in the presence and power of God; it can inhibit the growth of the word.[67] The second verb means to be troubled, distracted, even to create an uproar.[68] Martha, then, is far too troubled and anxious; she is exaggeratedly concerned. She is losing the right perspective. It is not really necessary to 'go over the top', to prepare such an elaborate *cordon bleu* menu. Perhaps she could cut back a little, and then she would also have time to listen. What Jesus needs is not a generous table but a listening ear.[69]

There are two aspects to discipleship: there is service, kindness, practical living; and there is listening to Jesus, hearing the word of the Lord. As Caird puts it so well, Martha "has not yet learned that unselfishness, service, and even sacrifice can be spoiled by self-concern and self-pity, that good works which are not self-forgetful can become a misery to the doer and a tyranny to others."[70] Jesus continues: "Mary has chosen the good portion, which shall not be taken away from her."

After the story of the Samaritan's generous response to a traveller's need, which Jesus proclaims should be a permanent way of living, his comment here comes as a surprise. It has also proved something of a problem for subsequent readers, as the manuscript variations testify.[71] The good or better part, portion, course or dish (a little wordplay is evident here), the thing which is most essential, the right choice, is to make space for Jesus and to listen to his word. Besides, the one thing necessary for hospitality is attention to the guest, and if the guest is a prophet, the appropriate way to express welcome is to listen to his message. This is what he would wish for.[72] Listening is service too. In the scale of values, it is listening to the word that has priority.[73] Jesus defends Mary; she has made the correct choice. Martha should have been content to prepare one dish, the normal form of hospitality, and join Mary in a different form of hospitality.[74] Mary will not be deprived of this opportunity to listen to Jesus. "This rhythm of listening quietly and acting decisively is the very rhythm Jesus has displayed in his own working."[75]

Reflections

To love God with whole heart and mind and the neighbour as one's self demands both compassionate and effective entry into the world of the neighbour as well as undistracted attentiveness to the word of the Lord. Far from exalting one mode of discipleship above the other, the two narratives say that one cannot authentically exist without the other.[76]

For Luke, it is important both to listen and to do.[77] Receiving the Lord's teaching and serving, hearing and doing belong together in discipleship. Receptive attention to the word must keep company with faithful action, and vice versa.[78]

The two sisters of this narrative invite us to examine the priorities in our lives. Most of us take ministry and mission seriously and try genuinely to reach out to others in care and compassion. But there are times when we become aware that we are becoming too busy, and such overactivity induces tension, anxiety and stress into our lives. Symptoms of workaholism, incipient or verging on the chronic, become evident. The quality of our service begins to deteriorate and relationships become a little fraught. We can lose perspective and focus. "Frenetic service, even service of the Lord, can be a deceptive distraction from what the Lord really wants."[79] In many ways, Martha is exactly like us, and we warm to her.[80]

In the busyness of everyday life, we realise that somehow, we are neglecting to make time to reflect prayerfully on the Lord's word.[81] Such reflection centres our lives on Jesus. It is Jesus who is our inspiration, whose life enlivens our vision, reveals true values, informs our style of serving. Mary models a crucial and single-hearted style of hospitality. Without regular times of prayer in which we listen to God's love, our apostolic ventures can become jobs or careers rather than ministries, and we run the risk of building our own kingdoms rather than that of Jesus. Values other than those of the Gospel can influence our decisions and actions. Selfishness, individualism and pragmatism and the seeking of success, instead of the Spirit, can determine the outcome of our discernment.

The Jesus of this story is not unwilling to be served but is conscious of a message that he desires to share, and this clarifies his priorities. His normal affection and care are again evident, but he is gently assertive. He makes his point in unambiguous terms. His friends come to know his mind and priorities; they know where he stands. It is a point that he probably needs to make with us repeatedly. The balanced integration of reflection and action is an ongoing challenge. His manner of dealing with this situation can serve as an example for us, too, in other situations that we frequently face. He addresses the issue with sensitivity and with clarity. His leadership style is worth pondering and following.

Notes

1   This is the view of Donahue, *Gospel,* 134–139; Marshall, *Luke,* 450–451; Carroll, *Luke,* 42, 246; Green, *Luke,* 433–434. Reid, *Parables,* 106, disagrees, claiming that there is nothing in the text that warrants such a link. But I believe that Luke's juxtaposing the two stories is sufficient indication of his mind.

2   9:51. References to the movement of the journey punctuate the next ten chapters (9:57; 10:1, 17, 38; 11:1; 13:30; 14:1, 25. Jerusalem is the goal: (9:51; 13:22, 33; 17:11; 18:35; 19:1, 11). See Donahue, *Gospel,* 127.

3   Lambrecht, *Astonished,* 59, asks whether dialogue and parable were together from the beginning; whether a specific dialogue in Jesus' life led to the story; or whether the combination was made later, possibly the result of Luke's redactional activity. He believes, p. 62–65, that Luke used Mark 12:28–34, where Jesus gives the answer and the two commandments are separate. Luke has changed these two points. Luke 18:18 contains the same question, and Jesus refers the young man to the commandments (see Mark 10:17). There are items in which Matthew's version (22:34–40) and Luke's agree over against Mark: shorter, no "Hear, O Israel", Jesus is addressed as "teacher", the question is put by a lawyer (not one of the scribes), and the question is a test. This suggests that Luke knew a 'Q' version, and in his redaction, drew on both sources. He believes that v. 28 is redactional ("do" and "live", as v. 25). Likewise, v. 29: the idea of self-justification occurs also (and only) in 16:15; the question in v. 29 is in tension with

the parable in v. 36. On p. 66, he concludes that the whole of the first dialogue is Luke's redaction, which introduces the parable. On p. 68, he suggests that the parable probably came to Luke without any specific indications as to the occasion on which it was spoken by Jesus. The background is probably not historical. Levine, *Stories*, 81, while referring to Luke's repackaging traditional material elsewhere, is open to the possibility that the current context "neatly fits what we can take to be Jesus' own agenda." Evans, *Luke*, 464, suggests that it is not impossible that Luke has removed Mark 12:28–34 to occupy this more prominent position, and reformulates it with the parable in mind. Marshall, *Luke*, 440–441, discusses these issues, observing that Luke knew Mark; he refers to the possibility of a 'Q' version. McBride, *Parables*, 156, notes that the question and double quotation were present in Mark and 'Q'; Luke used his editorial freedom to add the parable to the controversy. It is the conclusion of Meier, *A Marginal Jew*, 5: 207, that the parable and the introduction are thoroughly Lukan, and is not the reworking of a pre-redactional parable, and probably does not go back to the historical Jesus.

4   Bailey, *Through Peasant Eyes*, 34, suggests that here there are two dialogues; each comprises two questions and two answers; the sequence in each is lawyer, Jesus, lawyer, Jesus.

5   Green, *Luke*, 425.

6   Bailey, *Through Peasant Eyes*, 35.

7   An expert in Mosaic Law, a theologian (*nomikos*), asks the question. Byrne, *Hospitality*, 99, sees the question as hostile, to "test" Jesus, perhaps by getting him to suggest an alternative route than fulfilment of the Law. In Mark and Matthew, the question concerns the greatest commandment; it is Jesus who provides the answer. Johnson, *Luke*, 172, also sees it as hostile, not neutral. Carroll, *Luke*, 244, writes: "Hidden within what may be a sincere religious question, concerning the path to enduring life (pictured as property one inherits), is a challenge to Jesus' authority as a teacher, a test of his approach to the Torah." Green, *Luke*, 427, observes that Luke uses "lawyers", "teachers of the law" and "scribes" interchangeably. Priests also served as experts on the law when not performing their duties in the temple. On p. 428, he sees the lawyer as challenging Jesus; "the encounter as a whole is formulated along antagonistic lines." Levine, *Stories*, 83, notes that calling Jesus "Teacher" shows lack of respect for who Jesus really is (7:40; 8:49; 9:38); for Luke, "Lord" is better. Reid, *Parables*, 107, detects hostility (the verb *ekpeirazein* means "to test"). On p. 109–110, she notes how in Luke a whole spectrum of Jews address Jesus as "teacher"; the issue is whether he is competent to offer interpretations of the Law.

8   Eternal life is a prize to be won by meticulous observance of religious rules (Caird, *Luke*, 148). He wants duties limited and defined with rabbinic thoroughness. Levine, *Stories*, 82, notes Luke's antipathy towards lawyers (7:30; 11:45), but believes that the audience would probably have a positive attitude towards them. Evans, *Luke*, 465, notes that "eternal" does not mean everlasting, but the life characteristic of the coming (final) age.

9   Levine, *Stories*, 84, suggests he is thinking of a checklist rather than a way of life. The quote is from p. 85. On p. 86 she points out that Jews do not follow Torah to gain eternal life; they follow it in response to the gracious gift of the covenant. The lawyer

is also focusing on his own salvation rather than loving God and neighbour. He asks obnoxious questions to which he knows the answers already.

10   Levine, *Stories*, 87, notes that Jesus evades the trick and plays to the lawyer's ego, enabling him to display his knowledge in public.

11   "With all your mind" is an expansion of the Old Testament text. Levine, *Stories*, 89, notes that the combination was not original. To quote a verse recalls a whole chapter and context. McBride, *Parables*, 157, suggests that either the combination was a theological commonplace in rabbinic teaching, one which Jesus endorsed, or that the lawyer knew that Jesus originated it and was simply quoting what he had heard. Evans, *Luke*, 465, believes that it is still debated whether the combination of the two commandments comes from Jesus or had previously been made in Judaism. Luke runs the two together. Francis J. Moloney, *Love in the Gospel of John: An Exegetical, Theological and Literary Study* (Grand Rapids: Baker Academic, 2013), 2, maintains that the combination of the two texts most likely goes back to Jesus himself; he refers to Meier, *A Marginal Jew*, 4:478–646, who concludes that this is the case.

12   Levine, *Stories*, 91, notes that this refers not to a single action but an ongoing relationship; and the focus is on living now. Bailey, *Through Peasant Eyes*, 38, notes that "you shall live" means primarily the immediate future ("you shall come alive"); it can also refer to the next life.

13   Caird, *Luke*, 148.

14   Bailey, *Through Peasant Eyes*, 38.

15   Johnson, *Luke*, 172, refers to Luke's collapsing the two into one; on p. 174, he asserts that now love of neighbour has the same force as love of God.

16   Lambrecht, *Astonished*, 76, notes that the discussion leading up to the parable orientates our understanding; Jesus is not giving an example of mercy in general, but what "love of neighbour" involves.

17   Green, *Luke*, 429, sees the second question as a reminder of the initial antagonism; he is bent on self-justification. Levine, *Stories*, 90, states that "he proves his malevolent intent toward Jesus by posing another, even more inappropriate question."

18   McBride, *Luke*, 139, refers to a "cerebral clarification"; in *Parables*, 157, he notes that the meaning of "neighbour" was not uncontested in the tradition. Green, *Luke*, 426, believes the point of the lawyer is to calculate the identity of those to whom we need not show love.

19   Lev 19: 18, 34; 47:22–23. Levine, *Stories*, 92, notes that "proselyte" does not mean convert; it means someone who chooses to live among a different people and share their lives. For Leviticus, love has to extend beyond the people in one's group. She maintains, 93, that the question is misguided; it is really a polite way of asking "Who is not my neighbour?" The lawyer had not been listening to Jesus' words in the Sermon on the Mount (Matt 5:43–45; 6:32). Leviticus does not require Jews to love their enemy.

20   Green, *Luke*, 429, observes that different attitudes to foreign intrusions (Hellenistic and Roman) developed into a fractured social context in which boundaries distinguished not only Jew and gentile but also between Jewish factions. Marshall, *Luke*, 444, suggests that there was a tendency among some Pharisees to exclude the ordinary people too.

21   Byrne, *Hospitality*, 100; see also Levine, *Stories*, 81.

22   As does Johnson, *Luke*, 175, and Green, *Luke*, 424 (his heading). Evans, *Luke*, 467, believes that Luke is using a more literary source than usual.

23   The person is not identified; he is everyman. Marshall, *Luke*, 447, notes that the audience would presume he was a Jew; also, McBride, *Parables*, 159; Bailey, *Through Peasant Eyes*, 42.

24   Jerusalem is 2,500 feet (762 m) above sea level, Jericho 800 (244 m) below. (See 2 Sam 15:23–16:14; 2 Kings 25:4). Evans, *Luke*, 470, comments that half the priests resided there; it was the "chief priestly city". Similarly, Marshall, *Luke*, 448.

25   The term (*lēstēs*) is used in 19:46 and 22:52; also, Mark 11:15–19; John 10:7–8; in Mark and Matthew the men crucified with Jesus are called by this term. It means member of an armed gang; they tend to act without mercy. Reid, *Parables*, 111, notes that because of exploitation of the peasants and landless labourers by the ruling elite, the latter were often the targets of social banditry.

26   Bailey, *Through Peasant Eyes*, 42; Donahue, *Gospel*, 130; Green, *Luke*, 429. Levine, *Stories*, 96, has some interesting comments about modern allegorical (mis)interpretations!

27   McBride, *Parables*, 159.

28   Byrne, *Hospitality*, 100, notes the threefold pattern which cumulatively builds up expectation in the hearer. Bailey, *Through Peasant Eyes*, 41, mentions the pattern of the action: in each case the verbs are "come, do, go". Johnson, *Luke*, 173, observes that priests and Levites were not among the wealthy aristocracy, but did symbolically represent the leadership of the people; they were restricted by purity regulations that limited their contacts with others. Levine, *Stories*, 8, refers to stereotypical negative interpretations that go beyond the justified critique of their failure to act. The priest and Levite are not elite; they may have had neither wealth nor status; their positions were inherited.

29   Carroll, *Luke*, 245, agrees. The text is not explicit about this.

30   Bailey, *Through Peasant Eyes*, 43, holds that the natural assumption of the parable is that he is riding, given his social status. Otherwise, he could have given some form of first aid, but would have had to wait for someone with an animal to come along. The Samaritan too has a mount.

31   Bailey, *Through Peasant Eyes*, 44–45. Byrne's view, *Hospitality*, 100, is that the first two pass by "to avoid the defilement from contact with the dead—or soon to be dead—which would prevent them, according to the Law, from carrying out their religious duties." McBride, *Luke*, 140, sees this as a possibility. Johnson, *Luke*, 175, notes the shock that Jews esteemed for their place in the people and dedicated to holiness before the Lord would allow considerations of personal safety or even a concern for ritual purity to justify them not even crossing the road to look. They cannot be bothered. Green, *Luke*, 430, is doubtful: they have completed their temple duties; they had an obligation to bury a neglected corpse. The fact is that they do nothing. Lambrecht, *Astonished*, 71, sees the ritual purity line as unconvincing. Levine, *Stories*, 99, dubs this view "pervasive" (with examples) and "misguided". Torah expects corpses to be respected and buried (Tobit 1:16–20). The priest should have checked; if he found him alive, he should have helped him. Besides, he was going away from Jerusalem and temple. Marshall, *Luke*, 448, is sceptical about the ritual ideas; "it is the heartlessness of the priest which is at issue".

32   Carroll, *Luke*, 245, sees this as possible, Marshall, *Luke*, 448, the simplest explanation. Carroll thinks it unlikely that they are concerned to avoid ritual impurity. It is not their motives but their actions that judge them. McBride, *Parables*, 160, mentions fear as a possibility, or concerns with ritual impurity, or the advice of Ben Sirach.

33   Marshall, *Luke*, 448. On p. 449, he suggests the same kind of motives were in his mind.

34   Bailey, *Through Peasant Eyes*, 46. Reid, *Parables*, 113, suggests the Levite would follow the priest's lead. Levine, *Stories*, 100, notes the distinction between priests and Levites regarding purity laws to this day; but Samaritans were also bound by laws concerning corpse contamination. On p. 101, she quotes Josephus who sees Jews as expected to attend to a corpse on the roadside; burying the dead is an important commandment. Luke is not interested in purity laws here; when he is, he mentions Pharisees and scribes.

35   Donahue, *Gospel*, 131–132. He notes the rhythm "when he sees, he passed by on the other side", the final verb changing with the Samaritan (has compassion). See and have compassion occurs also in 7:13 and 15:20. Green, *Luke*, 430, notes that they had high status because of their birth; they were legitimated by the world of the temple; their worldview was concerned with status. They would be evaluated as righteous and holy.

36   Levine, *Stories*, 102. They were thinking about themselves, not the man in the ditch.

37   Lambrecht, *Astonished*, 62.

38   Levine, *Stories*, 102, reminds us of the "rule of three"; the first two anticipate the third. Similarly, McBride, *Parables*, 162, "a storytelling device common in popular tales". Tannehill, *Luke*, 183, refers to a "folkloric triad".

39   Evans, *Luke*, 469.

40   Donahue, *Gospel*, 130; Carroll, *Luke*, 245; Levine, *Stories*, 105–111. On p. 111 she refers to the 2 Chron 28:8–15 text; as does McBride, *Parables*, 159; (in the text, the Samaritans help the Jews; many aspects of the description of their help are present in the parable). See also Raymond E. Brown, *The Gospel according to John*, Anchor Bible, 2 vols (London: Geoffrey Chapman, 1971), 1:170; Bailey, *Jesus Through Middle Eastern Eyes*, 203; Reid, *Parables*, 113–114. For a good history of the Jewish-Samaritan relationship, see McBride, *Parables*, 152–155.

41   Donahue, *Gospel*, 131.

42   Donahue, *Gospel*, 132. Green, *Luke*, 431, notes that what distinguishes him is not Jew/Samaritan, religious/merchant, but his compassion, leading to action, in face of their inaction. In n. 125, he observes that the verb is the centre of the unit (68 words before, 67 after). Levine, *Stories*, 104, says that it signals the drive to restore wholeness.

43   Levine, *Stories*, 112, notes that the man has money, freedom to travel, the ability to find lodging, and leverage with the innkeeper. He provides long-term care and shows trust. Reid, *Parables*, 115, suggests he may have been a merchant in oil and wine; both were commonly used medicinally.

44   Bailey, *Through Peasant Eyes*, 49. Donahue, *Gospel*, 131, notes that oil and wine are elements of the daily temple sacrifice. Hos 6:6: "I desire mercy and not sacrifice". Isa 58:5–9 suggests that true religious observance consists of deeds of mercy and loving

kindness. The priest and Levite knew all about pouring wine and oil in liturgy, but did not show mercy.

45   Bailey, *Through Peasant Eyes*, 51. Green, *Luke*, 432, notes that inns had a negative image; the monetary arrangement could lead to extortion.

46   Bailey, *Through Peasant Eyes*, 51–53.

47   Bailey, *Through Peasant Eyes*, 53–54. Donahue, *Gospel*, 133, notes that it is not enough to enter the world of the neighbour with care and compassion; one must leave it in such a way that the neighbour is given freedom along with the help.

48   Caird, *Luke*, 148–149.

49   Green, *Luke*, 431.

50   Lambrecht, *Astonished*, 57–58, notes the shift of meaning, the change from neighbour as object to neighbour as subject. Later, 67, he supposes that the original parable ended with a neutral question, like "Which of the three showed mercy to the man who fell among robbers?" Luke probably introduced the use of the second person, and mention of "neighbour", in order to adapt the conclusion to his introduction. He therefore brought the parable to a climax with the theme of 'becoming a neighbour', and does so due to the influence of the parable that concerns the active expression of compassion. 37b is also probably redactional.

51   Carroll, *Luke*, 246, does not agree that the scholar is reluctant to credit a hated Samaritan with neighbourly love. The emphasis is on performance. He notes the frequent usage of the verb "to do" during the whole episode, as does Green, *Luke*, 425. Levine, *Stories*, 113, notes that the lawyer is unable to voice the hated name "Samaritan"; similarly, McBride, *Parables*, 164. Reid, 116, notes the significance of the term "mercy" (*eleos*): "by doing mercy, God's people most faithfully keep the covenantal law."

52   Levine, *Stories*, 113, states that the issue for Jesus is not the "who" but the "what", not the identity but the action. The lawyer speaks of "mercy" rather than compassion; the latter is felt in the gut and needs to be enacted in the body. She notes the use of mercy in the Infancy Narrative.

53   McBride, *Luke*, 139. Carroll, *Luke*, 244, writes that Jesus explodes the notion that the imperative of loving action has boundaries that include some persons (kin, friends, ethnic group) but exclude others (outsiders, enemies); he radicalises the twofold love command that is at the heart of the Law of Moses (though in a manner anticipated by the command to "love the alien as yourself" in Lev 19:34).

54   Compassion is found in 1:78 (concerning God's covenant faithfulness); 7:13; 6:17–49 (where Jesus eliminates the lines drawn between friends and enemies). Green, *Luke*, 427, notes that this could destabilise the world of the lawyer and challenge him to embrace the new world propagated through Jesus' ministry.

55   Donahue, *Gospel*, 134. McBride, *Parables*, 164, "neighbour means possessing the human capacity to identify with the one in need and meet his need with mercy." Neighbourhood does not create love; love creates neighbourliness.

56   Walter Kasper, *Pope Francis' Revolution of Tenderness and Love*, trans. William Madges (New York: Paulist Press, 2015), observes that for Pope Paul VI, the example of the Good Samaritan was the model of spirituality for Vatican II.

57   Byrne, *Hospitality*, 102, shares my experience. He also doubts whether here

Luke's main point is to say something—positive or negative—about the status of women.

58   Donahue, *Gospel*, 134–135. He describes this story as a parabolic narrative.

59   For Green, *Luke*, 433, the basic theme or issue is welcome.

60   Barbara E. Reid, *A Retreat with Luke: Stepping Out on the Word of God* (Cincinnati: St Anthony Messenger Press, 2000), 92.

61   Marshall, *Luke*, 451, notes the view that she may have been a widow; she is the mistress of the household. Byrne, *Hospitality*, 102, sees her as the dominant figure; Caird, *Luke*, 150, the central figure, "a stronger figure and more mature disciple."

62   Johnson, *Luke*, 173; see 7:38; 8:35, 41; 17:16. Green, *Luke*, 435, speaks of her "submissiveness". Tannehill, *Luke*, 186, believes she is not portrayed as passive, for she has taken bold action in leaving a serving role to listen to Jesus.

63   Green, *Luke*, 435, suggests that normally women were excluded from learning. N.Tom Wright, *Surprised by Scripture: Engaging Contemporary Issues* (London: SPCK, 2014), 71, notes that Mary is sitting in the male part of the house; this was the real problem for Martha; she had cut across one of the most basic social conventions. Jesus declares that she is right to do so! Reid, *Retreat*, 96, holds that Jesus was not the only Jew who thought women should be allowed to study the Law.

64   *Perispaomai*. See Marshall, *Luke*, 452, and 1 Cor 7:35. Johnson, *Luke*, 173, observes that her being overwhelmed is an objective fact, not a case of neurotic obsessiveness. Wright, *Luke*, 130, points out that the main problem is that Mary is behaving like a man, crossing an important social boundary; the kitchen was the space where women belonged. Tannehill, *Luke*, 186, suggests Martha is trying to force her sister back into the expected woman's role.

65   Green, *Luke*, 437, notes Martha's threefold use of "me"; "she is concerned to engage his assistance in her plans, not to learn from him his." Similarly, Resseguie, *Spiritual Landscape*, 84, refers to her "self-referential and self-absorbed posture" which prevents her from focusing on Jesus. She accuses him of failing to help *her* achieve *her* goals, and seeks to tell *him* what *he* must say.

66   12:13; see 15:28–29.

67   8:14; see 12;29; 21:34.

68   Johnson, *Luke*, 174: the verbs are *merimnaō* and *thorybazō* (make an uproar like a crowd in an assembly.) Resseguie, *Spiritual Landscape*, 85, observes that the doubling of her name and alliteration draw attention to her anxious behaviour (*Martha, Martha, merimnas*). Marshall, *Luke*, 453, opts for "to be troubled, distracted".

69   McBride, *Luke*, 142–143 ("a gastronomic extravaganza"). Byrne, *Hospitality*, 103–104, notes that, as in 7:36–50, Jesus first admonishes the critic and then defends the one attacked. Green, *Luke*, 437, observes that Martha's behaviour is negatively assessed, Mary's positively. Mary need no longer be defined by socially determined roles; the priority is to attend to the guest.

70   Caird, *Luke*, 150. Green, *Luke*, 434, states that the manner of Martha's practices exposes them as ill adapted to the sort of hospitality that Jesus seeks. "The welcome Jesus seeks is not epitomized in distracted, worrisome domestic performance, but in attending to this guest whose very presence is a disclosure of the divine plan."

71   Caird, *Luke*, 149, notes that there are five variants; he maintains that reference

to the one or few things needful ought to be omitted, given the evidence of the western text. "Martha, Martha, you are troubled; Mary has chosen ..." This removes comparison between the sisters; Mary is defended, not praised to the disparagement of Martha. Byrne, *Hospitality*, 103, n. 8, prefers "only one"; likewise, Johnson, *Luke*, 174: in hospitality, the only thing necessary is to pay attention to the guests. Evans, *Luke*, 473, believes the original may be: "Martha, Martha, you are anxious and troubled about many things, but one thing is needful." Marshall, *Luke*, 454, finally opts for one; Luke probably understood the saying in a spiritual sense.

72   Johnson, *Luke*, 175; Resseguie, *Spiritual Landscape*, 85. Several commentators stress that active and contemplative styles of spirituality are not being compared or evaluated here: Caird, *Luke*, 149; Green, *Luke*, 433; Marshall, *Luke*, 451. Thus McBride, *Luke*, 142, calls this kind of interpretation "a cartoon".

73   McBride, *Luke*, 142, states that it is about the primacy of the word of God in the Christian life.

74   Tannehill, *Luke*, 187, notes the importance of hospitality towards missionaries in the early Church; the story cautions against allowing it to distract one from the message and the community's real purpose.

75   Carroll, *Luke*, 248; see 6:46–49; 11:28.

76   Donahue, *Gospel*, 136–137, linking the story of the sisters with the parable of the Good Samaritan.

77   8:21; 11:28; 12:47.

78   Carroll, *Luke*, 247.

79   Byrne, *Hospitality*,103.

80   Resseguie, *Spiritual Landscape*, 85.

81   Fitzmyer, *Luke*, 2:892, notes that a *diakonia* that bypasses the word is one that will never have lasting character.

Chapter Nine
On Riches and Poverty

In the last chapter, we considered the theme of "Listening and Doing". This chapter encourages us to do just that, as we hear the words of Jesus about riches and poverty offered in the parable of the Rich Fool (12:13–21) and its sequel, which concerns trust in God's providential care (12:22–34). This will be followed by a further parable on the topic: Dives and Lazarus (16:19–31). One of Luke's concerns with regard to the Christian community of which he was part was the danger posed by wealth and a mistaken attitude towards possessions; the issue of the relationship between possessions and discipleship was of singular importance to him. This passage occurs quite early in Jesus' journey to Jerusalem, after sayings concerning hypocrisy on the one hand and fearless confession on the other.

The Introductory Incident (12:13–15)

Jesus finds himself surrounded by a large crowd, so numerous that they are trampling on one another (12:1). Jesus has been focusing his attention on instructing his disciples when someone from the crowd suddenly interrupts him. He addresses Jesus respectfully as "teacher", and voices a problem that he wants Jesus to sort out:

> Someone in the crowd said to him, "Teacher, tell my brother to divide the family inheritance with me." But he said to him, "Friend, who set me to be a judge or arbitrator over you?" And he said to them, "Take care! Be on your guard against all kinds of greed; for one's life does not consist in the abundance of possessions."

The issue seems to be a dispute over the family estate, and it was not unusual for plaintiffs to bring their case to a religious leader, who was knowledgeable concerning the Law and skilled in a wide range of legal matters, and to seek arbitration. The situation seems to be that on the death of their father, two sons have been left an inheritance in the form of joint ownership of an undivided property; property was always a sensitive issue in that culture. It was considered desirable for heirs to live together and keep the family property intact.[1] The petitioner, probably the younger of the two, wishes to enjoy his portion separately. The rabbis considered this kind of arrangement to be acceptable. However, it appears that this man is not really seeking arbitration; he has already decided what his rights are and what he wants. Basically, he is telling Jesus to carry out his plan; he is attempting to use Jesus to secure what he sees to be his right.

Jesus is unwilling to become involved, replying: "My friend, who appointed me your judge or the arbiter of your claims?"[2] The term "friend" or "man", which is confined to Luke in the Synoptics, is generally somewhat aloof, brusque or harsh, indicating a level of disapproval. There is clearly a broken relationship, and the man seems to be asking Jesus to finalise it. But Jesus does not promote division, nor see his role in terms of legal involvement.[3] In turning to address the wider audience, Jesus highlights the real underlying issue, an issue which can affect the lives of everyone: "Watch, be on your guard against avarice of any kind, for life does not consist in possessions, even when someone has more than he needs." The audience is wider than the two brothers. Jesus' words pinpoint the root problem; he identifies the reason why the two brothers were distanced in the first place: it is the result of greed, avarice, covetousness, the insatiable desire to have more.[4] This is a vice "that turns its victim away from both God and neighbour."[5]

After the warning comes the maxim, that human life does not consist in an abundance of possessions ("in what is more than enough").[6] "It is not the mere possession of material goods that will spell the downfall of the rich man, but his constant desire for more which leads to surplus possession, which today we might call 'conspicuous consumption'—the modern world's insatiable desire for a higher standard of living."[7] The genuine aliveness of a human being does not depend on the abundance or superfluity of one's material possessions. "It is much more important to *be* rather than to *have*—to be one who listens to God's word and acts on it than to live in an unnecessary abundance of wealth."[8] The saying leads into the parable and suggests its meaning.

The Parable of The Rich Fool (12:16–21)

Then he told them a parable: "The land of a rich man produced abundantly. And he thought to himself, 'What should I do, for I have no place to store my crops?' Then he said, 'I will do this: I will pull down my barns and build larger ones, and there I will store all my grain and my goods. And I will say to my soul, Soul, you have ample goods laid up for many years; relax, eat, drink, be merry.' But God said to him, 'You fool! This very night your life is being demanded of you. And the things you have prepared, whose will they be?' So, it is with those who store up treasures for themselves but are not rich towards God."

The parable illustrates the wisdom saying.[9] The man in the story is already extremely rich. There is no intimation of how his wealth was acquired. Without any effort on his part, his wealth is increased by a bumper harvest. This windfall he does not need. It does, however, present an unexpected logistical problem. That is the basic scenario. The parable continues in the form of soliloquy, a literary feature frequent in Luke.[10] It does not occur to the man that he might thank God for this stroke of good fortune; nor does the possibility of sharing the produce with those in need cross his mind. The focus of his attention and calculating is how best to preserve it all for himself. The pressing problem is the lack of storage space. Normally in that culture a man would discuss such matters at considerable length with his family, friends, peers and village community. This man ponders in total isolation, talking to himself, trusting no one.[11] The word "my" punctuates his musing, which becomes "a monologue of obsession with himself."[12] His wealth imprisons him.

The solution, which emerges from his pondering, is to pull down the barns that he has and build bigger ones in which to store his abundant crops; this would also be an investment.[13] Continuing to talk to himself, he suggests that the best way forward is to take things easy, to eat and drink and have a really good time. After all, he has copious supplies for many years to come.[14] His smug security is interrupted, presumably some time later, by his God, whom he has excised from his life and plans: "You fool! This very night your life is being demanded of you. And the things you have prepared, whose will they be?"

God does not usually enter so explicitly into Jesus' parables.[15] The word that Luke chooses for "fool" suggests being devoid of spirit, emotions or mind.[16] "This very night" is emphatic and is sudden and shocking. The word translated "demand" is often used in the context of collecting a loan. In Jewish thought, an individual was a living person because of God's creative goodness, and so one's earthly existence could be pictured as a loan to be repaid; God now wishes that loan to be returned.[17] The interrogative "whose will it be" links with the question that initially gave rise to the parable. The rich man's covetousness has so isolated him that he has not made provision for his heirs, which will create a situation not unlike that with which the parable began. Isolated in the midst of his plenty, he will die utterly alone and will bequeath to his family a legacy of bitter dispute over the inheritance.[18] Despite his wealth, his life is empty and bankrupt. He dies in the most abject poverty.

To the parable is appended an application: "So it is when someone stores up treasure for himself instead of becoming rich in the sight of God." The alternatives are stark. Amassing property and wealth, relying on the security and power that this can bring, is a mindless and worthless exercise.[19] What really matters is to live in a way that is pleasing to God. Riches of this kind birth a new form of security and are of everlasting worth; death cannot take them away. For Luke, this means a response of faith and the using of possessions in accordance with faith, which means sharing them generously with others rather than accumulating them for oneself only.[20] As happens frequently with the parables of Jesus, we are not informed how the two brothers or the crowd responded.

Sayings About Anxiety and Trust in Providence (12:22–32)

Jesus now switches his focus to the disciples, and in a beautiful little discourse highlights human anxiety and God's generous care:[21]

> He said to his disciples, "Therefore I tell you, do not worry about your life, what you will eat, or about your body, what you will wear. For life is more than food, and the body more than clothing. Consider the ravens: they neither sow nor reap, they have neither storehouse nor barn, and yet God feeds them. Of how much more value are you than the birds! And can any of you by worrying add a single hour to your span of life? If then you are not able to do so small a thing as that, why do you worry about the rest? Consider the lilies, how they grow: they neither toil nor spin; yet I tell you, even Solomon in all his glory was not clothed like one of these. But if God so clothes the grass of the field, which is alive today and tomorrow is thrown into the oven, how much more will he clothe you—you of little faith! And do not keep striving for what you are to eat and what you are to drink, and do not keep worrying. For it is the nations of the world that strive after all these things, and your Father knows that you need them. Instead, strive for his kingdom, and these things will be given to you as well.
>
> "Do not be afraid, little flock, for it is your Father's good pleasure to give you the kingdom. Sell your possessions, and give alms. Make purses for yourselves that do not wear out, an unfailing treasure in heaven, where no thief comes near and no moth destroys. For where your treasure is, there your heart will be also."

With his peasant village background, Jesus is aware that as human beings we are concerned about life (food) and the body (clothing), and that this concern can develop into anxiety and worry. In fact, anxiety and fear can often lead to the tendency to accumulate, which was criticised in the parable. He encourages his disciples to avoid this, for life, which is God's gift, has further dimensions than food and clothing, necessary though these may be. Anxiety can cause us to lose sight of these deeper aspects of authentic existence. With a poetic flourish, Jesus turns to nature to illustrate his point, inviting his disciples to use their imagination and learn from the ravens, which neither sow crops nor reap the harvest. Unlike the man in the parable, they have no storehouses or barns, but God takes care of them.[22] The disciples are worth far more than the birds of the sky.[23] God will take even greater care of them. Jesus moves to a different area of human anxiety, the moment of death. For all our worry and anxiety, we cannot add even a small quota of time to our lifespan; in fact, anxiety can bring on premature old age (Sir 30:24)! However much we worry, we cannot postpone the moment of death.[24]

Switching imagery, Jesus turns to the flowers of the countryside. The lilies grow; they need not spin nor weave. But even the renowned King Solomon, in all his royal splendour, could not match the beauty of the Galilean crocus or purple anemone.[25] Such clothing in rich colour and beauty is God's work, God's gift, and this even though the wild flowers blossom for only a short time before being cut down and used to heat the oven. If God is so painstaking in his creative care for these fleeting flowers, then how thorough and all-embracing will be his care for the disciples, despite their lack of trust. To see God's providential hand at work in nature and in ordinary life requires a faith vision; Jesus is inviting his audience to embrace that vision more completely.

The earlier theme of preoccupation with food and drink (no longer with clothing) returns, with an underlining of the level of anxious concern, as Jesus categorically and emphatically enjoins the abandoning of all worry. Human beings need food and clothing and shelter, they look for security, but being overanxious about all this can divert from life's main purpose. It is natural for the gentiles of the world, who have no knowledge of God, to worry about these things. But the disciples must not be like this, for they know God, and God is "Father", and God is well aware of their needs. Rather than focusing time and energy on material concerns, becoming obsessive and anxious about things that are perishable, what really matters, what is of crucial importance, is commitment to furthering the Kingdom, "God's restorative project".[26] God will see to the provision of everything else; they can rest secure about that.[27]

Imagery and focus shift again, as Jesus with great gentleness addresses his disciples as his "little flock", assuring them that the Father has chosen to give them the Kingdom. Therefore, there is no need for them to fear. The shepherd imagery of the Bible races into view. God is the shepherd, Israel is God's flock (Ezek 34:11–24).[28] That shepherd role is made present through Jesus, as he reaches out in compassion and goes out in search of the lost. The disciples, by God's free gift, have been caught up in the burgeoning reality of God's reign through their association with Jesus. This liberates from fear and anxiety and alters the complexion of everything. Imagery of treasures, wealth and possessions returns, as Jesus exhorts them to sell their possessions and give to people who are poor. This becomes a less daunting prospect because of their trust in God and God's care.[29]

With earthly treasures, there is always the threat of burglary, which can cause anxiety. Possessions are perishable. Moths attack expensive clothes and destroy cloth purses containing cash. Security cannot reside there. Finally, Jesus sums up: "For wherever your treasure is, that is where your heart will be too." Amassing earthly treasure is an indication of a heart distant from God, whereas the seeking of heavenly treasure, by making God central to life and being generous to others, indicates a God-focused heart and life. The statement is a forceful ending to the whole section.[30]

The Rich Man and Lazarus (16:19–31)

This parable, found only in Luke's Gospel, follows the three parables of seeking and finding (15:1–32), which we shall examine later in Chapter Ten, the parable of the dishonest manager (16:1–13) and a number of disparate sayings of Jesus (16:14–18). It is the only parable of Jesus in which one of the characters has a proper name, Lazarus, meaning "God helps" or "has helped"; Dives, which has for centuries been treated as a name, simply means "wealthy man". The parable can be understood as a narrative expression of the beatitude and woe concerning poverty and riches, which is found in the Sermon on the Plain (6:20, 24), a role reversal that echoes the *Magnificat* (1:51–53). As it stands, the story is addressed to the Pharisees who, alleged to be lovers of money, have ridiculed Jesus because he has emphasised the impossibility of serving both God and wealth (16:14).[31]

> There was a rich man who was dressed in purple and fine linen and who feasted sumptuously every day. And at his gate lay a poor man named Lazarus, covered with sores, who longed to satisfy his hunger with what fell from the rich man's table; even the dogs would come and lick his sores. The poor man died and was

carried away by the angels to be with Abraham. The rich man also died and was buried. In Hades, where he was being tormented, he looked up and saw Abraham far away with Lazarus by his side. He called out, "Father Abraham, have mercy on me, and send Lazarus to dip the tip of his finger in water and cool my tongue; for I am in agony in these flames." But Abraham said, "Child, remember that during your lifetime you received your good things, and Lazarus in like manner evil things; but now he is comforted here, and you are in agony. Besides all this, between you and us a great chasm has been fixed, so that those who might want to pass from here to you cannot do so, and no one can cross from there to us." He said, "Then, father, I beg you to send him to my father's house— for I have five brothers—that he may warn them, so that they will not also come into this place of torment." Abraham replied, "They have Moses and the prophets; they should listen to them." He said, "No, father Abraham; but if someone goes to them from the dead, they will repent." He said to him, "If they do not listen to Moses and the prophets, neither will they be convinced even if someone rises from the dead."

The story takes the form of a two-act drama; the action takes place in two phases and two locations. It concerns two individuals alive in this world, and then alive after death in the next. The human players are described in vivid, graphic, perhaps exaggerated terms. One, who remains anonymous, is extremely wealthy. This finds expression in his highly fashionable dress: he habitually wears expensive purple outer garments or woollen mantles, purple being the colour of royalty and the elite, and also fine linen, usually a luxury import.[32] "White garments under a purple robe—this was the sign of the highest opulence."[33] It finds expression also in his lifestyle, especially his dining in sumptuous style every single day. He seems the epitome of wealth and self-indulgence.[34] His counterpart is a poor man who has been left (literally thrown down or 'dumped') outside the gateway of his mansion, a destitute beggar, probably disabled, clearly visible.[35] He is covered with sores, possibly ulcers, and obviously quite ill.[36] He is also hungry and longs to eat the scraps that might fall from the rich man's table, indicating the pita bread that the banquet guests used as napkins and then threw on the floor for the dogs to eat. His longing goes unrequited. The dogs scavenging in the neighbourhood come to lick his sores, adding to his indignity.[37]

The scene is thus set. The original audience would not necessarily consider the rich man as evil and Lazarus as virtuous. Abundant possessions were often seen as a gift from God, and the condition of people like Lazarus was popularly interpreted as an expression of God's disfavour. The rich man, however, is aware of Lazarus but fails to respond to his needs and offer help. "The 'gate' which should be a public space for rendering justice, particularly compassionate justice for the vulnerable (Amos 5:12, 15), has become a site for dehumanising injustice."[38]

Death suddenly intervenes for both of them; their situations are dramatically reversed. This is the turning point of the parable. This time it is Lazarus who is mentioned first. Without mention of a funeral, he is carried immediately by angels into Abraham's embrace.[39] The imagery of angels accompanying a soul to the next life is unusual, and is a later development in Judaism (150 CE).[40] The other aspect of the image, Abraham's embrace or bosom, is found only in Luke. It could refer to a child on Abraham's lap and denotes great intimacy. Or it could denote the place of honour next to Abraham in the heavenly banquet.[41] Marshall opts for a combination of the two ideas.[42] A third option is derived from the ancient biblical idea of being gathered to one's people at death.[43] Abraham is the father of the Jewish people. It is not because of any virtue that Lazarus is welcomed, but simply that his poor and neglected condition is the object of God's action.[44] The parable may comfort the poor, but it is primarily designed to challenge the rich.[45]

The rich man has a decent burial, as would be expected, but, surprisingly, he is now to be found in Hades, a place of torment. Instead of his gourmet feasting, he is racked with thirst; instead of fashionable clothes, he is engulfed by flames.[46] In the midst of his suffering, he catches sight of Lazarus in Abraham's bosom. So, somewhat audaciously addressing Abraham, the model of hospitality to strangers, as "Father Abraham", presuming to emphasise his status as a member of Abraham's family, he asks, ironically, as an expression of mercy[47] that Lazarus should be sent to dip the tip of his finger in water and cool his tongue. It is he who is now doing the begging, and it is his longing that remains unfulfilled. For him, Lazarus is no stranger; he knows his identity and still selfishly thinks that he is there to serve his needs! In reply, Abraham renders explicit the divine reversal promised in the Sermon on the Plain: "Child, remember that during your lifetime you received your good things, and Lazarus in like manner evil things; but now he is comforted here, and you are in agony."

The term "son" or "child" could be merely formal, or it could connote Abraham's acknowledgement of kinship. However, as John the Baptist had intimated, being a descendant of Abraham carried no guarantee if not accompanied by conversion (3:8). Abraham goes on to elaborate the changed circumstances, the new situation, indicating the chasm or gulf separating the two sides, which prevents anyone from crossing either way.[48] In life, there was a gate that separated them, a gate which the rich man chose not to open in order to help Lazarus; now in death, there is a yawning chasm separating the two men, fixed by God, and this is irreversible.[49]

Some scholars are of the opinion that the original parable could have ended here, and consider the rest a Lukan addendum.[50] The rich man is condemned because of his failure to respond to the needs of Lazarus at his gate; this is to neglect the demands of the Torah. However, as Levine puts it, "Jesus is just as capable of speaking of Moses and the Prophets and post-mortem judgement as any other Jew."[51] The parable text continues with a dialogue between the rich man and Abraham. Whereas his first request had been to ask Abraham to send Lazarus to his own aid, Dives now requests that Lazarus be sent to warn his brothers, who probably enjoy a similar lavish and selfish lifestyle, not to continue to neglect the Law.[52] Repentance is, theoretically, still a possibility for them. He implies that if he had had sufficient information, he would have acted differently. The situation envisages the five brothers living at home on the family estate, which has not been broken up.[53] Dives is still arrogant and has an exalted sense of his privileged position. He still presumes to treat Lazarus as a lackey to serve his own ends.

Abraham[54] replies, not without irony, that his brothers have Moses and the prophets, that is, the scriptures that contain prescriptions about care for the poor, the orphan, widow and stranger, which is a fundamental obligation of covenantal fidelity.[55] "Let them listen to them." Listening is a favourite Lukan motif; the verb includes a positive response of obedient action (10:25–37). The rich man is aware that his brothers do not give serious thought to what the scriptures say. More is required. He suggests that they would be moved to repentance by someone returning from the dead, a special envoy. But Abraham rejects the request: "If they will not listen either to Moses or to the prophets, they will not be convinced even if someone should rise from the dead." The Torah is abundantly clear. If the brothers have no intention of serving God by response to his existing revelation, the return to them of Lazarus will not suddenly work a transformation. "Miracles in themselves cannot melt stony hearts."[56]

In the text, there is a significant change of wording, in that it is no longer someone "returning from the dead" who will fail to convince but someone "rising from the dead". Here, the technical Christian language of resurrection is used, indicating an allusion to the 'Risen One'.[57] The risen Jesus, as we shall see in the final chapter of this book, twice explains to his disciples how his passion and death were predicted by Moses and the prophets. He was comfortable referring his audience to them. But Luke has another audience in mind, and, both warning and encouraging, "directs the final verse to those in his community who, by neglecting the poor, do not heed the teaching nor follow the example of Jesus who rose from the dead."[58]

Reflections

This material dealing with the teaching of Jesus concerning wealth and poverty is as challenging for us today as it must have been for his original hearers, who were perhaps becoming accustomed to a more settled and rather bourgeois lifestyle. It is also carefully nuanced. We have already seen the demands that Jesus makes on those wishing to follow him and share in his mission in the radical terms of leaving homes and family and possessions. But other followers, like Levi and Zacchaeus, do not dispossess themselves completely, and generous women use their wealth to support Jesus and his disciples during the ministry. "Luke does not provide a monochrome picture of poverty and wealth, a quality of the narrative that hints at some measure of heterogeneity within Luke's earliest communities of readers with regard to wealth and social status."[59] The texts of this chapter serve as a warning of potential dangers and an exhortation to compassionate and generous concern for those in need by sharing resources.

In the first parable and its introductory setting, Jesus highlights the basic human tendency to want more, for which we tend to use the terminology of greed, acquisitiveness, covetousness, an obsession with possessions. Others see it as market forces, economic astuteness. However, it is a pervasive fashion of our day, a preoccupation fostered by media bombardment and extremely clever advertising, fuelling desires that soon become needs and compulsions. This is the world of the more, bigger, better, faster, latest, and of upward mobility. It is a world with a highly developed and sophisticated focus on 'having': competitive, aggressive, individualistic. This compulsion can be operative at all levels: individuals, corporate entities and businesses, nationally and internationally. Though the rich fool in the parable was a farmer, as Fitzmyer points out, he stands for human beings seduced by "every form of greed", whether peasant or statesman, craftsman or lawyer, nurse or doctor, secretary or professor,[60] banker, politician or churchman. This is our world; we are all part of it; aspects of this mentality and way of living inevitably have an influence on all of us. "The domain ruled by wealth is a dangerous habitat, for attachment to wealth entangles one in concerns that run counter to the values and commitments of the realm of God."[61] Jesus would wish us to be alert and self-critical here, to be aware of our dreams and tendencies as we plan and shop and celebrate.

As with the rich fool and with Dives, too, obsession with wealth and the power, security and comfort it may bring, can lead to the sidelining of God; God is airbrushed out of life's equation. God is no longer needed in our human endeavours; God is an irrelevance. In his sayings after the first parable, Jesus reintroduces God into the frame. With remarkable realism and common sense, he addresses our fundamental anxieties about food and clothes, our basic concern about our survival and well-being as human beings. This he had lived with each day in his village community. He was aware that it is often anxiety and fear that lie at the root of our preoccupation with possessing, before other factors intervene. Jesus urges us to keep things in perspective, to get our priorities right, to develop a real and deep trust in God's providential and loving care for each of us. He would also wish us to realise that the demands of the Kingdom are paramount.

Possessions in themselves are not evil. Biblical tradition understands wealth as blessings flowing from God's love.[62] It is the selfish amassing of them, the insatiable thirst for more, which is reprehensible. The rich man in the first parable never thought of using his goods for others. Dives was blind to the needy person outside his gate. As we look around our town, our country or our world, and see the widening gap between rich and poor, the increasing number of folk living on the streets, sleeping on park benches, the increase in food banks, rising destitution, shanty towns in other parts of the world, institutionalised and structural injustice and oppression, we have to stop and think; we have a responsibility. Contrasting extremes is a breathtaking phenomenon of our world. Luke wanted the members of his community to stop and think too. Wealth, understood as God's gift, has been given also for the benefit of the poor and needy, not for the economic benefit and status enhancement of its possessors alone. Luke was aware that inequalities can be destructive of community. Jesus announces Good News to the poor; his Kingdom dream includes the liberation of the oppressed, the banishing of injustice, the sharing of goods, compassionate outreach to the needy; it is a message of hope.[63] "Luke thus places many twenty-first-century readers in an uncomfortable position among those opposed to—and opposed by—the values, commitments and practices of the divine realm as Jesus pictures and enacts it."[64]

Notes

1   Evans, *Luke*, 521; Marshall, *Luke*, 522. Inheritance laws are found in Deut 21:15–17; Num 27:1–11; 36:1–9. It was a sad day for Abraham when he and Lot were obliged to separate (Gen 13:5–7). Ps 133:1 praises the situation when brothers and sisters live together in unity on ancestral property. Clearly that is not always what happens in any culture!

2   Jesus' response echoes that of Moses in Exod 2:14.

3   Bailey, *Through Peasant Eyes*, 61. The word translated as "arbiter" (*meristēs*) literally means "divider"; Jesus is about reconciliation (*mesitēs*).

4   The Greek word is *pleonexia*. It is equated with idolatry in Col 3:5; see Rom 1:29; 2 Cor 9:5; Eph 4:19: 5:3; 2 Peter 2:3; it is scorned by Hellenistic moralists (see Green, *Luke*, 489, n. 32). Reid, *Parables*, 137, observes that in first-century Palestine, the operating assumption was that if someone's share gets larger, someone else's decreases; greed was destructive of village solidarity; Carroll, *Luke*, 268.

5   Donahue, *Gospel*, 177.

6   Fitzmyer, *Luke*, 2:968, sees this as an appended saying, which may reflect an early Christian attitude rather than an authentic logion of Jesus.

7   Donahue, *Gospel*, 177. Manson, *Sayings*, 271, writes that it is true that a certain minimum of material goods is necessary for life; but it is not true that greater abundance of goods means greater abundance of life.

8   Fitzmyer, *Luke*, 2:969.

9   Bailey, *Through Peasant Eyes*, 58, maintains that there is a wisdom saying before and after the parable, and the parable falls into five stanzas. The theme of the parable is well known to his audience (Eccl 2:1–11; Job 31:24–28; Ps 49).

10   Green, *Luke*, 490–91, notes that persons engaged in soliloquy are usually portrayed negatively by Luke. His good business practice will have detrimental consequences for his peasant neighbours.

11   Bailey, *Through Peasant Eyes*, 65.

12   G.H.P. Thompson, *The Gospel according to Luke* (Oxford: Clarendon Press, 1972), 185.

13   Green, *Luke*, 490, points out that building additional barns would take up agricultural land, hence his plan to knock the old ones down and rebuild on the same land. He also intends to hold his produce until the markets are better.

14   This proverbial expression of hedonism is found also in Isa 22:13; Qoh 8:15; Tobit 7:10; Sir 11:19; 1 Cor 15:32.

15   Donahue, *Gospel*, 178; the language recalls the Old Testament polemic against "folly": (Ps 14:1; 53:1; 49:10; Sir 11:19–20). In Matt 5:21–22, Jesus urges human beings not to use this term of one another.

16   The word here for fool is *aphrōn;* there is wordplay with *euphrōn*, used for the good life.

17   Bailey, *Through Peasant Eyes*, 67; Thompson, *Luke*, 185; Green, *Luke*, 491.

18   Donahue, *Gospel*, 178. Reid, *Parables*, 139, notes that according to the biblical mentality, ownership, particularly if involving land, belongs to God; the rich man

has completely ignored God. Tannehill, *Luke*, 206, notes the social conviction that accumulation of goods should be condemned because it deprives others, unless the rich person is generous to others.

19   Bailey, *Through Peasant Eyes*, 68–69, maintains that the use of *eis* suggests the translation: "So is he who treasures up for himself, and is not gathering riches for God." We should labour in God's service so as to offer gifts to God. Gifts from God are returned to God. McBride, *Luke*, 163–64, highlights the difference between having and being. If having defines our identity, if possessions are the focus of our existence, we are foolish indeed.

20   Carroll, *Luke*, 268; Johnson, *Luke*, 199. Reid, *Parables*, 136, notes the relationship between one's attitude toward material inheritance in this world and heavenly inheritance in the next. Byrne, *Hospitality*, 115, notes that the problem is not possession of riches in itself, but the desire to increase them, which can lead to neglecting God and lacking in concern for others.

21   Much of this material is similar to that of Matthew's Sermon on the Mount (6:25–34). Green, *Luke*, 492, observes that although the focus is now on the disciples, the crowds remain as a secondary audience, for they too need guidance in the area of possessions.

22   Matthew, rather than "ravens", has "birds of the air". Ravens, as scavengers, were thought to be unclean (Lev 11:15; Deut 14:14). For God's care for them see Ps 147:9. Tannehill, *Luke*, 208, comments that the choice of ravens may accent God's indiscriminate goodness.

23   In 12:7 Jesus assures his disciples that they are worth more than many sparrows.

24   The word used here in Greek (*hēlikia*) can refer both to stature and age, so some translations speak of adding an inch to one's height. In this context age seems more appropriate.

25   The Greek word (*krinon*) can be used for flowers in general; Evans, *Luke*, 528, observes that it has been identified with the lily, the anemone, etc. Matthew here has "toil and spin"; Luke prefers "spin and weave", perhaps as an indication of higher skills in keeping with the splendid (purple) clothing of the proverbial Solomon (2 Chr 9:13). The flowers are feminine, the birds, masculine; the occupations of each are appropriate gender-wise in the culture of the day.

26   Green, *Luke*, 494. He notes that the verb (*meteōrizomai*), normally translated as "worry" can also mean "to be arrogant"; Jesus may be referring to the human pursuit of autonomy that expresses itself in anxiety and independence from God.

27   Carroll, *Luke*, 269, refers to "a life shaped by trust in God's gracious provision." There are echoes of the Martha episode here; the same verb is used (*merimnaō*).

28   For an interesting treatment of this theme, see Kenneth E. Bailey, *The Good Shepherd* (London: SPCK, 2015).

29   Tannehill, *Luke*, 209, believes that Luke has in mind members of believing communities who do not leave home for mission; they are challenged to sell their properties. Evans, *Luke*, 531, believes that these two verses illustrate Luke's concern with the question of wealth and poverty in the church.

30   Carroll, *Luke*, 272, says that the human heart attuned to the divine ways and

commitments will in generosity of spirit open itself to others who have need and invest resources in them. This is what it means to be rich in relation to God. Johnson, *Luke*, 202, notes that Jesus teaching here about lack of anxiety is all of a piece with what just precedes this section, when he tells them about facing death (12:4–12). Tannehill, *Luke*, 210, refers to investing one's heart in earthly things or in God.

31   Fitzmyer, *Luke*, 2:1125; Green, *Luke*, 610. Donahue, *Gospel*, 169, notes the folkloric atmosphere of the parable, evocative of Egyptian tales about fate reversal after death, and a midrash concerning Abraham's servant Eliezer. He believes that the parable does not go back to the historical Jesus, but originated in those groups that brought to Luke traditions about wealth, which he adopts and sharpens. Levine, *Stories*, 277, thinks it more likely that Lazarus' name evokes the second son of Moses and Zipporah (Exod 18:4), than Abraham's servant. Jesus, a good storyteller and Aramaic speaker, probably gave the poor man his name, rather than Luke, who shows no affinity for Hebrew or Aramaic terms, nor would his audience! Byrne, *Hospitality*, 136, n. 5, notes that similar stories involving reversal of fortune and retribution in the afterlife circulated in the wider milieu in the time of Jesus. It is possible that he or the early Church tradition took up and adapted a pre-existing folk tale of this kind. Carroll, *Luke*, 335–36, mentions the Jerusalem Talmud and writings in the Greco-Roman world. Johnson, 255, adds 1 Enoch 94:8; Reid, *Parables*, 209–10, gives similar examples, concluding that it is possible that Jesus composed his parable along the lines of known popular folk tales. Evans, *Luke*, 612–13, notes parallels in Egyptian and Jewish sources; such stories are widespread and well-known folk tales. (Also, Marshall, *Luke*, 633). It is difficult to discern how far Jesus, early Christian tradition, or Luke himself is responsible for the story in its present form. For Caird, *Luke*, 191, Jesus is using a familiar folktale and adapting it. He believes that the rich man is a Sadducee because of his social standing and lack of belief in the afterlife. He acted irresponsibly because he did not believe in a judgment. Fitzmyer, *Luke*, 2:1127, after listing various folktales, comments that "if the Lukan parable echoes such folktales, it has refashioned them, and there is no reason to think that this refashioning was not done by Jesus himself." Marshall, *Luke*, 634, comments that the present parable probably rests on tradition traceable to Jesus himself.

32   See Judg 8:26; Sir 45:12; Esth 1:6; 8:15.

33   Green, *Luke*, 605.

34   Reid, *Parables*, 211, suggests that he clearly belongs to the urban elite, who control the political and economic lives of the city and surrounding countryside. Levine, *Stories*, 273, calls his style of life "obscene".

35   Donahue, *Gospel*, 170; McBride, *Parables*, 67; Carroll, *Luke*, 336; Byrne, *Hospitality*, 69; Johnson, *Luke*, 252. Green, *Luke*, 605, sees Lazarus as numbered among society's "expendables", a man who had fallen prey to the ease with which, even in an advanced agrarian society, persons without secure landholdings might experience devastating downward mobility. The name Lazarus is derived from the Hebrew Eleazar, meaning "he whom God helps". This was the name of Abraham's servant and messenger (Gen 15:2–4). Levine, *Stories*, 275, maintains that not all poor are beggars; a real beggar actively begs (see Mark 10:46, as opposed to 12:42–43; John 9:8). But the people who left him at the gate expected the rich man or his visiting friends to see him and act. She prefers to

take the Greek verb as "lying there" (Matt 8:14; Mark 7:30).

36   Levine, *Stories*, 280–82, notes that his sores are not leprosy; he is not ritually unclean; the saliva of dogs was thought to have healing properties and is not a source of uncleanness, so the dogs do him a service; some Jews kept dogs as pets.

37   Byrne, *Hospitality*, 136, n. 7, maintains that this canine attention was not benign; it adds to the indignity of his situation and highlights the lack of human relief. Dogs were considered unclean. Similarly, Johnson, *Luke*, 252; Green, *Luke*, 606; Fitzmyer, *Luke*, 2:1132.

38   Carroll, *Luke*, 337; Green, *Luke*, 609. On p. 606, he notes that the rich man is active in the ensuing story, whereas Lazarus is entirely silent and passive. Levine, *Stories*, 274, maintains that the Jewish audience would have known that a rich man who did not give alms to the poor man at his door, would suffer in the afterlife; they would not have regarded his wealth as a sign of righteousness (see Tobit 4:7–10).

39   Levine, *Stories*, 282, reminds us of the firm Jewish tradition of treating dead bodies with respect and burying corpses. Fitzmyer, *Luke*, 2:1132, believes he was left unburied by human beings, but was carried off by heavenly beings.

40   Marshall, *Luke*, 636.

41   McBride, *Parables*, 70, prefers this idea; his whole section emphasises table fellowship. Lazarus is welcomed to a table fellowship which he was so consistently denied in life. Carroll, *Luke*, 337, speaks of the intimate association and care that he was deprived of previously; Tannehill, *Luke*, 252, to warm welcome and continuing care.

42   Marshall, *Luke*, 636; Reid, *Parables*, 213; Green, *Luke*, 607, "intimacy and honour", care and comfort, paradisal bliss. Levine, *Stories*, 282, speaks of intimacy and feasting (appropriately for the parable).

43   Johnson, *Luke*, 252 (Gen 49:33; Num 27:13; Deut 32:50).

44   Byrne, *Hospitality*, 137. Levine, *Stories*, 285, suggests that poverty is unjust and therefore those who suffer from it must receive recompense.

45   Tannehill, *Luke*, 252.

46   Evans, *Luke*, 613, considers that the language reflects a popular, unsystematic and partly un-Jewish eschatology. The picture is not that of Sheol, (an underworld to which all went without bodies until the final judgement), nor Gehenna, (the permanent abode of the wicked). Marshall, *Luke*, 636–37, observes that Jewish representations of the afterlife were fluid and developing; pictures are not consistent. Reid, *Parables*, 214, thinks Hades is roughly equivalent to Sheol, though the latter is not a place of punishment. Green, *Luke*, 607, suggests that both are in Hades, though in separate sections; Hades is the universal destiny of all humans, sometimes with the expected outcome of the final judgement already mapped out through this separation. He notes lack of precision in statements about the afterlife. Fitzmyer, *Luke*, 2:1132, also thinks that two different locales in Sheol are meant.

47   There is wordplay in Greek: mercy is *eleos*; merciful almsgiving is *eleēmosunē*. In John 8:39 the people say, "Abraham is our father". Levine, *Stories*, 282, notes that as father, Abraham provides food. By the Second Temple period, his hospitality had become one of his dominant characteristics; he was also associated with the afterlife (4 Maccs 7:19; 13:17; Luke 13:28). On p. 288, she notes he knows Abraham's name and role,

but has failed to extend hospitality to the poor man, who is also a child of Abraham. He will receive what he gave to Lazarus.

48   McBride, *Parables*, 69, notes the double shift in fortune: the rich man moves from having to not having and longing; the poor man from not having and longing to having.

49   Carroll, *Luke*, 338; Green, *Luke*, 608.

50   Donahue, *Gospel*, 171; he adds that the final verses, showing strong Lukan redaction, give a deeper understanding to the text. Johnson, *Luke*, 252, writes that this is an appendix that complicates the simple story and gives it a polemic ring. Byrne, *Hospitality*, 136, calls it a kind of epilogue.

51   Levine, *Stories*, 290. "Even if the words are from Luke, the ideas fit what we know from multiple other sources about Jesus of Nazareth."

52   Green, *Luke*, 609, notes that the idea of the dead returning to visit the living was common in the ancient world; also, Marshall, *Luke*, 639. Levine, *Stories*, 292, recalls 1 Sam 28; Luke 24:39; a first-century audience would not have seen the request as odd.

53   Marshall, *Luke*, 638; the rich man seems to have had his own establishment.

54   McBride, *Parables*, 71, notes that Abraham too was a rich man (Gen 13:2), his riches interpreted as a sign of God's favour (Gen 14:13–24) and was buried with honour (Gen 25:7–11). Now he is the advocate of the poor and excluder of the rich.

55   See Exod 22:21–22; Lev 19:9–10; Deut 10:17–19; 24:19,21; 27:19; Ps 94:6; Amos 2:6–8; Isa 1:7; 5:7–10; 30:12; 58:3; Jer 5: 25–29; 22:3; Zech 7:10.

56   Marshall, *Luke*, 632.

57   Evans, *Luke*, 615, calls this a Christian reflection, since only on the Christian background of the resurrection of Jesus is the resurrection of an individual before and apart from the general resurrection conceivable. For Fitzmyer, *Luke*, 2:1128, an allusion to Jesus' own death and resurrection is unmistakable. Similarly, Johnson, *Luke*, 253, n. 31.

58   Donahue, *Gospel*, 172.

59   Carroll, *Luke*, 375.

60   Fitzmyer, *Luke*, 2:972.

61   Carroll, *Luke*, 374.

62   Levine, *Stories*, 295, notes that neither Torah nor prophets condemn wealth *qua* wealth nor commends poverty *qua* poverty. But wealth is a danger. As Reid, *Parables*, 216, puts it, it is the way we use possessions that matters.

63   Donahue, *Gospel*, 179; Wright, *Luke*, 199–200.

64   Carroll, *Luke*, 377.

Chapter Ten

Mercy

Luke's Gospel has long been recognised for its presentation of God's mercy made present in Jesus. The theme runs throughout his Gospel story, and the next three chapters will be devoted to it. In this chapter, we shall examine several narratives in which this theme is reflected. In the following chapter, we shall reflect on the three parables of seeking and finding found in Luke 15, and then, in Chapter Twelve, the theme of meals will be our subject.

Some Background

Luke's Infancy Narrative, as we have seen, can be viewed as an overture to his Gospel, carefully crafted to introduce many of the main themes. From the outset, God's loving and faithful mercy is one such theme. For instance, when the two pregnant mothers, Mary and Elizabeth, meet, the youthful Mary responds to the older woman's greeting by proclaiming the hymn that we know as the *Magnificat,* in which she twice refers explicitly to God's mercy: "His mercy is for those who fear him from generation to generation" (1:50); "He has helped his servant Israel, in remembrance of his mercy, according to the promise he made to our ancestors" (1:54). After the birth of Elizabeth's child, her neighbours and relatives "heard that the Lord had shown his great mercy to her, and they rejoiced with her" (1:58). And Zechariah, speech and hearing restored, blesses God who "has looked favourably on his people; who has shown the mercy promised to our ancestors." And later in the canticle: "By the tender mercy of our God, the dawn from on high will break upon us" (1:68, 72, 78).

Of course, this idea of a merciful God was not new. It is rooted in the experience of God, which Israel had throughout her long history, and in the words and concepts that Israel used to articulate her reflection on that experience. Luke and/or his source are drawing heavily from Old Testament texts.[1]

Israel's insight springs from the confluence of two main streams of thought. First, there is the significance that clusters around the Hebrew word *rahamin* or *rachamin;* it denotes the attachment of one being to another. It comes from the same root as the words meaning bowels, mother's womb, our deepest innards. So, it captures shades of meaning proper to the relationship of particular love that a mother has for the child of her womb: tenderness, pity, understanding, protection, nourishing, patience, a readiness to forgive. It means to be moved to the depths of one's being.

Secondly, there is the Hebrew word *hesed* (usually rendered in Greek by *eleos*). This word implies friendship, favour, trust and faithfulness. Used of Yahweh, it normally refers to God's faithfulness to the covenant choice, God's pledge to Israel. God can be relied upon, can be trusted, whatever happens. When Israel sins, God's *hesed* takes the form of forgiveness and pardoning grace. When there are situations of distress and misfortune, it finds expression in concrete acts of protection, deliverance, restoration.

A wonderful expression of the depth and richness of such reflection is provided in the following text from the book of Exodus; it almost amounts to a definition of God's identity: "Lord, O Lord, God of tenderness and compassion, slow to anger, rich in steadfast love and faithfulness" (Exod 34:6 NJB). Similar expressions are found elsewhere in the psalms: "God is tenderness and pity, slow to anger and rich in faithful love" (Ps 103:8). "But you, Lord, God of tenderness and mercy, slow to anger, rich in faithful love and loyalty, turn to me and pity me" (Ps 86:15). "Our God is mercy and tenderness" (Ps 111:4). And in the prophets: "Because you are a forgiving God, gracious and compassionate, patient and rich in faithful love, you did not abandon them" (Neh 9:17). "How can I give you up, Ephraim ... My heart recoils within me; my compassion grows warm and tender" (Hos 11:8). "In overflowing wrath for a moment I hid my face from you, but with everlasting love I will have compassion on you ... For the mountains may depart and the hills be removed, but my steadfast love shall not depart from you, and my covenant of peace shall not be removed, says the Lord" (Isa 54:7–8). Among them there is a beautiful little passage in Jeremiah (31:30)[2]: "Is Ephraim (Israel) my dear son? My darling child? For the more I speak of him, the more do I remember him. Therefore my womb trembles for him; I will only show motherly compassion upon him."

And there is that wonderful parable or literary meditation called the book of Jonah, written after the exile. Jonah is the reluctant prophet who struggles to come to terms with the mercy of God for the Ninevites, Israel's enemies.

Displeased and angry with God for changing his mind about punishing them, he prays: "O Lord! Is this not what I said while I was still in my own country? That is why I fled to Tarshish at the beginning; for I knew that you are a gracious God and merciful, slow to anger, and abounding in steadfast love, and ready to relent from punishing" (Jon 4:2).

God's 'Godness' is revealed in his freedom to forgive, in mercy. God's mercy is seen after the fall in clothing Adam and Eve, then in marking Cain to protect him, then in the new beginning after the flood, then in the call of Abraham. God's mercy is seen in the liberation from Egyptian oppression. After the molten calf incident, when Moses seeks to intercede for the unfaithful people, God says: "I will be gracious to whom I will be gracious and will show mercy to whom I will show mercy" (Exod 33:19). God's mercy is an expression of God's freedom and otherness. The Old Testament is an unfolding story of God's mercy, and there is always a strong orientation to the needy, the weak and the poor.

Jesus dramatically rekindled and deepened this vision, this understanding of God and of our humanity. In Luke's presentation of the ministry of Jesus, there are many stories in which Jesus responds to people in need; sometimes they or their friends come to him with a request, sometimes Jesus takes the initiative himself. These episodes are all examples of the way in which Jesus fulfils the mission statement that he made in the Nazareth synagogue, when he quoted Isaiah: "He has sent me to bring release to the captives and recovery of sight to the blind, to let the oppressed go free, to proclaim the year of the Lord's favour" (4:16–30). The ministry of Jesus is indeed Good News for the poor. In this chapter, I have made a selection from the many incidents that Luke presents.

The Leper (5:12–16)

After casting out a devil in the synagogue at Capernaum, and then healing Simon's mother-in-law and many others in the town, Jesus calls Simon to be a disciple, along with his fishing partners, James and John.[3] The next person he calls is Levi, but before this takes place there are two stories that illustrate Jesus' mercy: the cure of a leper and the healing of a paralysed man. Both stories are found in Mark;[4] Luke's version of the first reads:

> Once, when he was in one of the cities, there was a man covered with leprosy. When he saw Jesus, he bowed with his face to the ground and begged him, "Lord, if you choose, you can make me clean." Then Jesus stretched out his hand, touched him, and said, "I do choose. Be made clean." Immediately the leprosy

left him. And he ordered him to tell no one. "Go," he said, "and show yourself to the priest, and, as Moses commanded, make an offering for your cleansing, for a testimony to them." But now more than ever the word about Jesus spread abroad; many crowds would gather to hear him and to be cured of their diseases. But he would withdraw to deserted places and pray.

The man in question is "covered with leprosy". He falls on his face before Jesus and begs him: "Lord, if you choose, you can make me clean." The man clearly recognises the power of Jesus, for his reputation as healer has gone before him, and, perhaps uncertain whether Jesus will be prepared to respond to one in a condition like his, entrusts himself to his mercy.[5] Lepers were unfortunate individuals, banished to the margins of society, segregated from the social and religious life of the community.[6] A leper was obliged to wear his clothing torn and his hair dishevelled, and cry, "Unclean, unclean!" as he moved around. He had to live apart and was forbidden to enter any walled town or reside in a village.[7] He was thus denied access to Jerusalem and to the temple. This was not mainly for reasons of hygiene, but because leprosy was deemed to be evidence of and punishment for sin; a leper was considered unclean in the religious sense. If he entered a house, he rendered it unclean; even a chance encounter could entail ritual contamination. His life was thus a misery, a source of physical discomfort, mental anguish and spiritual guilt. It is small wonder that lepers were dubbed "the firstborn of death", living corpses.[8] And yet he encounters Jesus in the city centre, an indication of his boldness and desperation![9]

Jesus stretches out his hand and touches him,[10] saying with warmth and authority, "I do choose. Be made clean." The compassion of Jesus, mentioned explicitly in some of the manuscripts for Mark's version, is palpable. Jesus ignores the risk of contagion, and he incurs the stigma of ritual defilement according to the Law, something no rabbi would have been prepared to do. He makes whole this leper, publicly deemed to be a sinner, restores him to the life of the community, draws him into personal relationship and fellowship with himself and enables him to experience the dawning Kingdom, the presence of a gracious God. The compassionate response of Jesus in touching the untouchable and crossing the boundary between clean and unclean, was as scandalous as the leper's audacity in first approaching him.[11] Jesus tells the man to carry out the formality of presenting himself to the temple priest who, after examination, could officially declare him clean and thus facilitate his reintegration into society; the man could then offer the requisite thanksgiving sacrifice (Lev 14:1–32). In this way Jesus manifests his respect for the Law of Moses, as well as his concern for the individual's future in the community.

After this act of healing, Jesus' reputation spread more widely;[12] crowds gathered to hear him preach and to seek healing. But Jesus also sought space to be alone and to pray. As we have seen, both aspects are important for Luke.

Reflections

The leper is an interesting character. Obviously, he is suffering terribly. The disease presented not only physical problems but entailed a severe level of segregation from family, village community and friends. This would have caused a sense of loneliness and isolation. Furthermore, the affliction had a religious dimension, being considered an indication of sin and therefore a cause of guilt and alienation from God. In his hopelessness, the man comes to Jesus. His need and desperation are such that he disregards the regulations. He takes a chance, takes the risk of exposing his situation to Jesus publicly. He shows faith, falling at Jesus' feet in supplication; but it is a hesitant faith because he is not sure that Jesus would be prepared to bring him healing. His later ignoring of Jesus' injunction to silence is probably understandable, but it does create problems for Jesus.

Jesus comes across as a man of great compassion, as he reaches out warmly and touches the sufferer. As in other stories that we have considered, he ignores taboos for the sake of a person in need. He touches the unclean and restores wholeness. He draws the man back into society, restoring his relationships while assuring him also of God's acceptance. He offers him a new life. Just as evil affects many areas of our lives simultaneously, the Kingdom of God is a multifaceted reality, embracing all dimensions of an individual and of human experience. It has to do with healing, wholeness and connectedness in every aspect of life.

This story can serve as a paradigm of human experience. The man's condition is an invitation to us to acknowledge occasions and situations when we experience fragmentation within ourselves, levels of isolation and exclusion, when relationships have broken down, including our relationship with God. It can help us locate a whole spectrum of feelings as we seek to cope with our situation. Disconnectedness is, I believe, the fundamental expression of our basic human sinfulness, our need for God. God in Christ Jesus is offering us reconciliation, healing and integration for every dimension of our being and our living. Jesus restores us to God, to one another, to our world. As disciples of Jesus, we are called to reach out to others as instruments of wholeness, to seek to overcome whatever divides and fragments, whatever separates one person or group from another. The story is not only a paradigm of human experience, it also reveals the meaning of the Kingdom and is a cameo of the mission of Jesus.

The Paralysed Man (5:17–26)

The next story describes the encounter of Jesus with a paralysed man; for me, this episode, too, is paradigmatic. Luke, again probably adapting Mark, describes it this way:

> One day, while he was teaching, Pharisees and teachers of the law were sitting nearby (they had come from every village of Galilee and Judea and from Jerusalem); and the power of the Lord was with him to heal. Just then some men came, carrying a paralysed man on a bed. They were trying to bring him in and lay him before Jesus; but finding no way to bring him in because of the crowd, they went up on the roof and let him down with his bed through the tiles into the middle of the crowd in front of Jesus. When he saw their faith, he said, "Friend, your sins are forgiven you." Then the scribes and the Pharisees began to question, "Who is this who is speaking blasphemies? Who can forgive sins but God alone?" When Jesus perceived their questionings, he answered them, "Why do you raise such questions in your hearts? Which is easier, to say, 'Your sins are forgiven you', or to say, 'Stand up and walk'? But so that you may know that the Son of Man has authority on earth to forgive sins"—he said to the one who was paralysed—"I say to you, stand up and take your bed and go to your home." Immediately he stood up before them, took what he had been lying on, and went to his home, glorifying God. Amazement seized all of them, and they glorified God and were filled with awe, saying, "We have seen strange things today."

In the immediate context, as he sets the scene, Luke includes for the first time the presence of the Pharisees and teachers of the Law, an official delegation coming even from the religious centre of Jerusalem.[13] The indication of their presence as Jesus conducts his ministry of teaching makes their later critical intervention less abrupt than it is in Mark.[14] Luke mentions that the "power of the Lord" or "Spirit of the Lord" was with Jesus in his healing ministry, recalling the baptism and Nazareth synagogue scenes.[15] Through the quoting of Isaiah in the Nazareth synagogue, Jesus clarified his mission as entailing the release of those held captive, and the freeing of the oppressed, a ministry of liberation. This takes place in the current story, where healing and forgiveness are closely interwoven, illustrating dramatically that Jesus has both power to heal and authority to forgive, the twin aspects of the Old Testament picture of mercy. His liberating response to human need becomes the occasion for conflict.

Our attention is focused first on a group of men who approach the place carrying a paralysed individual "on a bed". The first obstacle that they encounter in their quest to bring the man to Jesus is the thronging crowd, which blocks their access. But they are determined, and with practical imagination they climb the stairs onto the roof, remove the tiles (a Lukan adaptation to an urban style of architecture) and lower their friend on his bed into Jesus' presence.[16] Their kindness and firm commitment are impressive; nothing seems too much trouble. This is friendship at its best. They also manifest a deep faith in Jesus, in his ability and willingness to help their friend and bring him healing. They take the risk of appearing quite foolish if Jesus fails to respond positively to their quest.

Jesus immediately recognises their faith, and presumably that of the paralysed man himself.[17] The man's physical condition and his need for healing are obvious. Jesus would be aware of accompanying disabilities: the man cannot live a normal family life; he cannot work and earn a living; nor can he take part in the political, social and religious life of the community to which he belongs. In Israel, a person with disabilities was seriously marginalised and was in fact an outcast. In that culture, physical misfortune was often popularly considered to be the result of sin or a punishment for it; this was a further burden for an individual to carry. But Jesus is aware of a more fundamental need, a greater disability. When approached for a cure, it is to this more fundamental and urgent need that, with intuitive empathy, he turns his attention first.

With authority and warm affection, he speaks the word of forgiveness: "Friend, your sins are forgiven", the prophetic announcement of the inbreak of the Kingdom, God's reign in love, into the contorted frame of the paralysed man's life, assuring him of the gift of God's unconditional, saving acceptance.[18]

The religious leaders, who are present on the sidelines, take umbrage at this apparent subverting of the prerogative of God. In their view, this amounts to blasphemy. Jesus is aware of their thinking and their antagonism.[19] He rounds on them and poses a counter question, rhetorical, whether it is easier to pronounce a word of forgiveness or of healing. As incontrovertible evidence that he has authority to forgive sins, he turns to the paralysed man and tells him to pick up his bed and go off home.[20] Immediately, he does so. He is healed, released from his paralysis. He can stand erect, bend and carry; he can hike, work in the fields and saw wood; he can stand to his waist in the water and cast a net. And his feelings of guilt, inadequacy, frustration, anger, failure and resentment, feelings which must have weighed heavily or torn him apart, are dissipated like the early morning mist on the lake. He is restored to his family and the life of the local community. A new day has dawned. He knows at first hand the full reality of the Kingdom. The cure confirms the truth and effectiveness of Jesus' word of forgiveness. The liberation from the dominion of evil, the salvation that Jesus brings, embraces the whole person, physical, psychological, spiritual. Both forgiveness and healing are the expressions of mercy.

As he walks home, the man praises God. The onlookers, aware that something unusual is taking place, are filled with awe and wonder at the unexpected things that have occurred, and they, too, praise God, thus recognising that God is at work in Jesus. The religious leaders, deeply upset, Jonah-like, are left confused and challenged by Jesus' activity and claim.

Reflections

While Jesus and the paralysed man are the key players in this story, it is important not to overlook the role of the man's friends. The quality of their friendship and concern for the poor sufferer is quite special. This is friendship at its best, its most beautiful. They go to extraordinary lengths to get the man to Jesus, showing strong determination, creative, practical imagination and ingenuity. It seems that nothing is too much trouble, so firm is their commitment. They also manifest a deep faith in Jesus, in his ability and willingness to help their friend and bring him healing. They take the risk of appearing quite foolish if Jesus should fail to respond positively to their quest. The faith of the paralysed man himself is not highlighted in the narrative. Yet, his willingness to go along with their plan, to suffer the additional pain and inconvenience of being carried along, taken up the staircase and then lowered down into the house, suggests that he, too, hoped and trusted that all would not be in vain. When told by Jesus to pick up his mat, he responds immediately and does so.

Luke does not inform us about the owner of the house in which Jesus was speaking, or who fronted the repair work! Jesus seems unruffled by the sudden interruption and its rather unusual style. He takes it all in his stride. He must have been impressed by the determination, lateral thinking, genuine care and concern of the man's friends and their confidence in him. Jesus focuses his attention on the individual at his feet. He is sensitive to the whole person before him, aware of the different dimensions of his affliction and its effects on his life. Perceiving the man's need for forgiveness and reconciliation, he freely offers this gift with no demands or preconditions. Then he makes him whole, restoring him to family and friends, enabling him to rebuild his life again. This is what the

Kingdom is about, and as his ministry develops, this kind of response to need is typical of Jesus.

We can perhaps identify with the paralysed man in some ways. Some of us are physically impaired and long for relief and healing. We all need forgiveness. There can be other areas of paralysis in our lives; we can be held bound by guilt, low self-esteem, fear, selfishness, feelings of inadequacy, anger and frustration; we can have allowed ourselves to get stuck in a rut, without vision or enthusiasm, content with mediocrity and boredom. We can be carrying around inner hurts, which fester and occasionally erupt. Reaching out and involvement with others can be a challenge. We need to be set free and made whole and become more fully alive. We need to be liberated by the compassion of Jesus.

Finally, the paralysed man's remarkable friends may lead us to consider the quality of our own friendships. We might wonder just how sensitive we are to their feelings and needs, how ready we are to really put ourselves out to support and help them, what is the level of our commitment and generosity, especially when they are in difficulties of one kind or another. One element of their friendship is their realisation of their limitations; they know that they cannot bring a cure but realise that Jesus can. They bring their paralysed friend to Jesus. That is a beautiful aspect of Christian friendship—helping our friends to grow closer to Jesus so that they can experience his healing, forgiving, life-giving love. It is also important for us not to get in the way of such an encounter.

The Healing of The Centurion's Servant (7:1–10)

The next story in which the mercy of Jesus is evident is the call of Levi, which we have already considered in Chapter Four. After the call of Levi, Luke follows Mark in presenting four controversy stories. Several issues are raised: the sharing of table with sinners, laxity with regard to fasting, breaking the Sabbath and healing on the Sabbath (5:29–6:11). Next, after some time in prayer on a mountain, Jesus chooses The Twelve as his "apostles" (6:12–16). This is followed by a powerful summary:

> He came down with them and stood on a level place, with a great crowd of his disciples and a great multitude of people from all Judea, Jerusalem, and the coast of Tyre and Sidon. They had come to hear him and to be healed of their diseases; and those who were troubled with unclean spirits were cured. And all in the crowd were trying to touch him, for power came out from him and healed all of them. (6:17–19)

Jesus then proclaims the Sermon on the Plain, a shorter form of Matthew's Sermon on the Mount (6:20–49).[21] It is at the conclusion of Jesus' teaching, given to all the people, that we pick up the storyline with two further incidents that illustrate the mercy and compassion of Jesus. The first concerns a gentile centurion, the second a Jewish widow.[22]

The story of the soldier and his servant is found in a slightly different form in Matthew (8:5–13); there is also a version in John, which may be an independent tradition (4:46–54). Luke's narrative has echoes of Elisha and Naaman but also makes explicit what Jesus implied at Nazareth concerning God's help extending beyond Israel.[23] It links, too, with Jesus' words in the Sermon on the Plain that one should love one's enemies, showing that Jesus' gracious ministry does reach even the gentiles.[24] It reads:

> After Jesus had finished all his sayings in the hearing of the people, he entered Capernaum. A centurion there had a slave whom he valued highly, and who was ill and close to death. When he heard about Jesus, he sent some Jewish elders to him, asking him to come and heal his slave. When they came to Jesus, they appealed to him earnestly, saying, "He is worthy of having you do this for him, for he loves our people, and it is he who built our synagogue for us." And Jesus went with them, but when he was not far from the house, the centurion sent friends to say to him, "Lord, do not trouble yourself, for I am not worthy to have you come under my roof; therefore I did not presume to come to you. But only speak the word, and let my servant be healed. For I also am a man set under authority, with soldiers under me; and I say to one, 'Go', and he goes, and to another, 'Come', and he comes, and to my slave, 'Do this', and the slave does it." When Jesus heard this he was amazed at him, and turning to the crowd that followed him, he said, "I tell you, not even in Israel have I found such faith." When those who had been sent returned to the house, they found the slave in good health.

Jesus returns to the frontier town of Capernaum, which he seems to have made his base early in his ministry. A centurion is introduced, a man of considerable standing, presumably from the military garrison that was manned by soldiers in the service of Herod Antipas.[25] He probably hails from Syria and is a gentile.[26] He has a servant for whom he has a deep regard, who is severely ill and near death.[27] Having come to hear about Jesus as a healer, and aware of his presence in the town, he decides to seize his opportunity and seek help.[28] The slave is clearly too ill to be brought to Jesus. The centurion believes himself unworthy to approach Jesus himself and uses some local community elders as intermediaries to make the request on his behalf that Jesus should come to his house and heal the servant.[29] On reaching Jesus, these men plead earnestly with him, adding as motivation that the centurion is worthy of being helped because he loves the Jewish people and has even built the local synagogue for them.[30]

After hearing their request, Jesus agrees to accompany them to the home of the gentile centurion. He is prepared to have dealings with a gentile and even enter his home, thus incurring ritual defilement and, inevitably, some local displeasure. The centurion must have caught sight of Jesus approaching and has second thoughts, sensitively sending other friends to meet him with an alternative suggestion that would enable Jesus to avoid defilement. Addressing Jesus respectfully as "Lord" or "Master", with great humility and an awareness that he has no claim on Jesus, he expresses his unworthiness that Jesus should enter his house, whatever the earlier delegation had intimated, and acknowledges that Jesus need only say a word.[31] That would be sufficient to bring healing and new life to his servant. He clearly recognises the authority of Jesus and defers to him. For, in his position and with his army experience, the centurion knows what authority is all about and is well acquainted with the power of a word of command. If he can command with a word, all the more so can Jesus.[32]

On hearing this further message, Jesus is amazed and, turning to the crowd around him, observes emphatically that he has not found insight and faith of such quality among the people of Israel.[33] The man has shown some awareness of Jesus' closeness to God. He has also sensed that as a gentile, he is not entirely excluded from Jesus' care.[34] Jesus must then have turned away and continued his business. He does not, in fact, speak a healing word. Meanwhile, those who had met with him on the road, on returning to the house, find the servant restored to health. Jesus has met neither centurion nor servant; his act of mercy in healing the servant has been carried out quietly from a distance. The emphasis in the story is more on the centurion's faith than on the miracle. This gentile outsider has become a model for the faith of the Kingdom; role reversal is under way.[35] "Faith and the healing power of Jesus overcome socio-religious barriers."[36]

Reflections

This episode occurring early in Jesus' ministry highlights both the trust or faith of the centurion and the generous openness and freedom of Jesus. This is a compelling combination. One suspects that Jesus would be surprised at the request communicated by the village elders on behalf of a gentile. Unusual as this is, and contrary to the normal thrust of his ministry, he responds with great openness, even spontaneously setting off down the street in the direction of the centurion's home in order to cure his servant. He does not baulk at the probability of incurring criticism and hostility from the townsfolk for his trouble. There is a remarkable freedom about him. When the second delegation comes to meet him, friends this time rather than officials, with a message evincing great humility and profound trust, Jesus is quick to acknowledge the qualities of the man, publicly praising his faith, a faith which he has not previously encountered.

In commenting so favourably on the gentile's faith, Jesus puts him forward as an exemplar.[37] This is the case not only for the Jews of the town in which the incident took place; it is true for us today. There is something engaging and attractive about the man's humble awareness that he has no rights, no claims; he knows that he cannot demand a cure for his servant. This is what poverty of spirit really means. Such poverty of spirit must be ours when we approach Jesus with our hopes, dreams and needs. The man's words, slightly adapted, have been included in the new form of our eucharistic celebration prior to the reception of communion.[38] They sum up the dispositions that are appropriate for our welcoming of the Lord into our hearts. They also express our trust in the love and acceptance of Jesus, and his power to heal and bring life to the whole of our being.

The Widow of Nain (7:11–17)

While developing the theme of the mercy of God made real in the person and ministry of Jesus, Luke surprisingly explicitly attributes to Jesus the quality of compassion (using the technical verb *splanchnizesthai*) only once. It is found in his moving description of the raising to life of the widow's son at Nain, an episode not recounted by the other evangelists, giving substance to the earlier beatitude "blessed are you who weep now, for you will laugh." Nain, which is not mentioned elsewhere in the Bible, was a small town some six miles (9.6 km) from Nazareth and five (8 km) from Capernaum, where Jesus had just healed the centurion's servant, who was seriously ill.[39]

> Soon afterwards he went to a town called Nain, and his disciples and a large crowd went with him. As he approached the gate of the town, a man who had died was being carried out. He was his mother's only son, and she was a widow; and with her was a large crowd from the town. When the Lord saw her, he had compassion for her and said to her, "Do not weep." Then he came forward and touched the bier, and the bearers stood still. And he said, "Young man, I say to you, rise!" The dead man sat up and began to speak, and Jesus gave him to his mother. Fear seized all of them; and they glorified God, saying, "A great prophet has risen among us!" and "God has looked favourably on his people!" This word about him spread throughout Judea and all the surrounding country.

Jesus goes to the town accompanied by his entourage and a large crowd. As they approach the gate, they meet a funeral procession moving out to the place of interment, probably a cave on the hillside.[40] It was the custom for burials to take place outside town and as soon as possible after death. Our attention is focused throughout on the sad plight of the woman: she has lost her husband and is therefore a widow, and now her only son, the support and hope of her life, has also died. She is therefore alone, without economic support or social status, and very vulnerable. A life of hardship, loneliness and poverty beckons.[41] The woman is accompanied by a large crowd of mourners, for it was considered meritorious to attend funerals and share in the grieving. Besides, a death in a small town touches everyone. Mourning was greater for an only child. The professional mourners would also be noisily present.[42]

No request is made of Jesus to intervene; again, the initiative is entirely his. "When the Lord saw her, he had compassion for her, and he said: 'Do not weep'." Jesus, described here as "the Lord", is deeply concerned and is "moved to compassion" for the woman.[43] First, he tells her that she need weep no more. In showing such care in public for the woman, Jesus once again crosses the boundaries of religious propriety and custom.[44] He then ignores the risk of incurring ritual defilement by approaching and touching the bier on which the corpse lay in a linen shroud. The bearers halt, and Jesus, speaking to the corpse with a word clearly audible to the crowd, raises the man to life again: "Young man, I say to you, get up!" The man sits up and begins to speak. Then, showing his deep concern for the woman, Jesus "gave him back to his mother."[45] Jesus' action in restoring life to the deceased young man is clearly remarkable, but it is subsumed into his care for the grieving mother.[46] Jesus restores life to her too.[47] In the story there is no mention of the woman's faith, nor that of the onlookers. The focus is entirely on Jesus' compassion, on liberating mercy freely bestowed.

The witnesses to what has occurred are numerous. Their initial reaction is one of fear and awe. Jesus has done what only God can do. Then they burst into praise of God, chorus-like, recognising that "a great prophet has arisen among us", and concluding with words that closely echo the words of Zechariah's *Benedictus:* "God has shown his care for his people."[48] The compassion of Jesus, his deep concern for human suffering, reveals the presence among them of God's saving mercy.

Reflections

The woman in this story has no active role. She represents the many bereaved and vulnerable in our world, people whose lives are in shreds, whose futures look grim. In her emptiness, she can only receive. Her inner poverty is a catalyst. In her need, she moves Jesus to compassion, a compassion that transforms her life. And yet she is a valuable reminder to us of our own inner poverty, our poverty of being. Awareness of our poverty, our areas of inadequacy and need, can open us to the healing and life-giving presence of Jesus. It is when we find ourselves in situations of loss that we can be found by him, loss of health (of sight, hearing, mobility), loss of independence, loss of friends and family, loss of position or job, loss of confidence. In our lives, there are many death experiences that we have to embrace and work through. Jesus comes as the compassionate one who will be supportively with us, sustaining us in our struggle. He can also open up new possibilities, transforming death into life.

Concerning Jesus, Denis McBride observes that Jesus is the one who takes the initiative, who speaks first, who notices suffering and desolation, and who does not bypass them along the road. He is not afraid of getting his hands dirty, of being regarded as unclean, in his movement of compassion. When he meets suffering at the crossroads, he does not take the route of least resistance and flee from the face of pain. He transforms it by his touch and by his word.[49]

An Interlude (7:18–24)

Before moving on in his narrative and following Mark's Gospel outline a little more closely, Luke includes a small section that enables the reader to pause and take stock of what has been happening.

> The disciples of John reported all these things to him. So John summoned two of his disciples and sent them to the Lord to ask, "Are you the one who is to come, or are we to wait for another?" When the men had come to him, they said, "John the Baptist has sent us to you to ask, 'Are you the one who is to come, or are we to wait for another?'" Jesus had just then cured many people of diseases, plagues, and evil spirits, and had given sight to many who were blind. And he answered them, "Go and tell John what you have seen and heard: the blind receive their sight, the lame walk, the lepers are cleansed, the deaf hear, the dead are raised, the poor have good news brought to them. And blessed is anyone who takes no offence at me."

It is implied that the disciples of John the Baptist have been present for the previous miracles of Jesus and so have gleaned a great deal of information to communicate to their master, now in prison, concerning what Jesus has been saying and doing and the way in which people are responding to him.[50] Presumably, they have been able to visit him in prison and inform him about Jesus' activity and message. It is clear that there is a discrepancy between the style and outlook of the Baptist and that of Jesus. Earlier in the story, the reader is informed about the preaching of the Baptist near the Jordan, in which he refers to "the wrath to come" and "the axe lying at the root of the trees". As the precursor, he describes the one coming after him as baptising, not with water like him, but with the Holy Spirit and fire. "His winnowing fork is in his hand, to clear the threshing floor and to gather the wheat into his granary; but the chaff he will burn with unquenchable fire."[51] John is expecting imminent judgement, the overthrowing of wrong. The tone and emphasis in the words of Jesus are different, as is evident in his inaugural sermon in Nazareth.[52] The activities he is engaged in, healing and exorcising, are also different. This puzzles the Baptist and spurs him to seek clarification as to whether Jesus is the figure he envisaged. So, he sends two of his disciples[53] to put the crucial question concerning Jesus' identity in blunt terms: "Are you the one who is to come, or are we to wait for another?" Two was the normally accepted number for genuine witnesses. The disciples do what they have been asked to do, repeating John's question *verbatim*.

In the meantime, Jesus has been continuing his healing activity, and so in answer, rather than a simple "yes" or "no", he points his visitors to what has been happening and what they themselves have witnessed: blind people see, the lame can now walk, lepers are cleansed, folk who were deaf can hear again, the dead are raised to life. These phrases strongly echo the messianic expectations of the prophet Isaiah.[54] They are also examples of the way in which Jesus is fulfilling his mission statement issued in the Nazareth synagogue. The evidence is clear and indicates the presence of the promised eschatological salvation. And he adds in the place of emphasis that the poor and ordinary people have been brought Good News. His final comment, while couched in general terms, is something of a challenge to his interlocutors: "Blessed is anyone who has taken no offence at me." Jesus is aware that John is struggling to come to terms with the unexpected style of his ministry; he is sensitive to his perplexity.[55] The messengers are left to draw their own conclusions and report back.[56]

The response of Jesus throws the burden of accurate discernment back to the Baptist. One issue is to clarify the kind of "coming one" he was expecting or hoping for. If the message and activities of Jesus measure up, the Baptist has his answer: he need not wait for another. If there is a discrepancy, Jesus indirectly invites him to think again before dismissing him and not be put off by his quite different approach and style. The prophecies really are being fulfilled. In the storyline there is no reply, only the silence of the prison cell. Perhaps John went to his death still questioning, still unsure about Jesus.[57]

Reflections

In this passage, we find a deeply religious and committed man in a state of some confusion and perplexity. He has very clear ideas about God and God's ways. The arrival of Jesus on the scene with different priorities and a different agenda has thrown him into turmoil. He needs and seeks clarification. Perhaps we can identify with him to some extent. The arrival of Pope Francis into the Vatican has created for many of our contemporaries a similar experience of uncertainty. Long established ways and styles and systems have been gently but strongly challenged. This kind of thing can happen to all of us less dramatically on a regular basis. We are called to reassess our priorities, examine our values.

One writer states: "Another attractive facet in the personality of Jesus is seen in his dealings with John the Baptist. In spite of the deep gulf that separated his radiant friendliness from John's forbidding austerity, he had a profound appreciation of his grim herald."[58] By means of John's emissaries, Jesus lays before him the evidence, evidence with a solid scriptural pedigree. In a gentle way, Jesus is showing John that some of his expectations need to be revised quite radically; only then will he be able to answer his own questioning. With us that is often the case too. We can create expectations of ourselves, our loved ones, colleagues, those for whom we work. We need a reality check, a motivation check; we need to evaluate evidence dispassionately; we need the freedom to adapt, to change, to move away and forward. Jesus has a deep appreciation for each of us, but he may want us to be alert and sensitive enough to discern the need for modification, perhaps even a radical reappraisal and change of direction.

The Ten Lepers (17:11–19)

The next episode that I wish to consider occurs late on during the journey to Jerusalem and follows a number of parables and a selection of Jesus' sayings (14:15–17:10). It is found only in Luke's Gospel and begins with a reminder that Jesus is "on the way to Jerusalem", the place of his destiny, his "exodus"; the journey motif, last explicitly mentioned in 13:22, continues.[59]

> On the way to Jerusalem Jesus was going through the region between Samaria and Galilee. As he entered a village, ten lepers approached him. Keeping their

distance, they called out, saying, "Jesus, Master, have mercy on us!" When he saw them, he said to them, "Go and show yourselves to the priests." And as they went, they were made clean. Then one of them, when he saw that he was healed, turned back, praising God with a loud voice. He prostrated himself at Jesus' feet and thanked him. And he was a Samaritan. Then Jesus asked, "Were not ten made clean? But the other nine, where are they? Was none of them found to return and give praise to God except this foreigner?" Then he said to him, "Get up and go on your way; your faith has made you well."

At this juncture in his itinerary, Jesus' route takes him and presumably his disciples through an area between Galilee and Samaria, a border area, "a liminal zone".[60] On entering an unnamed village, presumably Jewish,[61] he is approached by a group of lepers, ten in number, who probably base themselves on the village outskirts, near enough to be able to beg. Whatever the nature of their skin disease, here designated as leprosy, these men were ostracised from normal society,[62] living on the margins; they were considered cursed by God and ritually unclean. However, observing the regulations of the Law, they keep their distance and shout out to Jesus with respect and trust: "Jesus, Master, have mercy on us."[63] They are not seeking alms, but merciful healing.

Jesus responds immediately, simply dispatching them and urging them to fulfil the Law by going to show themselves to the priests for verification of a cure (Lev 13:49), as he had told the individual leper earlier.[64] So they follow his instructions and set off, which is a further expression of their faith. While *en route* and now some distance from Jesus, they come to the realisation that they are healed.[65] At this, one of them turns back, loudly praising God as he goes. On reaching Jesus, he falls at his feet and expresses his gratitude. It is at this point in the story that we are informed for the first time that he is a Samaritan.[66] This is something of a bombshell for the reader, as Luke "seems deliberately to challenge notions of the privileged position of the Jewish people within the redemptive economy of God."[67]

Faced with this situation and the implied presence of the disciples, Jesus asks three staccato questions. He is clearly disappointed, maybe hurt, that none of the other nine, presumably members of the Jewish people, have taken the trouble to come and offer thanks and praise to God and to the one through whom God's mercy has touched them. The only one to have done so is a "foreigner", someone on the fringes of Israel.[68] Jesus then addresses the former leper, telling him to stand up and go on his way, adding that it is his faith that has saved him (also 7:50; 8:48; 18:42). Again, Jesus is crossing boundaries; the leper joins other outsiders who have been healed, accepted and saved by Jesus.[69] As well as the initial bold approach to seek Jesus' help and his setting off to see the priests at Jesus' word, the Samaritan's faith includes his return to thank Jesus and honour God.[70] His being saved entails more than a physical cure and restoration to his community; it includes a new awareness of God's presence in the ministry of Jesus, and brings a new relationship with God and the Kingdom.[71] "He models the thankfulness and the acknowledgement of God's glory—and the faith—that such an act of gracious deliverance should evoke."[72]

Reflections

This story highlights the issue of gratitude and ingratitude. The Samaritan returns to Jesus to express his thanks for being cured and restored to normal life. Perhaps the other nine felt grateful but did not take the trouble to say so. There are, then, two aspects to thankfulness.

Along with the word "yes", I believe "thanks" is one of the most significant words in our language. It conveys the recognition that we are not rocks or islands,[73] that we depend on others in so many dimensions of our existence. So many people have contributed to making us who we are, people within our family and people beyond that circle, like educators, doctors, pastors and friends. Countless others, the majority of whom are anonymous, contribute to our daily welfare, producing and marketing the food we eat; inventing the cars and electronic gadgetry we have become dependent upon for transport, communication and entertainment; creating the buildings and infrastructure on which we rely. I'm particularly grateful to those who have forged walking routes and created maps. So many others have written books that have influenced our thinking and understanding, or have brought joy and satisfaction through music and art and entertainment. The list could go on and on. I believe it is so important not to take anything or anyone for granted, and each day to stop and acknowledge this and commend all these people to our God.

As well as feeling gratitude in our hearts, it is important to express it. Jesus in the story was clearly delighted with the Samaritan who returned and disappointed with the nine who did not. A word of thanks can make such a difference to someone's day, even if someone is doing a job for which they get paid. A phone call, an email, a text, too, can communicate our appreciation for what someone has done for us. Gratitude is an expression of poverty of spirit, a recognition that we are not self-sufficient but interdependent beings; it is an indication that we do not take people and life for granted.

Of course, we need to be grateful above all to our God. So many of the psalms turn to God in thanksgiving. Daily, I thank God for the immense beauty and unfathomable wonder of the world, for the gift of life and health, for the network of sustaining relationships about me, for sending Jesus into the world and into my life with the saving gift of his abiding presence and the commission to promote the Kingdom. Even here, there is the danger of taking God for granted, of becoming bogged down in busyness, of allowing our problems and concerns and projects to dull our sensitivity to the awesome mystery of God's loving presence and providential care. Let us continue to develop the art of gratitude.

The Blind Beggar (18:35–43)

The journey of Jesus to meet his "exodus" in Jerusalem is nearing its terminus. After his discussion with the rich ruler, and subsequent challenging words about riches, he has again spoken to his disciples in some detail about his coming violent end in that city. They were unable to understand his message and were blind to its import.[74] Jesus, his disciples, probably among a pilgrim crowd, and the story move on as they arrive in the vicinity of Jericho, a prosperous city on the main route to Jerusalem, which was still some 15 or 16 miles distant (24 or 25 km).[75] It stood 6 miles (9.6 km) north of the Dead Sea and had the character of a 'garden city', a place with ready access to water and a good climate. It was an agricultural centre, a crossroads and a winter resort for the Jewish aristocracy. Herod the Great had built a winter palace there. At 850 feet (259 m) below sea level, it was the lowest inhabited place in the world, and had been inhabited since around 8,000 BCE; Jerusalem was 2500 feet (762 m) above sea level.[76]

> As he approached Jericho, a blind man was sitting by the roadside begging. When he heard a crowd going by, he asked what was happening. They told him, "Jesus of Nazareth is passing by." Then he shouted, "Jesus, Son of David, have mercy on me!" Those who were in front sternly ordered him to be quiet; but he shouted even more loudly, "Son of David, have mercy on me!" Jesus stood still and ordered the man to be brought to him; and when he came near, he asked him, "What do you want me to do for you?" He said, "Lord, let me see again." Jesus said to him, Receive your sight; your faith has saved you." Immediately he regained his sight and followed him, glorifying God; and all the people, when they saw it, praised God.

As Jesus reaches the city, he comes across a blind beggar seated by the roadside, probably near the city gate. Since this was on the pilgrim route to Jerusalem at Passover, a time for almsgiving, it was doubtless an advantageous spot. As a blind man, condemned to begging for survival, he was a nobody, an expendable, clearly one of the "poor".[77] But he hears the crowd as they pass by and asks what is happening.[78] They inform him that it is Jesus of Nazareth who is passing by.[79] On hearing this, he determines to seize his opportunity and cries out: "Jesus, Son of David, have pity on me!" It is unclear what he may have had in mind in calling Jesus "Son of David", though this title is important for Luke.[80] He may simply have been indicating Jesus' Davidic ancestry, or it could be the first public announcement of Jesus as the Davidic Messiah during his adult career.[81] This title was a fairly common messianic title in later Jewish literature (though not in the Old Testament). In contemporary Jewish traditions, it was associated with Solomon, the only reigning king to be called by this title in the Hebrew Bible, who was famous for his exorcisms and healing qualities.[82] As Son of David, Jesus is the one through whom divine blessings are manifest—a profound insight.[83]

The crowds, probably mainly pilgrims, who are milling around and less insightful than he, and possibly the disciples too, probably thinking he is asking for alms, tell him with some vigour to hold his tongue.[84] They consider the man an embarrassment, a nuisance, and presume that Jesus cannot be bothered with such folk. Far from being dissuaded, the man continues to cry out with strong faith for mercy all the more loudly and insistently, repeating the title but not the name Jesus.

Jesus stops and has the man brought to him (by some of those who were telling him to be quiet!);[85] he puts to him that gently provocative question, inviting him to articulate his need, which is also to express his faith:[86] "What do you want me to do for you?" And the reply comes unhesitatingly and predictably: "Lord, let me see again." The man is aware of his need and helplessness, and finds hope in the person of Jesus, turning to him for help, this time addressing him as "Lord", believing that Jesus can and will heal him, confident in his merciful compassion. It seems that at one time he had been able to see; only Jesus can bring fresh sight. Jesus says: "Regain your sight."[87] His sight is restored because of his trust, his energetic faith: "Your faith has saved you."[88] "Here that faith appears to combine insight into Jesus' role as divine agent of healing, a turn toward him in expectant trust (if not desperate hope) and especially persistence that overcomes obstacles."[89] The word of Jesus brings immediate and complete healing.[90] The man can now see Jesus face-to-face but also sees with insight, which leads him without delay to set off to follow Jesus as a disciple, and as he does so, he glorifies God; he has entered the Kingdom of God.[91] As so often happens in Luke's narrative, the people who see this wonderful occasion burst out in praise of God. They have recognised that God has visited his people and brought healing and liberation through Jesus, the prophet from Nazareth. This is the only occasion in Luke in which Jesus gives sight to a blind person, though this is included in some general summaries (4:18; 7:22).

Reflections

This blind man is presented as a man of considerable faith. The antagonism of the crowd does not deter him in his quest to meet Jesus and find healing. His dogged determination, in fact, grows. There is strong emotion in his response to Jesus' question. He longs to see again. His response to Jesus' cure in opting not to go home but to follow Jesus on the way to Jerusalem means that he has an ongoing role in the narrative. He is a model of what discipleship is about. And he is a challenge to us in our lives today.

The compassion of Jesus is again evident.[92] When he hears the man's impassioned cry, he stops and gives him his attention, overruling the crowd's attempts to silence him. Calling him to come to him, he immediately communicates his willingness to respond. In asking him what he wanted, he was acknowledging the man's responsibility for what lay in the future, the consequences of being healed. Jesus must have warmed to his single-mindedness and enthusiasm, as he fell in behind him on the journey.

I'm deeply grateful to God for the gift of sight. Last year a member of staff was suffering with cataracts. After the operation, I phoned her and was almost blown off my feet by the excitement in her voice as she described being able to distinguish colours again, read the paper clearly, watch the TV in comfort. It was an insight into what the blind man must have felt. It really is wonderful to be able to see the beauty of the world around us in its bewildering variety of hue, shape, texture and movement. What a blessing to be able to scan people's faces, sensitive to details of uniqueness and mood, to catch the warmth in a smile, the twinkle in an eye, the sadness on a brow. The opportunities for wonder, excitement and growth are endless. We have a multitude of reasons for gratitude.

We can still be blind, however, at least sometimes and in some areas of life. We can see without seeing. This was a problem that Jesus encountered frequently, not only with the authorities, but also with his disciples. We can have selective sight; we can close our eyes and pretend not to notice. Selfishness, fear, prejudice can cause our eyes to grow dim. To see clearly can be dangerous and demanding, challenging and even life-changing. Often, we opt to be a little blind; paradoxically, it can be safer and more comfortable that way, even if it is life-diminishing. To say to Jesus: "Lord, let me see", and really mean it, takes much courage.

This story also invites us to ponder our understanding of Jesus, our faith in him, expressed in our practical living. In our lives, we have listened to sermons and attended lectures. We have read articles and books, received counsel and advice. We have spent time in prayer. We have engaged in conversation and discussion. Opportunities for enlightenment have been numerous. How rich is our vision, how deep our understanding, how strong our commitment? Perhaps, like the disciples, we stumble along, sometimes in the light, sometimes in the shadows. There are things about Jesus that perhaps are something of a puzzle. There are aspects of discipleship with which we struggle. Though we are not blind, our sight is impaired and partial still. Like him, we ask Jesus to enable us to see, to see more clearly and more truly. We pray for firmer faith and stronger commitment in following him.

Zacchaeus (19:1–10)

My final story in this chapter is also found only in Luke; this time the person concerned is given a name, a Jewish name, Zacchaeus. He is literally one of the 'little people' of the New Testament![93] In its current location, the story of Zacchaeus is the final episode in Luke's journey narrative and the climax in Jesus' ministry of mercy to the outcast.[94] The text reads as follows:

> He entered Jericho and was passing through it. A man was there named Zacchaeus; he was a chief tax-collector and was rich. He was trying to see who Jesus was, but on account of the crowd he could not, because he was short in stature. So he ran ahead and climbed a sycamore tree to see him, because he was going to pass that way. When Jesus came to the place, he looked up and said to him, "Zacchaeus, hurry and come down; for I must stay at your house today." So he hurried down and was happy to welcome him. All who saw it began to grumble and said, "He has gone to be the guest of one who is a sinner." Zacchaeus stood there and said to the Lord, "Look, half of my possessions, Lord, I will give to the poor; and if I have defrauded anyone of anything, I will pay back four times as much." Then Jesus said to him, "Today salvation has come to this house, because he too is a son of Abraham. For the Son of Man came to seek out and to save the lost."

After the cure of the blind beggar on the outskirts of Jericho, Jesus has entered the city itself and is passing through *en route* for Jerusalem.[95] Another significant encounter is about to take place. A citizen named Zacchaeus is quickly introduced and is described as the "superintendant of taxes", an unusual term, found nowhere else in Greek literature.[96] He has evidently benefited from the financial possibilities that such a post in a city like Jericho offered, for he is said to be extremely wealthy. Like Levi in a different town, he would have been very unpopular, hated and despised as a collaborator, and, from the religious viewpoint, considered unclean.[97] So far in Luke's story of Jesus, tax collectors have responded positively to Jesus; but Jesus has also spoken with some severity about the rich. We wonder how this Jericho encounter will unfold.

Zacchaeus, however, "was eager to see what Jesus looked like", having heard no doubt of his reputation in his treatment of people like him, and possibly aware that one of his disciples had been a member of his profession. We might speculate that he may have wished to escape from his self-imposed loneliness, the social ostracism that went with the job, to break free from a profession now burdening his conscience.[98] Given his social situation as an outcast, he risks ridicule and violence from the crowd, who are deliberately getting in the way and blocking his view. So, he runs on ahead, something which adults do not do in that culture, and to get a clear view unimpeded by crowd or stature, climbs up a tree.[99] Rich and powerful people do not climb trees! This was an extravagant gesture, which illustrates the intensity of his desire.[100] Apparently, sycamore fig trees have low branches and are easy to climb; they have large, thick leaves, and thus provide good cover for someone wishing to hide. The regulations insisted that they should not grow within the city.[101]

The spotlight now focuses again on Jesus. It is he who, in response to Zacchaeus' interest, seizes the initiative. Jesus is aware of his presence; he stops, looks up at him in the tree and calls him by name. Perhaps he knew his name because of the insults being levelled against him by the crowd, who are relishing the opportunity afforded them. Jesus, to everyone's surprise and shock, bursts through religious prejudice and, presuming on the man's generosity, invites himself to a meal and lodging in his home, the house of a rich man, popularly regarded as a sinner: "Zacchaeus, be quick and come down, for I must stay at your house today." There is a note of urgency in Jesus' words; and the "must" draws what is happening into the ambit of God's saving plan.[102] Zacchaeus is delighted with the turn of events. This is more than he has ever envisaged. So, he climbs down with alacrity and welcomes Jesus gladly. He is obviously touched by the graciousness of Jesus and his spontaneous offer of fellowship, and all that this implies. There is great joy in his offering hospitality.

By contrast, the bystanders, possibly including the disciples,[103] are scandalised by the fact that Jesus has chosen to be the guest of a "sinner". They begin to murmur and voice their disapproval. Jesus seems to have incurred the hostility of the whole town.[104] For to their way of thinking, to share this man's unclean table and home is to share his sin and emerge ritually defiled, and this shortly before Passover. Jesus frequently breaks through the barriers of religious prejudice with great freedom, and such freedom always creates a problem for others. Jesus does not lock people in their past; he can see beyond the present; he can see what is in the human heart; he has a vision of what is possible for the future.

As far as Zacchaeus is concerned, this freedom "awakened to vibrant life impulses that had long lain dormant and revealed to him the man he was capable of becoming."[105] In response to Jesus' graciousness, and also to exonerate him from the crowd's suspicion and to deflect their anger, Zacchaeus stops[106] and publicly declares that he turns his back decisively and without delay on his past: "Here and now, sir, I give half my possessions to charity; and if I have defrauded anyone, I will repay him four times over." Without any prompting from Jesus, Zacchaeus implicitly acknowledges his guilt, professing his intention to offer alms beyond the normally expected twenty per cent and to pay restitution far in excess of the legal prescription.[107] In Judaism, repentance involved restoration. This is a clear illustration of conversion, the change of heart and ways that is the genuine response to Jesus. He declares his intention to live a new life, "shaped by the values and commitments of God's realm",[108] and illustrates what this might entail.[109] The financial oppression of the Jericho community will now be relieved considerably. This comes after Jesus has taken the initiative and reached out to him; it isn't a precondition.

Jesus, in his final words, acknowledges and affirms Zacchaeus and his attitude, as he addresses Zacchaeus and the crowd as well: "Today salvation has come to this house—for this man too is a son of Abraham. The Son of Man has come to seek and save what is lost." Salvation has come to him and his household that very day, "today". It is not a thing of the future, a distant dream. And it has come in the person of Jesus, who in an expression of costly love, has shifted to himself the crowd's opposition and hostility.[110] Zacchaeus accepts Jesus' love; he accepts being found and accepted so completely by Jesus. He is a man transformed. He is drawn into the hospitality of the Kingdom community.[111] He is no longer an ostracised outsider but is accepted in God's eyes, a genuine son of Abraham and heir to the promise of salvation. But salvation entails living day by day in Jesus' way; it is a transforming experience. The final comment of Jesus sums up the scene, as it sums up his whole ministry. The language is that of the parables of the shepherd and of the compassionate father: "lost and found".[112] The response of Zacchaeus in placing his wealth at the service of the poor and righting the wrongs he had committed stands in contrast with that of the rich ruler (18:18–24), for whom "the allure of riches was stronger than the call to discipleship."[113]

Reflections

Zacchaeus, this unpopular citizen of Jericho, experiences the transforming and liberating effect of Jesus' forgiveness. A social and religious outcast, he longs to see Jesus. Such a desire suggests that he wishes to be set free. He goes to great lengths in order to catch sight of Jesus, risking the antipathy of those around. On encountering the gracious acceptance of Jesus, he responds generously, an indication of a new beginning.

Jesus shows his typical awareness of what is happening around him. Probably the crowd's reaction to Zacchaeus alerts him to his presence in the tree and also his name. Jesus reacts to the situation by stopping, calling his name, and becomes himself a seeker by requesting hospitality in his home. It is a creative and sensitive move, acknowledging his own need, opening up for Zacchaeus the possibility of experiencing the presence of God's Kingdom. But it inevitably incurs the wrath of the onlookers and their antagonism and critique. This, Jesus is obliged to absorb. His words are affirmation and defence for Zacchaeus and challenge for the onlookers, inviting them to embrace a different way of understanding God and God's ways.

One of scripture's most beautiful themes highlights our yearning for God: "As a deer longs for flowing streams, so my soul longs for you, O God. My soul thirsts for God, for the living God. When shall I come and behold the face of God?" (Ps 42:1–2)[114]

Like Zacchaeus, deep in our hearts, we wish to see Jesus, we desire to become more involved with him and more a part of what he stands for. This longing surfaces in different ways at different times. And Jesus is aware of it. We trust that he will identify our tree and invite us down. On the other hand, like the disciples and crowd, we can be adept at labelling people, using words and phrases that are dismissive and negative and hurtful. Such strategies stifle compassion, and often betray attitudes and prejudices that are destructive, and which imprison us, and blind us to the remarkable transformations that Jesus can make possible.

Conclusion

Each of these Gospel stories reveals a quite remarkable Jesus, who reveals a remarkable God. They invite us to come to know better this God of mercy and compassion. They invite us to align our thinking and living and ministering with that of Jesus in its inclusiveness and barrier-shattering freedom. In compassion and mercy Jesus heals, forgives, invites to friendship, reaches out, liberates, gives life; and he does so with amazing freedom. He does so because he knows the heart of his Father. In our prayer, we need to listen to God's love, God's love for us personally and God's love for others, and allow it to touch us deeply. Let us accept joyfully the mercy that the Father continually offers us in Jesus.

And of course, in the stories there are many Jonah lookalikes in the background among the religious elite and others, who just cannot come to terms with the God of Jesus. Maybe there are sometimes similar judgemental, negative and harsh traces in our own hearts. These we must combat ruthlessly, for mercy stands at the heart of the Gospel and is the fundamental attribute of God.[115] Jesus puts the issue clearly: "Be compassionate as your heavenly Father is compassionate" (Luke 6:36).

Notes

1   See Chapter One.

2   Wisdom 15:1 reads: "But you, our God, are kind and true, patient, ruling all things in mercy."

3   For the call of Simon Peter and Levi, see Chapter Four.

4   See Winstanley, *Jesus and the Little People*, 135–138 and 49–55 respectively.

5   Tannehill, *Luke*, 103. Marshall, *Luke*, 208, comments that for the rabbis the cure of a leper was as difficult as raising someone from the dead.

6   The term covers a variety of skin diseases. The NJB refers to "a virulent skin disease". The term would include psoriasis, lupus, ringworm, favus. Leprosy, now known as Hansen's Disease, was found in India in 600 BCE. It had become a common disease by Greek and Roman times, and may have begun to appear in Palestine by the time of Jesus. Stephen Voorwinde, *Jesus' Emotions in the Gospels* (London: T&T Clark, 2011),

69, n. 17, is of the view that the leper cured by Jesus could have been suffering from leprosy as we know it; similarly, Donahue & Harrington, *Mark*, 88. On the other hand, he could have been afflicted with one of the skin diseases described in Lev 13–14, whose symptoms are not consistent with modern leprosy. Green, *Luke*, 236, is adamant that the "leprosy" of Luke's story is unrelated to the disease identified in this way in modern times. The disease was foremost a social disease, causing segregation.

7   See Lev 13:45–46.

8   See also Donahue & Harrington, *Mark*, 88.

9   In 4:43, Jesus has stated his intention to proclaim the Good News to other cities in the area. Green, *Luke*, 236, suggests that far from the temple and Pharisaic scrutiny, legal requirements may have been relaxed locally.

10   Marshall, *Luke*, 209, links Jesus' stretching out his hand with the action of God (Exod 6:6; 14:16; 15:12; Jer 17:5).

11   Voorwinde, *Emotions*, 71. In the Old Testament there are only two accounts of the healing of leprosy: the cases of Miriam (Num 12:10–15) and Naaman (2 Kgs 5:1–14).

12   In Mark's version (1:45) the leper himself freely proclaims to all and sundry what has happened.

13   The "Pharisees" (separated ones) were deeply religious men who observed the Law and oral tradition strictly, especially in matters of ritual purity. They tended to form groups of "associates". They kept their distance from other people and were the defenders of strict Jewish orthodoxy. The "teachers of the Law", often referred to as the "scribes", were the professional interpreters of the Law; they were both theologians and lawyers; most of them were Pharisees. The Pharisees and scribes are Jesus' chief opponents in Galilee.

14   Johnson, *Luke*, 93, also makes this point.

15   Green, *Luke*, 240, observes that in Luke the "power of the Lord" is equivalent to the "Spirit of the Lord".

16   In Mark, the roof would probably have consisted of branches and hardened mud. Luke seems to have a Roman-type house in mind; see Carroll, *Luke*, 130, though Marshall, *Luke*, 213, suggests that tiled roofs were in use in Palestine by this time.

17   This is the first mention of "faith" in the Gospel; for Johnson, *Luke*, 93, it denotes hope, trust and perseverance.

18   Carroll, *Luke*, 131, states: "As God's Son, commissioned and empowered by God's own Spirit, Jesus acts with divine authority." Johnson, *Luke*, 93, notes that the perfect passive of the verb indicates that forgiveness is an accomplished fact, and is done by God.

19   The ability to perceive inner thoughts and attitudes is typical of a prophet (see Byrne, *Hospitality*, 59). Carroll, *Luke*, 130, refers to "prophetic discernment". As Simeon states (2:35) "the thoughts of many will be revealed." Jesus is also bypassing the normal temple system with regard to forgiveness.

20   This is the first use of "the Son of Man" in Luke. The phrase is found only on Jesus' lips in the contexts of his ministry, his suffering and his future judging role; for this, see Johnson, *Luke*, 94.

21   Most people are familiar with Matthew's "Sermon on the Mount" (5:1–7:29). Luke, 6:20–49, locates the discourse of Jesus "on a level place"; Jesus stands rather than sits, and he addresses a large crowd as well as his disciples. Luke relocates much of Matthew's material to the journey narrative (9:51–19:44).

22   Marshall, *Luke*, 276, entitles this section (7:1–50) "the compassion of the Messiah".

23   Carroll, *Luke*, 159, 162.

24   Green, *Luke*, 283–284.

25   Caird, *Luke*, 108; Marshall, *Luke*, 279. Meier, *A Marginal Jew*, 2:721, notes that most centurions were ordinary soldiers who progressed through the ranks; the number of troops they commanded varied; it could be 30 or 60 men. They exercised more than simply military duties, including building and diplomatic roles. They are not a homogeneous group. Herod Antipas had a private army, probably consisting mainly of gentiles, and had adopted Roman military nomenclature. Their role was to control Galilee. Levine, "Luke: Introduction and Annotations", 114, states that Rome stationed no troops in Galilee in the time of Antipas; he could be a pensioned officer. Evans too, *Luke*, 343, notes that Galilee was not occupied by the Romans until 44 CE. Carroll, *Luke*, 160, n. 23, suggests that whatever the historical situation in Galilee at the time of Jesus, the Roman imperial context for Luke's narrative as a whole, and for a late-first-century audience, does point to a leadership position in the Roman army.

26   In John's version, he is called a "royal official" *(basilikos)*. Francis J. Moloney, *The Gospel of John*, Sacra Pagina 4 (Collegeville, MN: The Liturgical Press, 1998), 157, 160–161, maintains that he is a gentile.

27   In John, he has a fever; in Matthew, he is painfully paralysed but not near death. Luke calls him a servant/slave *(doulos)*, John a son *(huios)*, Matthew a *pais*, which can mean son or servant. Green, *Luke*, 286, comments that the centurion not only regarded the slave as useful, but esteemed him.

28   McBride, *Luke*, 94, observes that he is not concerned with his reputation as a public figure, but with the well-being of his sick slave.

29   Gentiles use intermediaries in John 12:20. Tannehill, *Luke*, 124, observes that in the patronal system of the time, his patronage requires reciprocal support from his beneficiaries; also, Carroll, *Luke*, 161; Green, *Luke*, 285. For Marshall, *Luke*, 280, these men also acted as a disciplinary body for the synagogue.

30   Johnson, *Luke*, 117, calls him a "God-fearing Gentile" like Cornelius in Acts 10:1, 22. He provided funds for the construction of the synagogue. On p. 120, he notes echoes of the story of Elisha and Naaman the Syrian in 2 Kgs 5:1–14; also, Carroll, *Luke*, 159,162, who mentions that, like Elisha, Jesus heals from a distance and responds to the request of a gentile for help, aided by the Jewish servant girl; similarly, Green, *Luke*, 284. Marshall, *Luke*, 280, suggests that their pressing their case "eagerly" may indicate that they felt Jesus might not be willing to help a gentile. Carroll, *Luke*, 160, comments that the fact that this outsider is a friend of Jewish people and has funded the construction of their synagogue, indicates that the boundaries between Israel and the nations have begun to blur. Green, however, *Luke*, 287, maintains that their words betray their captivity to a world system whose basis and practices run counter to the mercy of God.

31   The Greek (*kyrios*) is a sign of respect; it is the gentile equivalent of "rabbi"; but a Christian reader would see a deeper significance. Carroll, *Luke,* 159, believes that "the focus on command and obedience in the passage suggests that with this address the centurion is deferring to Jesus' authority as Lord."

32   Voorwinde, *Emotions,* 19, notes that the centurion has authority because he is under (imperial) authority; Jesus is similarly under divine authority. Jesus is backed by God's authority. Similarly, Caird, *Luke,* 108: Jesus derived his authority from a higher source; Marshall, *Luke,* 282. Tannehill, *Luke,* 125, mentions a chain of authority. Green, *Luke,* 99, also notes the analogy. Ulrich Luz, *Matthew* 3 vols (Minneapolis, MN: Augsburg Fortress, 2001, 2005, 2007), 2:10, "If even I, a minor officer, can give commands, how much more can you!"

33   Tannehill, *Luke,* 125, states that his faith consists in his surmounting the social barrier between Jew and gentile, his willingness to lay aside his personal honour, his trust in Jesus' healing power and perhaps his insight into Jesus' divine authority.

34   Luke omits the severe warning of Jesus found in Matthew (8:11–12): "I tell you, many will come from east and west and will eat with Abraham and Isaac and Jacob in the kingdom of heaven, while the heirs of the kingdom will be thrown into the outer darkness, where there will be weeping and gnashing of teeth." Similar words are found later in Luke 13:28–30.

35   McBride, *Luke,* 94; Carroll, *Luke,* 160; on p. 163 he notes how remarkable in Jesus' eyes is the centurion's bold trust.

36   Green, *Luke,* 288.

37   Luz, *Matthew,* 2:11, sees him as the first member of the gentile church (referring in the footnote to Aquinas).

38   "Lord, I am not worthy that you should enter under my roof, but only say the word and my soul shall be healed."

39   The two incidents are carefully paired by Luke; they also illustrate his male/female penchant. Although found only in Luke, the story about the widow of Nain is not a Lukan creation, but is derived from his special source material, which he has edited. Meier, *A Marginal Jew,* 2:797, notes that the anchoring of the story in the obscure Galilean town of Nain (now shown by archaeology to have had a gate), as well as the presence of some possible Semitisms in the text, argues for the origin of the story among Jewish Christians in Palestine. With some hesitation, he inclines to the view that the story goes back to some incident involving Jesus at Nain during his public ministry. Mark, Luke and John have each only one story of Jesus raising someone from the dead. Meier acknowledges the influence of the Elijah-Elisha stories and the story of Jairus' daughter on the way Luke's story is written. Carroll, *Luke,* 164–165, likewise (Elijah in 1 Kings 17:8–24 LXX; Elisha in 2 Kings 4: 32–37).

40   McBride, *Luke,* 95, refers to a crowd following life and a crowd following death.

41   Also, Fitzmyer, *Luke,* 1:658; Johnson, *Luke,* 118; Evans, *Luke,* 346; Carroll, *Luke,* 165. Care for widows is a prominent theme in the Old Testament (Deut 10:18; 14: 28–29; 24:17–21; 27:19; Job 24:3; Ps 146:9; Isa 10:1–2).

42   Marshall, *Luke,* 285; Wright, *Luke,* 83.

43   This is the first time that Luke uses the title "Lord" for Jesus, a title common

in the early Church; it is appropriate in this life-giving context and becomes a distinctive feature of the narrative of this Gospel. See Johnson, *Luke*, 118; Fitzmyer, *Luke*, 1:659; McBride, *Luke*, 96; Marshall, *Luke*, 285. Luke also uses the technical verb for compassion (*splanchnizesthai*) in two parables, as he describes the reaction of the Samaritan and of the father of the two lost sons (10:33; 15:20).

44 Francis J. Moloney, *This is the Gospel of the Lord (C)* (Homebush: St Paul Publications, 1991), 134.

45 This phrase echoes 1 Kgs 17:23, the story of Elijah and the son of the widow of Zarephath; there are a number of parallels and verbal echoes. The other Old Testament instance of raising someone to life is the case of Elisha and the Shunamite woman's son (2 Kgs 4:32–37). The two prophets pray fervently to God; Elijah stretches himself over the child three times. Jesus simply speaks a word; he is in a different league. See Voorwinde, *Emotions*, 127. Luke tells the story with deliberate echoes of these prophets: thus Wright, *Luke*, 83; Fitzmyer, *Luke*, 1:659; F. Mosetto, *Lettura del Vangelo secondo Luca* (Rome: LAS, 2003), 156; Johnson, *Luke*, 120; Evans, *Luke*, 346; Green, *Luke*, 290.

46 Byrne, *Hospitality*, 70; Green, *Luke*, 290, observes that here the healing is the restoration of the woman within her community.

47 Green, *Luke*, 292.

48 1:68; in 1:78 *splanchna* is used.

49 McBride, *Luke*, 96.

50 John's being in prison is not mentioned here as it is in the Matthaean parallel; Luke has mentioned it in 3:20. Green, *Luke*, 294, notes the close link with what has just been narrated.

51 3:7–17; in 3:16 the Baptist speaks of the "one more powerful than I" who is coming.

52 4:16–21. Green, *Luke*, 295, notes that "John's interest lies on the fault line between his eschatological expectations and the realities of Jesus' performance."

53 Caird, *Luke*, 111, maintains that the presence of disciples who are aloof from the movement of Jesus is an indication that the Baptist is not convinced of Jesus' role.

54 Isa 61:1; 35:5–6; 26:19; 29:18–19; 42:18; 43:8. Green, *Luke*, 297, observes that the "overlap with Jesus' inaugural sermon and his answer to John provides a powerful sanction for the integrity of his mission: he is doing what the Spirit of the Lord anointed him to do." Marshall, *Luke*, 291, notes that the list refers to the ministry of Jesus as a whole, and is couched in the language of the Old Testament.

55 Byrne, *Hospitality*, 71; Caird, *Luke*, 112. McBride, *Luke*, 98, calls this "a delicate plea for understanding".

56 Marshall, *Luke*, 287, observes that "the person who recognises the fulfilment will know that Jesus is the Coming One, and will not be put off by his failure to live up to the traditional—or Johannine—expectations."

57 Meier, *A Marginal Jew*, 2:136.

58 Caird, *Luke*, 111.

59 Green, *Luke*, 620, details similarities between this story and that of Naaman in 2 Kgs. Luke is not only linking Jesus with the Old Testament prophets, but noting that outsiders can receive the benefits of salvation.

60   Carroll, *Luke*, 343. Evans, *Luke*, 624, emphasises Luke's inadequate geographical awareness of Palestine. Green, *Luke*, 621–22, notes that Jesus is following the circuitous pilgrim route that bypasses Samaria, but, given the ambiguity of moving "along the border", Luke may also be indicating the possibility of status reversal. Fitzmyer, *Luke*, 2:1152, notes Luke's "geographical ineptitude". Carroll, *Luke*, 344, n. 101, notes the symbolic triangulation of the sites (Jerusalem—the destination; Galilee—Jesus' homeland and area of ministry; Samaria—cultural and religious border space and site of earlier rejection. "The spatial markers flow from meaningful rhetorical design, whatever the (im)precision of Luke's mapping of Palestine."

61   Green, *Luke*, 622.

62   Fitzmyer, *Luke*, 2:1151.

63   This is the only time Jesus is called "Master" by someone who is not a disciple.

64   This may entail travelling to Jerusalem (or Gerizim), but, according to Marshall, *Luke*, 651, they could approach priests living locally. But at some stage a sacrifice was required.

65   Evans, *Luke*, 623, notes that the healing of several people simultaneously is unique in the Synoptic tradition.

66   Early in Jesus' journey, a Samaritan village refused to welcome Jesus (9:51–53). Later, Jesus told the parable in which a Samaritan is the star (10:29–37). Acts 8 presents the mission to Samaria. Green, *Luke*, 619, sees Luke as here dropping a bombshell. This is his punch line. We discussed the difficulties between Jews and Samaritans earlier in Chapter Eight.

67   Green, *Luke*, 620.

68   Evans, *Luke*, 625, says that the word (*allogenēs*) means a religious alien; it was found on the barrier in the temple warning non-Israelites to go no further. Green, *Luke*, 626, adds that the leper is therefore not classified as a child of Abraham, and yet has behaved in a manner appropriate to the authentic children of Abraham.

69   Carroll, *Luke*, 344, notes the progression: mercy, cleansing, healing, cleansing, salvation.

70   Carroll, *Luke*, 344. Tannehill, *Luke*, 257, comments that all ten had sufficient faith to respond to Jesus' command but his blossomed into praise of God and gratitude to Jesus. Fitzmyer, *Luke*, 2:1151, refers to his conversion to God and his agent, Jesus.

71   Caird, *Luke*, 195. Evans, *Luke*, 623, refers to the genuine piety of a non-Israelite that manifests itself in gratitude.

72   Carroll, *Luke*, 342. Green, *Luke*, 626, comments that Luke presents Jesus in the role of the temple, the one in whom the powerful and merciful presence of God is realised.

73   Contrary to Paul Simon's famous song, "I am a Rock" (New York: Eclectic Music Co., 1965).

74   In Mark (10:35–45), this is illustrated by the request of the sons of Zebedee for the top jobs in the Kingdom. This episode Luke omits.

75   Luke is following Mark but has transferred this episode to the entry into Jericho rather than his departure, so that he can place the Zacchaeus story at that point. In Mark, the man is named as Bartimaeus. Matthew has two blind beggars in his version. Green,

Luke, 662, notes that the disciples have faded into the background.

76   McBride, *Mark*, 168–169.

77   Moloney, *Mark*, 208; Green, *Luke*, 663.

78   Bailey, *Jesus Through Middle Eastern Eyes*, 172, suggests that as well as the pilgrims from Galilee, the majority of the crowd would consist of locals who had gone out to meet a distinguished person who would spend the night in their town.

79   The Greek is *Nazōraios* rather than *Nazarēnos;* Luke uses it only here in the Gospel but frequently in Acts. Fitzmyer, *Luke*, 2:1215–16, suggests a possible added nuance of "consecrated one" or "sprout of David's line." See Chapter Three, n. 74 & 75.

80   Jesus' Davidic ancestry was mentioned in 1:32; 2:4; 3:31. The issue is raised in the controversy story (20:41–44); and also in Acts 2:29–32; 13:22–23. The man's cry for mercy echoes 17:13 (the ten lepers) and 16:24 (Dives in Hades).

81   Tannehill, *Luke*, 274; Peter's earlier confession was followed by a command to silence. Green, *Luke*, 663, too notes that this is the first public declaration. Marshall, *Luke*, 693, asks whether it was beyond the ability of the blind man to link the fact that Jesus was believed to work miracles, and that his mission could be understood in messianic terms? The title "Son of David" is used in Matt (15:22) by the Syro-Phoenician woman.

82   2 Sam 7:12–16; 1 Chr 17:11–14; Ps 89:29–38; especially the Psalms of Solomon, from 50 BCE. See Carroll, *Luke*, 370; Culpepper, *Mark*, 353; Meier, *A Marginal Jew*, 2:689–90; Martin, *Mark*, 281; Moloney, *Mark*, 209.

83   Green, *Luke*, 664.

84   The text actually states: "Those in front". Green, *Luke*, 664, notes that while this could be interpreted spatially, it could also refer to leaders, maybe disciples; they consider the man "outside the boundaries of God's grace."

85   Luke omits the Markan detail of the man casting aside his cloak.

86   Bailey, *Jesus through Middle Eastern Eyes*, 174, notes that a beggar normally has no education, training, employment record or marketing skills, so if healed, self-support would be difficult. Jesus is asking him if he is ready to accept the new responsibilities that will come to him if healed.

87   Fitzmyer, *Luke*, 2:1213, translates "regain" rather than simply "receive"; the imperative verb is *anablepson.*

88   Healing and faith have been linked in 7:50; 8:48. In Matthew (20:34) Jesus is "moved to compassion" and reaches out and touches the eyes of the two blind men; mention of their faith is omitted. Prior to this story in Luke, the issue of salvation was raised: "Who can be saved?" (18:26), a question partially answered in this and the subsequent stories.

89   Carroll, *Luke*, 370.

90   The verb (*sōzein*) often refers to both healing and salvation. Tannehill, *Luke*, 275, considers this the final healing event of Jesus' ministry, discounting 22:15.

91   Green, *Luke*, 665. Fitzmyer, *Luke*, 2:1214, notes that, prior to this episode, Jesus has spoken about the passion, but the disciples have failed to understand; the blind man does see more than they do.

92   In Matthew's version, in which two blind men are cured, this is specifically highlighted (20:34).

93   For a discussion of his name, see Fitzmyer, *Luke*, 2:1223.

94   Marshall, *Luke*, 694; Green, *Luke*, 668; Fitzmyer, *Luke*, 2:1222. Bailey, *Jesus Through Middle Eastern Eyes*, 170, sees the two stories as linked: the beggar healed by Jesus was one of the socially oppressed; Zacchaeus is an oppressor. He structures the story as nine cameo scenes in chiastic/inverted parallelism: Jesus, Zacchaeus, crowd, up tree, Jesus, down tree, crowd, Zacchaeus, Jesus.

95   Bailey, *Jesus through Middle Eastern Eyes*, 176, suggests that the Jericho community would be deeply disappointed that Jesus is not staying there for the night.

96   Caird, *Luke*, 207. The Greek term is *architelōnēs*. Green, *Luke*, 668, states that, though the job title is not clear, Zacchaeus is presented as a person of advanced status, if only among other tax collectors. His wealth came from his entrepreneurial activity. Tannehill, *Luke*, 275, comments that he is not an underling like Levi. Resseguie, *Spiritual Landscape*, 108, n. 44, refers to a district manager responsible for collecting taxes for a geographical area with assistant tax collectors working under him.

97   Wright, *Luke*, 222, describes his situation extremely well; see McBride, *Luke*, 244.

98   See Caird, *Luke*, 208; McBride, *Luke*, 244.

99   The Greek word here translated "of small stature" can also mean "young." Resseguie, *Spiritual Landscape*, 108, comments that the barricade of people adds to the indignity of his short stature.

100   Byrne, *Hospitality*, 150. Carroll, *Luke*, 373, speaks of "comic theatre of the absurd."

101   Bailey, *Jesus through Middle Eastern Eyes*, 178; Fitzmyer, *Luke*, 2:1224, notes that New Testament Jericho had parks, avenues and public squares where fine trees grew. Marshall, *Luke*, 696, points out that these oak-like evergreens (*sykomorea* or *ficus sycomoros* in Latin) are very different from our UK sycamores or planes. Carroll, *Luke*, 372, comments that the fact that he cuts such an undignified profile despite his wealth suits his marginal social position, and cues the reader that his riches will not have the last say.

102   Johnson, *Luke*, 285, notes that *dei* ("must") designates important turning points in the story as directed by God; Marshall, *Luke*, 697, also sees the necessity as imposed on Jesus by God; also, Green, *Luke*, 666, 670, who notes that "today" in Luke communicates the immediacy of salvation. Mosetto, *Luca*, 325, observes that the use of the verb *menō*, stay, recurs in the Emmaus story. Bailey, *Jesus Through Middle Eastern Eyes*, 180, notes how unusual it was for the guest to select the form of hospitality.

103   Johnson, *Luke*, 285; Fitzmyer, *Luke*, 2:1224; Green, *Luke*, 671.

104   Bailey, *Jesus Through Middle Eastern Eyes*, 180. Jesus "neither endorses the oppression nor ostracizes the oppressor. Instead he loves him."

105   Caird, *Luke*, 208.

106   Some, like Bailey, *Jesus Through Middle Eastern Eyes*, 181, believe that this takes place inside the house at a meal as a formal response; but that breaks the natural flow of the narrative. Marshall, *Luke*, 697, thinks it is probably outside in the presence of the people. Zacchaeus' words are not meant to sound like a boast; likewise, Fitzmyer, *Luke*, 2:1225. Green, *Luke*, 671, suggests that Zacchaeus lists behaviours "appropriate for those who have oriented themselves around the kingdom of God."

107   Also, Evans, *Luke*, 661; he notes, 663, that the Greek here does not convey any doubt. Bailey, *Jesus Through Middle Eastern Eyes*, 181, suggests that his words are exaggerated to indicate his sincerity, in traditional Middle Eastern style; his hearers would not expect him to fulfil what he says. Tannehill, *Luke*, 277, believes that such compensation will take all or most of his wealth.

108   Carroll, *Luke*, 373.

109   Marshall, *Luke*, 697; on p. 698 he expresses his view that the verb refers to the future. There is an alternative view that Zacchaeus in self-vindication is describing his customary lifestyle (see Winstanley, *Little People*, 64, referring to Byrne, *Hospitality*, 151; Fitzmyer, *Luke*, 2:1220–1221, 1225; Johnson, *Luke*, 257, 285–6). Green also, *Luke*, 671–672, does not see this episode as a story of conversion; similarly, Levine, "Luke: Introduction and Annotations", 139. Carroll, *Luke*, 371, 372, suggests that the disapproval of the crowd is hard to square with a tax collector who practises noble conduct! On either reading, Jesus defends Zacchaeus' public honour. Tannehill, *Luke*, 277, acknowledges this view but comments that it is hard to understand the antagonism of the crowd, or Jesus' word about "salvation" and reference to "the lost", if Zacchaeus is not indicating a fundamental change of life. Resseguie, *Spiritual Landscape*, 159, n. 54, maintains that the arguments of those favouring a customary present tense have been effectively refuted.

110   Bailey, *Jesus Through Middle Eastern Eyes*, 182, 185.

111   Johnson, *Luke*, 286, notes that the noun "salvation" is used only here after the Infancy Narrative; the verb, however, occurs frequently. Carroll, *Luke*, 372, sees Zacchaeus as another example of "inside-out reversal".

112   Fitzmyer, *Luke*, 2:1226 and 1222, also stresses the shepherd image and its background in Ezekiel 34 (also Green, *Luke*, 673). Further, Fitzmyer notes that the Son of Man title may have been added to an otherwise authentic saying of Jesus. Marshall, *Luke*, 695, makes the comment that the epitome of Luke's Gospel message is expressed here.

113   Resseguie, *Spiritual Landscape*, 114.

114   See also Pss 63:1; 143:6.

115   Kasper, *Pope Francis' Revolution of Tenderness and Love*, 35.

Chapter Eleven
Seeking and Finding

In the previous chapter, we examined several of the occasions when Jesus showed mercy and compassion in action. Now I propose to examine three of his parables that develop this theme. The wider context is the travel narrative, the journey of Jesus to Jerusalem. More immediately, it is an occasion when he is sharing his table with people who are on the margins of religious society, and he is criticised for it, not for the first time, by the religious elite. In the next chapter, we shall be reflecting more fully on the table fellowship of Jesus.

The Setting (15:1–2)

> Now all the tax collectors and sinners were coming near to listen to him. And the Pharisees and the scribes were grumbling and saying, "This fellow welcomes sinners and eats with them."

Though brief, this is a significant passage.[1] The religious outcasts and other outsiders, who bear the social stigma of "sinners", "persons living outside the structure of faithful Torah observance",[2] are drawing close to Jesus. Jesus is comfortable with people who would normally be excluded.[3] They obviously feel comfortable with him. Their purpose is to listen to him, which suggests a level of openness to him and his message.[4] In the background are the "Pharisees and scribes", who keep their distance to avoid contamination and shun table fellowship with sinners.[5] They "grumble" repeatedly and openly.[6] Their criticism is focused not only on Jesus' eating and drinking with these people, as on earlier occasions,[7] but also on his welcoming them, his offering them hospitality. To host or entertain sinners was a more serious offence in their eyes than simply to eat with sinners informally or to accept invitations, which was itself scandalous enough. In their eyes, Jesus was welcoming the dregs of society.[8]

The table fellowship of Jesus, as it is called, his sharing meals with others, seems to have been a key feature of his ministry. In the villages of Galilee, where hospitality was an essential aspect of life, it was quite natural that Jesus should frequently be invited to share table. Sometimes it would be an expression of gratitude, perhaps for his having healed someone, or an indication of respect; sometimes it would be an occasion for him to teach. In that culture, to share table was a very significant gesture. It was above all an expression of social inclusion.[9]

On this occasion, Jesus responds to the criticism levelled against him by recounting three parables.[10] There are two short parables presented in parallel and carefully matched in content and language: the parables of the lost sheep and the lost coin.[11] Then there is the longer and very familiar parable of the two lost sons, normally and misleadingly referred to as the parable of the prodigal son. In fact, I think that the usual emphasis on lostness in these parables is misplaced. In the Lukan context, I prefer to see them as parables of seeking and finding that which is lost, a seeking that is demanding and costly, and a finding that calls for joyful celebration.[12] Matthew has a version of the first of these parables; the other two are found only in Luke. Each evangelist is responsible for the choice of context in which he places the parables and for the particular interpretation or application he suggests at the end. The context chosen here by Luke probably reflects the original setting,[13] and in considering these parables, it is important to keep the context in mind: Jesus is in the company of sinners, and the Pharisees show contempt for him ("this fellow") and are indifferent towards and lacking in compassion for those with whom he dines. It is particularly to these that the parable is directed.

The Shepherd and The Lost Sheep (15:3–8)

The first parable concerns a shepherd:

> Which one of you, having a hundred sheep and losing one of them, does not leave the ninety-nine in the wilderness and go after the one that is lost until he finds it? When he has found it, he lays it on his shoulders and rejoices. And when he comes home, he calls together his friends and neighbours, saying to them, "Rejoice with me, for I have found my sheep that was lost." Just so, I tell you, there will be more joy in heaven over one sinner who repents than over ninety-nine righteous persons who need no repentance. (15:4–7)

The opening rhetorical question immediately draws us in, suggesting that we identify with the main character.[14] The image of a shepherd with a sheep on his shoulders has fired the imagination of artists and sculptors through the ages, going right back to the early Christian catacombs. But we have all had the experience of losing things that are important to us, and taking great efforts to find them. We have known the relief, joy and satisfaction that discovering them brings. I frequently misplace my glasses and occasionally my keys. I once mislaid a cheque for £10,000 given as a donation to the Salesians at Christmas time! On finding it, I certainly had a glass or two of wine in joyful celebration!

We are familiar with the storyline of the parable, but perhaps fail to appreciate its links with the classic Palm 23, "The Lord is my Shepherd". While the emphasis is on the shepherding element of the psalm, the context also recalls the meal element. We may not realise that Jesus follows a similar literary pattern (chiasm, ring composition, inverted parallelism) that goes back as far as the eighth century before him and is continued after him.[15] We might also overlook the fact that Jesus' choice of a shepherd as the hero of the story would upset the religious leaders in his audience. For, although shepherd imagery was applied to God in the Old Testament, in that culture, to tend sheep was a low-class occupation, a role avoided by religious people.[16] It was one of the proscribed trades; one carrying it out would be considered a sinner by the religious elite. It would, therefore, be a shock for the religious elite to be invited to think of themselves as shepherds.

The setting is the wilderness, an ominous place. The shepherd, not mentioned as such in the text but clearly implied, is possibly the owner of the sheep, a large flock of a hundred, or is looking after the sheep of several members of his clan.[17] He probably counts them in the late afternoon before settling them in a secure area for the night.[18] On realising that one is missing and that he has been careless, that he is at fault, he makes the decision to leave the rest in the wilderness[19] and go out in search of the stray, even though light is fading. It is important to him. The size of the herd would suggest that the shepherd has other helpers in whose care he leaves the other ninety-nine; the sheep would not be left alone. The search could prove lengthy and strenuous; it would be physically costly. A sheep that has wandered eventually gets exhausted, disoriented and lies down, afraid, and continues to bleat plaintively. The shepherd calls and hears the response, finds the sheep, puts it on his shoulders and carries it home.[20] He then organises a party for his friends[21] to celebrate his finding the sheep, for in a village culture all are involved. Saving face, he refers to the sheep that was lost, rather than admit that he had been careless and the loss was his fault.[22]

Having told the story, Jesus adds an interpretation.[23] Just as the shepherd rejoices at his finding the lost sheep, so God is delighted when sinners repent or are restored.[24] So the story is telling something about the shepherd God of the prophet Ezekiel (34). God desires to find the lost and bring them home. In the Old Testament, it was the flock that had wandered; here it is a single sheep, but the message is the same. Jesus knows the mind and heart of God; because God is like that, Jesus conducts his ministry in the way he does. Going a step further, Jesus puts himself in this parable. He is revealing to his hearers, both friends and foes, how he sees himself. His action in searching for the lost, which takes the form of his sharing table with them, is a fulfilling of the Old Testament promises. He is the shepherd God promised; he is acting out the role of God.[25]

The parable is also a critique and challenge to the religious elite, who have failed in their duty of care for the people and show no interest in saving them. In this, the parable recalls Ezekiel 34:1–16. Jesus is inviting them to change their attitudes. They probably consider themselves righteous through their observance of all the Laws and not needing to repent, but their understanding of God is defective, their self-awareness is skewed, and their care for others in need is sadly lacking.[26]

Finally, the interpretation at the end of the parable refers to sinners repenting, and we might ask where this takes place in the storyline. The emphasis is clearly placed on the searching action of the shepherd; all the sheep does is to respond to the shepherd's call by bleating, which is an acknowledgement of his plight, and allowing itself to be found, carried home and restored to the flock. The searching, Jesus' table fellowship, is an offer of rescue and salvation, freely given. Repentance is redefined as accepting the gift of salvation.[27]

The Woman and The Lost Coin (15:8–10)

The theme of losing, searching, finding and celebration is continued or repeated in the second parable of the trilogy:

> Or what woman having ten silver coins, if she loses one of them, does not light a lamp, sweep the house, and search carefully until she finds it? When she has found it, she calls together her friends and neighbours, saying, "Rejoice with me, for I have found the coin that I had lost." Just so, I tell you, there is joy in the presence of the angels of God over one sinner who repents.

The introductory phrase of the previous parable, "Which of you", is omitted. This time the chief protagonist is a woman. Jesus is being even bolder in his choosing a woman as an image of God, given that women had little social standing.[28] The religious elite would have been shocked.[29] But Jesus is sensitive to the fact that there are many women in his audience, and that some were genuine disciples. There were women in Israel's past who had acted heroically on behalf of their people, like Deborah and Judith.[30] There are other examples of Jesus presenting stories in pairs: modern-day equal opportunities.[31] The structure follows the prophetical rhetorical template.[32]

The setting is no longer a wilderness hillside but a village dwelling, probably a house built of basalt stones. The woman loses a coin, a "drachma", which amounted to a day's wages. The loss of one drachma out of ten is more serious than one sheep out of a hundred. While not destitute, her economic situation would not be secure.[33] This coin was taken out of circulation by Emperor Nero and replaced by the *denarius*, which maintained the same value; this is the only occasion that the term is used in the New Testament. The floor of the house may have consisted of basalt slabs, so the coin could have been lodged in one of the gaps. Light entered mainly through the door, as the windows were very narrow; this is why the woman has to light an oil lamp (unless we imagine that it is night). The woman's efforts are described in greater detail as she devotes time and energy in diligently searching for what she has misplaced, carefully sweeping the floor. On finding the coin, she calls together her female friends and neighbours for a celebration.[34] In this parable, too, the accent is on rejoicing, and a similar interpretation is appended: "there is joy in the presence of the angels of God over one sinner who repents."

The woman is put forward by Jesus as an image of God, the God who searches for what is lost and is delighted to find it. In this story, the coin does nothing; the accent is totally on the action of the woman, and therefore presents repentance or restoration as the free gift offered by God. Though lost, the value of the coin is not diminished; the same is true for the sinner. "As metaphors of divine action these two parables upset the way we normally think about God and shatter the barriers to God's mercy and love erected often by religious observance itself."[35] If human beings go to such lengths to find what is lost and then share their joy with others, wouldn't God? Our behaviour can tell something about God.[36] As in the earlier parable, Jesus is inviting his Pharisee hearers to understand his style of ministry, especially his inclusive table fellowship as reflecting the mind and heart of God, to rethink their own attitudes and views and to set about seeking the lost. Donahue emphasises the joy of finding and being found. "Applications of these parables which stress the need for repentance are really in tension with the parabolic narrative. Conversion or change of heart is not a condition but a consequence of God's love."[37]

The Searching Father (15:11–32)

It is this last point that leads us into a consideration of the parable of the two lost sons, one in a far, foreign pigsty, the other at home on the farm,[38] or the parable of a father, whose extravagant love leads him to search for them both. This is "one of the most touching and exquisite short stories in the pages of world literature."[39] The familiar text reads as follows:

Then Jesus said, "There was a man who had two sons. The younger of them said to his father, 'Father, give me the share of the property that will belong to me.' So, he divided his property between them. A few days later the younger son gathered all he had and travelled to a distant country, and there he squandered his property in dissolute living. When he had spent everything, a severe famine took place throughout that country, and he began to be in need. So, he went and hired himself out to one of the citizens of that country, who sent him to his fields to feed the pigs. He would gladly have filled himself with the pods that the pigs were eating; and no one gave him anything. But when he came to himself he said, 'How many of my father's hired hands have bread enough and to spare, but here I am dying of hunger! I will get up and go to my father, and I will say to him, "Father, I have sinned against heaven and before you; I am no longer worthy to be called your son; treat me like one of your hired hands".' So he set off and went to his father. But while he was still far off, his father saw him and was filled with compassion; he ran and put his arms around him and kissed him. Then the son said to him, 'Father, I have sinned against heaven and before you; I am no longer worthy to be called your son.' But the father said to his slaves, 'Quickly, bring out a robe—the best one—and put it on him; put a ring on his finger and sandals on his feet. And get the fatted calf and kill it, and let us eat and celebrate; for this son of mine was dead and is alive again; he was lost and is found!' And they began to celebrate.

"Now his elder son was in the field; and when he came and approached the house, he heard music and dancing. He called one of the slaves and asked what was going on. He replied, 'Your brother has come, and your father has killed the fatted calf, because he has got him back safe and sound.' Then he became angry and refused to go in. His father came out and began to plead with him. But he answered his father, 'Listen! For all these years I have been working like a slave for you, and I have never disobeyed your command; yet you have never given me even a young goat so that I might celebrate with my friends. But when this son of yours came back, who has devoured your property with prostitutes, you killed the fatted calf for him!' Then the father said to him, 'Son, you are always with me, and all that is mine is yours. But we had to celebrate and rejoice, because this brother of yours was dead and has come to life; he was lost and has been found'."

The parable divides naturally into three parts, each suggested by the text itself: the departure and fall of the younger son; his return and welcome by the father;

the father and the older brother. The father is the main character; his actions shape the way the narrative unfolds and provide the crucial turning points. The dynamics of human relationships and family life provide the field of comparison for the parable.[40]

Departure of The Younger Son

The opening statement recalls other men who had two sons: Adam with Cain and Abel; Abraham with Isaac and Ishmael; Isaac with the twins Jacob and Esau; Jacob's son Joseph with Manasseh and Ephraim; David was the youngest son of seven, and so on. In these cases, there is some sibling rivalry, and it is the younger son who is favoured. So, this would be the expectation of those listening to Jesus' parable, but parables don't usually follow expectations![41]

The father in the story is probably a farmer or landowner and quite well off. His younger son approaches him and asks for a share of the family estate. The legal situation in Jesus' time was complex. Some maintain that a father could dispose of his property during his lifetime, despite the cautions against such a course of action found in the book of Sirach (33:19–23), but it was highly unusual. Others believe that any transfer of the ownership of property normally took place after the father's death, so it was unusual for a son to ask for it. It has been suggested that the son's request may be considered as tantamount to wishing his father dead.[42] In that world, it was the family rather than the individual that was the source of identity; family loyalty was crucial. Solidarity with the village community was another key factor. Central to family identity was relationship to land, which should always remain in the family.[43] The implications of the young man's request are therefore considerable. On the other hand, given that younger sons often emigrated because of the precarious nature of the Palestinian agrarian economy, "the request should not be considered as rebellion or a desire for unwarranted freedom. It was legitimate, even if inappropriate."[44] In granting the request, which is couched rather like a command, the father demonstrates enormous love for his boy, and perhaps a little prodigality in giving the younger son half the estate rather than the usual one third.[45] But his reputation would suffer; he would lose honour and status in the village community; this he disregards.[46]

The father then probably sold some of the property "in order to provide the inheritance in liquid assets."[47] Some think that the father probably did not, at this stage, hand over the rest of the property to the older son but remained master of the house and owner of the remaining property.[48] Others take the opposite view, as the text suggests.[49] "If the father deeded the property to his sons during his lifetime, the sons would normally have the right of possession, but not the right of disposal, since the father retained the use and enjoyment of the property." [50] The younger son wastes no time in moving off. He leaves home and family, rejecting all that it stands for. He is prepared to sever his relationship with his father, showing no regard for his feelings or future well-being. Leaving his brother does not seem to pose a problem; it appears that they are not particularly close. The elder brother apparently makes no attempt to mediate, to reconcile, as might have been expected in that culture;[51] he may have been annoyed that he had received only half rather than the expected two thirds. The closely-knit village community would have been surprised and shocked at what had happened.

The young man sets off for the diaspora. There he irresponsibly squanders his money on a life of pleasure, self-indulgence and extravagance.[52] In doing so, he completely disposes of his capital, making it impossible for him to offer support to his father in his old age; he thus severs the relationship and dishonours the family. It is this that constitutes his sin.[53]

The situation changes dramatically with the onset of famine. Penniless and without friends, his freedom dream in tatters, he is obliged to hire himself out to a gentile landowner, who sends him to tend the pigs.[54] As a Jew, he is thus totally alienated, the epitome of lostness.[55] But his main problem is that he is starving to death, unable to eat the carob pods supplied to the pigs. No one bothers about his need. His hunger galvanises him into action.[56] "He came to his senses." He makes a snap decision to return home, where his father's "hired men have all the food they want."[57] He is prepared to acknowledge that he has done wrong in God's sight and has offended his father,[58] and there are signs of regret and remorse, but this probably does not amount to repentance. As he envisages a brighter future, though aware that he has forfeited his right to sonship and has no claims on his father, his plan is to ask his father to take him on as a hired servant. This would enable him to maintain his independence and social respectability living in the village. And he could use his income to fulfil the financial responsibilities to his father that he had selfishly abandoned. He seems to wish to return on his own terms, to do things his way. Some think that maybe this is not repentance so much as strategic conniving.[59] But he seems to assume that his father will look on him with a level of favour. "The hope of reconciliation, not restoration, brings him home."[60]

Return and Welcome

The spotlight switches and focuses on the father, who probably misses his son and worries about him, as would any father, and is on hopeful lookout. The key word in the whole parable, (or the key phrase in translation), is, I believe, the verb that describes the father's (extravagant)[61] response when he catches sight of the returning younger son in the distance: "But while he was still far off, his father saw him and was filled with compassion; he ran and put his arms around him and kissed him."

All that follows in the narrative springs from compassion. He is that kind of man. The delighted father runs to meet his son.[62] Normally an elder would not run; it was socially unacceptable.[63] But it also enables him to meet the young man outside the village boundary and protect him from the inevitable hostility of the villagers, who probably gathered quickly. A remarkable reconciliation takes place.[64] The father says nothing; there is no lecture or blame or criticism. The past is past. His actions express his profound paternal love, acceptance and welcome. He kisses him repeatedly in a firm embrace, a sign of forgiveness, a recognising that he is his son, and this is public, for all the villagers to see. None of them will cause him harassment now.

The son forgets the crippling hunger that prompted his decision to return. As he begins his rehearsed speech,[65] using the term "father", his father interrupts before he can announce his plan of maintaining his independence as a hired servant rather than a son. He comes to realise that what is at issue is a broken relationship, a relationship that he cannot heal. The possibility of that relationship being re-established, his being reinstated as son, can only come as a pure gift from his father. He perceives from his father's behaviour that such an offer is being made. The gift of the best robe, ring and shoes, which the servants are ordered to bring, are symbols of this; they are symbols of belonging and freedom, "emblematic of the son's honourable restoration to the family he had snubbed and abandoned."[66] The father's compassionate love brings about a change within him, and he graciously accepts the gift freely and generously offered, beyond his wildest dreams.[67] The father sets in motion the arrangements for a great celebration, to which the whole village community would be invited so as to participate in their rejoicing and share in the restoration and reconciliation that has occurred; it would also mend fractured village relationships.[68] The father sums up his view of things: "for this son of mine was dead and is alive again; he was lost and is found!"

To the lost and found language of the two shorter parables is added the appropriate image of death and resurrection. The son had cut himself off from the life of the family, his village community and his religion; he was as good as dead; now he is again alive. The family and community celebrate.

The Father and The Older Brother

The other son returns from the fields, which will be his when his father dies. He gets wind of the party, for there is music in the air. He plies one of the local children, or one of the servants, with questions. The youngster without guile, using kinship language,[69] informs him that his brother has returned home and that his father has killed the fatted calf to celebrate. The older brother's reaction is one of anger;[70] he refuses to participate in the celebratory meal that has been prepared. He remains outside, refusing to join in the meal and the fun and unwilling to fulfil his role as master of ceremonies. This is a public insult to his father.[71] The father reacts by coming out of the house and pleading with him.[72] Until now, he probably had not realised that the older son was lost to him; now he comes out searching for him. This was culturally quite shocking.[73] The latter's response reveals the extent of his alienation and resentment. There is no respect, no affection; he does not address his father as father. "Look here," he begins in an accusatory tone, and goes on to complain bitterly, betraying the attitude of a slave rather than a son.[74] He is resentful, self-righteous about his impeccable obedience, disparagingly critical of his father's other son, whom he accuses of wasting his money on "prostitutes", and refuses to acknowledge him as his brother. Obviously, he is quite incapable of understanding and entering into his father's joy.[75]

From the father, there is no outburst of anger, no criticism or rebuke, no recall to duty. Rather, he reaches out graciously with love and compassion, searching to bridge the gulf between them: "My son,[76] you are with me always and all I have is yours." He affectionately acknowledges his permanent and valued presence in the home, and reassures him that his rights and inheritance are still secure and protected, and finally reminds him that it really is right and necessary to celebrate.[77] He explains his joy in the terms used earlier—dead and alive, lost and found—but this time "your brother" replaces "my son".[78] It is an appeal for understanding, for brotherly reconciliation and acceptance, an appeal that he should join them, the family, and the whole community in fellowship and festivity. The parable ends at this point with an invitation, a fervent plea, and we never learn the sequel.[79] We do not know whether the elder brother joined the celebration, whether he was reconciled with his brother or whether he continued to live in alienation as a slave.[80] In this way we, the listeners/readers, are forced to think about our own reaction or response to this short story as it applies to our lives and experience.

The parable responds magnificently to the initial context. The sinners are sharing the banquet, found by the searching Jesus. The religious leaders stand critically aloof, refusing the invitation to accept the Good News and join the party.[81] The table fellowship of Jesus is a celebration of seeking and finding. Jesus' critics can "find themselves within the story and thereby be persuaded to embrace his practice of hospitality, enacting the welcoming grace of God's dominion."[82] The story challenges them to change their attitude to "sinners" and their understanding of God.[83]

Taken together, the three parables reflect the way in which Jesus understands his ministry, what he is about, as he daily seeks the lost and the needy but refuses to write off the righteous and religious elite. At the same time, these parables reveal a great deal about Jesus' understanding of God. Jesus operates in the way he does, shares table fellowship as he does, because he knows the compassionate heart of his Father, his all-inclusive, unconditional love, his unreserved acceptance and approval.[84] Table fellowship expresses it all.[85]

Reflections

These parables suggest to me several lines of reflection. First, there is the symbolic gesture of table fellowship, which, I believe, contains the whole Gospel in a nutshell. Through sharing table with those considered sinners and outcasts, Jesus revealed his understanding of God and of the nature of his mission. We cannot, therefore, avoid asking who the "sinners" and outcasts are in our society and our Church today, the despised, the written-off, the fringe members, the voiceless minorities. As disciples on mission, we are obliged to find ways of reaching out to them, ways of seeking and finding them and enabling them to see the face of the God of Jesus, and to experience God's closeness and love touching their lives. As individuals and as Church, we need to show vision, creativity and courage in fashioning ways of making present in our contemporary world the realities of which Jesus' table fellowship was a sign: unreserved acceptance, genuine respect, hospitality, forgiveness, friendship. Scripture poses disconcerting questions and offers an uncomfortable critique of our attitudes and responses and of some of our structures. We need to ask ourselves how accepting, inclusive and open we are as individuals, as families and communities, as Church.

The longer parable revolves around three actors: the prodigal son, the older brother and the compassionate father. We can identify with each of them. The younger son is wilful, self-centred, and thoughtless in initially asking for his inheritance and then leaving his father and community and doing his own thing. He seems to have sown his wild oats. Even his decision to return shows mixed motivation. We may not have been quite so dramatic in turning away from our Father, but we've probably at times made a bit of a mess of things and experienced the loss and hopelessness and confusion that our mistakes have engendered. On our return, we have known the Father's generous welcome and unstinting forgiveness, and have been able to celebrate. Perhaps the younger son is a member of our family or an acquaintance or someone in our school, parish or workplace. How do we enable a return? We may have to go out and search, reaching out in kindness, smothering our pain. Sometimes we may need just to sit patiently and wait, leaving the door open, alert for signs of movement and change. In either case, are we ready with a warm and generous welcome, with forgiveness, restoration, a celebration even?[86]

The older son is perhaps the one with whom religious people can more easily identify. He has kept the rules, done his duty, played it safe—and yet missed the point. He is self-centred too, critical, judgemental, joyless, self-righteous. In spite of his always being with the father, he doesn't really know his father's heart. The parable is unfinished, leaving us wondering whether he finally accepted the father's invitation to join the celebration, surrendering to his love, or did he remain sulking and disillusioned outside? Was he reconciled to his brother? I suspect we recognise some of his traits in our own hearts and lives. Is family or community reconciliation something we currently need to be involved in?

Finally, the parable reveals a great deal about the nature of the Father. He is a God who searches for both of his sons, a God of amazing patience, compassion and forgiveness. Is this the God we have come to know, love and serve? Is this the God whom we reveal to others, especially those with whom we live and those we seek to serve? It is so important to create space and make time to meet the God of Jesus, who gives us freedom and responsibility for our lives, who loves us whether we are near or far away, whose love is all-inclusive and unconditional, and who longs to give us all that he is and all that he has: "All I have is yours." This is an amazing statement, which invites much prayerful pondering; it opens the door on God's overspilling, utterly altruistic and infinitely abundant love for each of us.

Notes

1   The previous chapter of Luke's Gospel ends with the exhortation by Jesus: "he that has ears to hear, let him hear." Green, *Luke*, 569, notes the links with chapters 14 and 16, concerned with meals and hospitality (see 14:13; 14:21; 16:20). He sees the basic theme of chapter 15 to be Jesus' defence of his ministry, and an "implicit and open-ended invitation to his interlocutors to join him in reflecting in their practices God's own attitude towards sinners."

2   Carroll, *Luke*, 309. Green, *Luke*, 570, notes that in Luke the tax collectors and "sinners" have been presented as open to repentance (3:10–14; 5:27–32; 5:29–32; 7:35–60). The Pharisees, when presented *in tandem* with the scribes, consistently have the role of Jesus' foes (5:17–6:11; 7:29–30). McBride, *Parables*, 123, refers to the outcasts and the outraged! Evans, *Luke*, 583, comments on Luke's fondness for "all", which leads to a blurred picture.

3   Marshall, *Luke*, 599, suggests that the imperfect tense implies general circumstances rather than one incident.

4   This is important for Luke: 5:1,15; 6:17, 27, 47, 49; 7:29; 8:8–18; 9:35; 10:16, 24, 39; 11:28, 31.

5   The Pharisees were a fairly broad group with no particular membership requirements except a serious commitment to the Law and a concern to apply it to their day. Within them was a group called *haberim*, like a guild of friends or associates, who were very strict and who pledged to keep the Law very precisely. They avoided the "people of the land". See Bailey, *The Good Shepherd* (London: SPCK, 2015), 111–112; Reid, *Parables*, 181. They themselves, for fear of ritual defilement, had strict purity rules and food restrictions, and would eat only with their own.

6   The verb (*diegongyzon*) is stronger than 19:7 (Zacchaeus); it means "kept grumbling aloud". See Donahue, *Gospel*, 147; Carroll, *Luke*, 310.

7   5:30; 7:34.

8   Green, *Luke*, 571, notes that Jesus is rejecting the values and norms of the religious elite. They are the primary audience for the coming parables.

9   See the next chapter on table fellowship.

10   Lambrecht, *Astonished*, 25, observes that because these parables are well known, they may have lost their evocative power and be no longer able to make an impact. This challenges us to find a way of bringing the message to expression again.

11   Several key terms are repeated. Green, *Luke*, 573, notes the escalation: 1 out of 100; 1 out of 10; 1 of 2. Lambrecht, *Astonished*, 26, refers to them as "twin-similitudes". He suggests, p. 28, that they were told together on the same occasion and were in 'Q'; Matthew chose to omit the second.

12   Though, as Donahue, *Gospel*, 147, points out, the word "lost" appears five times in seven verses. McBride, *Luke*, 200, speaks of the experience of loss, the movement of search and the joy of discovery. Lambrecht, *Astonished*, 27, divides each into 3 sections: search; actions after the finding; application. Green, *Luke*, 573, reminds us that the finale of each refers to sinners and heaven, and so the parables are fundamentally about God.

13   Donahue, *Gospel*, 148. In Matthew (18:12–14) the parable is directed to his

disciples, not the Pharisees and scribes; it is an illustration of the type of leadership they should embrace.

14   Carroll, *Luke*, 310, notes that this means empathising with Jesus.

15   See Isa 5:1–7. The prophet and Jesus usually (though not always) leave their parables without an interpretation. Bailey, *The Good Shepherd*, 116–118, gives the pattern as three cameos (two are parables, one an interpretation): You, one, ninety-nine; lost, find, rejoice, restore, rejoice, find, lost; You, one, ninety-nine.

16   Donohue, *Gospel*, 148; Reid, *Parables*, 184. McBride, *Parables*, 128–129, claims that by the first century, shepherds were regarded as unclean and a threat to the property of the landed gentry. Levine, *Stories*, 41–44, contests this prevalent view. She objects (in general) to Christian attempts to make Jesus look good by making Judaism look bad.

17   Reid, *Parables*, 184. Green, *Luke*, 574, maintains that the average family would have had between 5 and 15 sheep. Evans, *Luke*, 585, comments that the man is not wealthy if he tends his own sheep; he sees his searching not because of care, but because he cannot afford the loss. Marshall, *Luke*, 601, accepts the view of Jeremias, *The Parables of* Jesus, that 100 would be a normal size for a small farmer. Tannehill, *Luke*, 238, suggests that the sheep may belong to the man's extended family. His behaviour is entirely appropriate.

18   Levine, *Stories*, 38, makes the point that, whereas it is easy to notice one sheep is missing when you have only five, to do so with a hundred is remarkable. Marshall, *Luke*, 601, mentions the evening counting.

19   Bailey, *The Good Shepherd*, 124, notes that a shepherd would probably not leave ninety-nine sheep unattended; usually there would be an assistant or apprentice who would bring the others home; also, Marshall, *Luke*, 601; Reid, *Parables*, 184.

20   Marshall, *Luke*, 601, considers this normal rural practice.

21   Bailey, *The Good Shepherd*, 128, observes that the word for friends is the same as that used for the guild of the Pharisees; the *haberim* come to the party! Levine, *Stories*, 40, wonders whether women were also invited, and whether mutton was served!

22   This is Bailey's comment, *The Good Shepherd*, 125; he links this with the "bad shepherd" tradition of the prophets; Jesus is much more gentle with his failure. He is encouraging them not to be entrapped in their past mistakes.

23   Some consider this line an addition by Luke, which perhaps distorts the original. Green, *Luke*, 575, sees the appendage as not strictly part of the parable; but within its local co-text, it should be interpreted as a response to the Pharisees. The celebration element is important for both parable and appropriation. Levine, *Stories*, 40, states that it is Luke who provides the first interpretation, allegorising the parable. The allegory fails to match the parable: ninety-nine who don't need repentance (!); no sin or repentance in the story; the owner lost the sheep! She notes, p. 41, that allegorical interpretations abound today. Lambrecht, *Astonished*, 28, notes the shift of emphasis that causes tension; the imagery emphasises the search, the application the response (conversion). After a comparison with Matthew's version, he concludes that there was probably an application in 'Q', which focused on the resulting joy (p. 40). The tension should not be overemphasised. Evans, *Luke*, 585, observes that repentance is a Lukan theme, but here it is artificial and involves allegorisation.

24   Bailey, *The Good Shepherd*, 133, notes the use of "return" (or "bring back") in the Old Testament texts, where it can be a return to a place, to a person or to God. Here, the verb *metanoiein* is used, but it is synonymous with *epistrephein*, the verb normally used to translate the Hebrew *shuv*.

25   Bailey, *The Good Shepherd*, 130, calls this "hermeneutical Christology" (how Jesus tells stories about God from the Old Testament and places himself at the centre, acting out the role of God); Green, *Luke*, 575, n. 215, suggests the possibility of a Christological understanding. Carroll, *Luke*, 311, also makes the link with Ezekiel, indicating that "this activity of Jesus is furthering the gracious activity of Israel's God." So does Green, *Luke*, 574.

26   In the prophets, the return was to the land of Israel from the nations; here the return is to God.

27   Reid, *Parables*, 186. Tannehill, *Luke*, 238, believes that Luke understands repentance as more an experience of being found than the product of human effort. Levine, *Stories*, 44–45, maintains that the owner is the main figure; the search and celebration are exaggerated. She asks whether *we* have lost folk, take responsibility for it and seek to find.

28   Donohue, *Gospel*, 149, refers to "a protagonist from a group which suffered religious and social discrimination in first century society." Carroll, *Luke*, 312, notes that "it is striking that Jesus casts himself, as it were, as a persistent woman householder so as to interpret and defend his gracious hospitality towards sinners." Tannehill, *Luke*, 239, notes that the housewife must be taken as an image of God and God's prophet-Messiah.

29   Donahue, *Gospel*, 149. McBride, *Parables*, 131, states that "it is going beyond what was socially and religiously acceptable." Levine, *Stories*, 45, questions this, noting a series of female characters in the Old Testament who are not offensive; we portray the context of Jesus too negatively.

30   Bailey, *The Good Shepherd*, 145–146, maintains that Jesus is also reclaiming the female component of Psalm 23, God's preparing a meal.

31   Matt 5:14–15; Luke 13:18–21; see also Isa 42:13–14; 51:1–2.

32   Bailey, *The Good Shepherd*, 144–145, gives this as: introduction; lost, found, rejoice, found, lost, conclusion; the central cameo is joy.

33   Carroll, *Luke*, 312. He notes how hearers and readers tend to fill in the gaps in the story. McBride, *Luke*, 201, observes that the coin could have been one of the drachmae from the precious headdress she received as a bride. Reid, *Parables*, 187, maintains that this practice was not the case for first-century Jewish women. Green, *Luke*, 576, presumes the woman is a village peasant living in an economy based on barter; her coins probably represent the family savings, so the loss would be catastrophic. Levine, *Stories*, 46, on the other hand, points out that she has her own home and friends and is relatively well off. While first-century Judaism was not an egalitarian paradise, it is not unusual for Jesus to tell stories about women; they have a significant role in the Gospel stories.

34   Levine, *Stories*, 47, notes that she needs no one's permission to do so!

35   Donohue, *Gospel*, 150.

36   McBride, *Luke*, 201–202. Levine, *Stories*, 48, notes that the emphasis in the

parable is on the shepherd and the woman, who had a problem and fixed it; in Luke's allegorisation, it is on the sheep and coin (and repentance and forgiveness) that are passive.

37   Donahue, *Gospel*, 151. Carroll, *Luke*, 313, comments that Jesus takes the divine initiative to persons in need of restoration: "God celebrates the recovery of the lost and their restoration to community through Jesus' ministry."

38   McBride, *Parables*, 133, says "lost in the wilderness of his own self-righteous hostility."

39   McBride, *Luke*, 203.

40   Donahue, *Gospel*, 152–153; Carroll, *Luke*, 315; Francis J. Moloney, *Reflections on Evangelical Consecration* (Bolton: Don Bosco Publications, 2015), 79. Marshall, *Luke*, 604, takes the father as the central figure. Green, *Luke*, 578, however, maintains that the younger son occupies centre stage and there are two responses to his recovery: compassion by the father and anger by the older brother. Lambrecht, *Astonished*, 31, suggests two sections, one dealing with the younger and the other with the older brother; both end in the same way (vv. 24 and 32: "lost and found"). The first part is similar to the two previous parables. On p. 46, he notes that the hearer is invited to enter into the drama of the (strange) family and approve the loving response of the father. He needs to decode its symbolic meaning and is then confronted with a choice. McBride, *Parables*, 134, speaks of a mixed human family in which tenderness, selfishness and hostility all vie with each other for possession. Marshall, *Luke*, 607, suggests that the son would be unmarried and about eighteen years old.

41   Levine, *Stories*, 50–51; Donahue, *Gospel*, 159; McBride, *Parables*, 137. Reid, *Parables*, 58, notes that in the Genesis stories, women play a significant role; in this story, there is no mention of a mother or daughter.

42   Reid, *Parables*, 59; Bailey, *The Good Shepherd*, 161–169; McBride, *Parables*, 136. Carroll, *Luke*, 315, comments: "even if in effect it means that the son is treating him as if he were already dead." Donahue, *Gospel*, 154 says: "he acts as if his father were dead" in squandering the inheritance. Green, *Luke*, 580, comments that the son's request is presumptuous and highly irregular; "read as the first of a series of actions that lead to his characterisation as 'dead and lost', his request clearly signifies his rejection of his family." In n. 230, he suggests that Bailey seems to have overstated the case. Levine, *Stories*, 51, maintains that there is no Jewish support for the view of such as Bailey. On p. 313, n. 33, she suggests that Bailey bases himself on medieval Arab Christian interpretation and contemporary Arab custom.

43   Reid, *Parables*, 59; McBride, *Parables*, 134–35. He reminds us that in the ancient Mediterranean world the family, not the individual, was the primary unit of importance and the psychological centre of life. Identity was family identity; individualism was shunned. Solidarity with the village came next in importance. "In the tightly knit community of the village, where you lived your life in close proximity to relations and neighbours, social conformity was a matter of survival." One's identity was largely determined by whether you commanded their respect or not. Nonconformity was a threat to cohesion. On p. 135, he notes that central to family identity was its relationship to land. "The father's house" (the extended family) was the basic kinship structure, providing a sense

of inclusion, identity and responsibility. The basic rule (tenaciously adhered to) was that land should remain in the family (Lev 25:25). The Old Testament gives no example of an Israelite voluntarily selling land outside his family. It would be an economic tragedy and social disaster.

44   Donahue, *Gospel,* 153–54; Fitzmyer, *Luke,* 2:1087.

45   The Greek uses the word *bios,* as in Mark 12:44, regarding the widow. For Carroll, *Luke,* 315, this means his entire means of sustaining life.

46   Reid, *Parables,* 59; Tannehill, *Luke,* 240; McBride, *Parables,* 137: "In dividing his property among his two sons, he is flaunting traditional values and custom; other families in the village would probably close ranks against him lest they be affected by his shameless example."

47   Levine, *Stories,* 53. Others (like Marshall, *Luke,* 607) believe that the son made a further request to dispose of his share, a request which was granted. Reid, *Parables,* 60, suggests that he converted his inheritance into cash; Tannehill, *Luke,* 240, that the son sells the land he has inherited.

48   Fitzmyer, *Luke,* 2:1087–1090.

49   Carroll, *Luke,* 315; on p. 318 he writes: "As the father observes, all the family's property belongs to his older son, though the father would retain his right to use it." Green, *Luke,* 580, says "the elder son receives his portion as well." Also, McBride, *Luke,* 206, adding that when the younger son leaves home he has no further claim on the home property, but he does have the obligation of supporting his father; similarly, Marshall, *Luke,* 607.

50   McBride, *Luke,* 206.

51   Reid, *Parables,* 59–60. Levine, *Stories,* 67, suggests that sibling rivalry is another biblical convention (Cain & Abel, Jacob & Esau, Leah & Rachel, Martha & Mary); and so the relationship between the two was probably dysfunctional. McBride, *Parables,* 137, believes the elder brother is culpable of standing by while his family breaks up. He is now the sole owner of what remains of the estate, although the father retains the right to enjoy the produce.

52   Levine, *Stories,* 54. She suggests that he engages in gambling, alcohol abuse, sexual indulgence, etc. She also thinks the father may be complicit in the son's debauchery by acquiescing to the son's request. However, it is the older brother who, only later, mentions inappropriate sexual activity.

53   Donahue, *Gospel,* 154. Green, *Luke,* 580, sees disposing of one's inheritance by turning it into transportable capital during the father's lifetime as a shocking breach of familial ties. Evans, *Luke,* 592, notes that it is the dissipation of the father's wealth which constitutes the wrong against him.

54   Levine, *Stories,* 56, observes that at the time of Jesus more Jews lived in gentile territory than in the Jewish homeland, and they did relate to gentiles. McBride, *Parables,* 138, sees him as a refugee and migrant worker; he depends on an "urbanite of some wealth".

55   Donahue, *Gospel,* 153, states that "he has lost his familial, ethnic and religious identity." Green, *Luke,* 581, notes that the practice of almsgiving was little observed among the Greeks and Romans. Marshall, *Luke,* 608, refers to "the nadir of degradation".

56   This is the turning point (*krisis*) of the story. Note the chiastic structure in McBride, *Parables*, 139.

57   The verb *anastas*, arise or get up, "anticipates the motif of new life with which his father will interpret his return and restoration to the family" (Carroll, *Luke*, 316). Green, *Luke*, 582, sees the verb as beginning to signal his return to life from death. McBride, *Luke*, 205, sees the experience of failure and hopelessness as the pivotal point of the story. Moloney, *Reflections*, 80, sees the moment when the son recognises the depths to which his wastefulness has led him as the turning point of the story. Reid, *Parables*, 60–61, sees no repentance here.

58   "Against heaven and against you" is a typical Old Testament expression; "heaven" is a circumlocution for God; the (empty) words are found in Pharaoh's mouth in Exod 10:16. Note the soliloquy.

59   Levine, *Stories*, 57–58, considers "coming to himself" as indicating that he knows that daddy will do what he asks: "I'll go to daddy and sound religious."Kenneth E. Bailey, "Poet & Peasant" in K. E. Bailey, *Poet & Peasant and Through Peasant Eyes: A Literary-Cultural Approach to the Parables in Luke* [Combined Edition] (Grand Rapids: Eerdmans, 1983), 173–180, refers to shrewdness and self-serving. Tannehill, *Luke*, 241, suggests that his return home may be motivated entirely by self-interest rather than any real feeling for the injury he has done to his father.

60   McBride, *Parables*, 139.

61   Carroll, *Luke*, 316, sees the father's reaction as "extravagant, prodigal, excessive." Reid, *Parables*, 61, as "most unexpected" of a patriarch grievously shamed.

62   Levine, *Stories*, 61–63, notes that Jewish fathers were not distant or wrathful; she quotes sayings and actions of Jesus in support (Matt 7:9; Jairus; the father of the epileptic boy). It would not be unnatural or surprising for a father to welcome back a wastrel son. "For the rabbis, the challenge is not in seeing God's love in a new way; the challenge—an inevitable challenge in any religious system—is to get the wayward to return."

63   Donahue, *Gospel*, 155; Green, *Luke*, 583; McBride, *Luke*, 207.

64   Carroll, *Luke*, 316, recalls Esau and Jacob (Gen 33:4). Marshall, *Luke*, 610, notes that the father's action is a sign of forgiveness and of the restoration of the broken relationship; the initiative is the father's.

65   Green, *Luke*, 582, notes that although the son acknowledges his sin and shame, it is his return that makes reconciliation possible. "The father's response, based solely on the return of his son, already undercuts the son's plans."

66   Green, *Luke*, 583. In n. 245, he notes that he is not being invested with his father's authority, as some suggest; the ring is not a signet ring; he probably needs clothing appropriate to his status in the family; they signify the restoration of his honour as a son. Lambrecht, *Astonished*, 32, believes that the forgiveness and restoration imply astonishingly more than the mere pardoning of offences. McBride, *Parables*, 142, recalls Gen 41:42. "The son is publicly restored to his position within the hierarchy of the household." Marshall, *Luke*, 610, sees ring and shoes as symbols of authority and freedom; Reid, *Parables*, 61, as symbols of "distinction and authority".

67   Levine, *Stories*, 66, believes this view is "generous"; she prefers to see the

favourite son as pampered and manipulative.

68   The slaughtering of an animal is a mark of the father's joy. Meat was not eaten often. With the reference to making merry, the first part of the parable ends (as did the two earlier ones). There is a double climax (Lambrecht, *Astonishes*, 32). He refers to "end stress", more emphasis placed on what comes last. The first part of the parable prepares for the second. McBride, *Parables*, 143, sees the invitation of the villagers to the celebration as also restoring village relationships. Reid, *Parables*, 62, considers the meal to be a gesture of reconciliation with the members of the village, and their acceptance of the invitation a sign of reintegration into the community.

69   Carroll, *Luke*, 317, uses this term.

70   Green, *Luke*, 584, stresses the contrast in affective states: compassion and anger; they give rise to contrasting behaviours. On p. 585, n. 252, he notes that his wish to celebrate with friends rather than family breaches the kinship values operative in his world; also, McBride, *Parables*, 145. McBride, *Luke*, 208, sees him now as the "separated one", far from home.

71   McBride, *Parables*, 144, notes that the elder brother's absence makes family rivalry a public issue; his absence will be interpreted as a reproach to the villagers.

72   The verb (*parakaleō*) can also mean to comfort.

73   Donahue, *Gospel*, 156. Reid, *Parables*, 63, notes that in a patriarchal world, a father rules over his sons and never entreats them to do what is obligatory. Tannehill, *Luke*, 243, states that the father ignores his own dignity and position.

74   Levine, *Stories*, 72, observes that the elder son's comment would not have rung true to one of the real slaves in the household. Green, *Luke*, 585, notes that the elder son has apparently lived in alienation from his father. Lambrecht, *Astonished*, 31, considers the language unusually harsh. McBride, *Parables*, 144–145, notes that his self-image is that of being a slave.

75   Carroll, *Luke*, 318, comments that self-interest and the integrity of the family inheritance, not to mention the favouritism apparently being shown to the younger son, provoke the older son's protest. McBride, *Parables*, 145, notes how he believes he has not received due recognition; he has been overlooked.

76   The Greek is *teknon*, child, conveying tenderness ("my dear son"). Levine, *Stories*, 73, observes that the father does not speak to the younger son; he communicates his love through his gestures. He expresses his love for the elder son in words, words that express their ongoing relationship.

77   The verb *dei* is used; Luke often uses this as indicating divine necessity.

78   Lambrecht, *Astonished*, 31, notes that the father repudiates the older brother's "this son of yours"; they are still brothers.

79   Moloney, *Reflections*, 81, suggests that the reason for this is that the main concern of Jesus is his presentation of the father.

80   Donahue, *Gospel*, 162. He stresses that the story does not convey a "patriarchal" father, concerned with authority and power. Quoting: "God is the one who respects our freedom, mourns our alienation, waits patiently for our return, and accepts our love as pure gift," Sandra M. Schneiders, *Women and the Word: The Gender of God in the New Testament and the Spirituality of Women (Madeleva Lecture in Spirituality)*, (New York:

Paulist Press, 1986), 47. Green, *Luke*, 579, writes: "Against the interpretive horizons of the Roman world, wherein the characteristic attributes of the father as the *paterfamilias* are remembered especially in terms of authoritarianism and legal control, the picture Luke paints is remarkable for its counter-emphasis on care and compassion." Moloney, *Reflections*, 80, stresses the surprising attitude of the father who does not wish to dominate or possess but gives them their freedom.

81   McBride, *Parables*, 146, notes that "the drama of the parable mirrors both Jesus' pastoral strategy towards sinners and the Pharisees' strategy of separation." There is an appeal to treat sinners with kindness, to move from a stance of separation to association.

82   Carroll, *Luke*, 313.

83   McBride, *Luke*, 204, writes: "Reaching out is more God-like than keeping away; association is more God-like than segregation." Lambrecht, *Astonished*, 33, suggests that the description of the indignant elder brother is given for the benefit of the Pharisees and fits them perfectly; they are invited to share the joy.

84   See Paul Tournier, *Guilt and Grace* (London: Hodder & Stoughton, 1962), 189. Moloney, *Reflections*, 82, notes that the parable questions the way God was understood and revered in the religion and culture of his time.

85   Moloney, *Reflections*, 79, sees this parable as a paradigm of the role of God and subsequently of his Son, Jesus, in shepherding. On p. 81, he states that Jesus lived the parable he told. Marshall, *Luke*, 604, states that Jesus defends himself and his attitude to sinners by appeal to the attitude of God.

86   Levine, *Stories*, 73–76. Reid, *Parables*, 64, notes the absence of a mother in the story, or a daughter. She maintains that female images are required that express equally well what the father image says of God. The second parable of the trio in which the woman householder is the protagonist, redresses this imbalance to some extent.

Chapter Twelve
Table Fellowship

One of the key features of Jesus' ministry is usually described as table fellowship. Of the three Synoptic writers, Luke gives greatest emphasis to this theme. It has been suggested that in Luke's narrative, Jesus is always going to a meal, present at a meal or coming away from a meal![1] This may be a slight exaggeration, but it is certainly true that sharing meals with others seems to have been a deliberate and significant aspect of his ministry. In the villages of Galilee, where hospitality was an essential aspect of life, it was quite natural that Jesus should frequently be invited to share table. Sometimes it would be an expression of gratitude, perhaps for his having healed someone, or an indication of respect for a prophet; sometimes it would provide an occasion for him to teach. While Jesus was invited on occasion to share table with the religious elite, invitations which he did not decline, his special and characteristic 'thing' was to dine with the outcasts and marginalised. This habit provoked raised eyebrows and critical comment.

In that culture, to share table was a very significant gesture. It was a sign of acceptance, respect and trust, an offer of peace, fellowship and friendship, an expression of inclusion. To share table indicated a being 'at home' with others, a willingness to share life, an identification and oneness with them; it was an expression of solidarity. Jesus' action bridged the social and religious divide in a culture extremely conscious of status and class, prestige and boundaries. It showed the sinners and outcasts that they mattered to him, that they had a value in his eyes. It was therefore a healing and liberating event. Since Jesus was looked upon as in some way a man of God, a prophet, his gesture of friendship communicated and experienced through table fellowship would have been understood as an indication of God's acceptance too. This gesture is, I believe, the most powerful parable of the Kingdom; it proclaims the message and makes present the reality of God's nearness in saving love and mercy. Meals are symbols of participation in the realm of God.[2]

The great scripture scholar Jeremias writes that "the inclusion of sinners in the community of salvation, achieved in table fellowship, is the most meaningful expression of the message of the redeeming love of God."[3] This symbolic gesture, I believe, contains the whole Gospel, the Good News, in a nutshell. It says it all—that in Jesus, God is freely and gratuitously reaching out in mercy and saving love, wanting to share life with us.

What fascinates me is that Jesus welcomes to his table anyone who wants to be there.[4] There are no exceptions, no blacklist. So, the indifferent or irreligious, the ordinary peasants who weren't able to observe many of the Laws, genuinely disreputable folk, people of questionable morality, people who lived outside the Law, the sick and the needy, men, women and children, all could have a place. One writer speaks of Jesus' "all-inclusive, unconditional love, his unreserved acceptance and approval."[5] No doubt Jesus hoped that the quality of his acceptance and the experience of his friendship and the listening to his message would enable those present to respond positively to the embrace of the Kingdom and to change their outlook and lives. But repentance and conversion would come after the experience, not as a precondition. Forgiveness and table fellowship are a gift, not a reward.

In this chapter, I propose to examine a number of episodes in which Jesus shares table with others: Levi's party, the meal with Simon the Pharisee, the multiplication of loaves and fishes, the meal in which the man with dropsy is healed, which is followed by teaching and a parable, the Last Supper. The meal with the Emmaus couple will feature in the final chapter, devoted to the theme of resurrection.[6]

Levi's Party (5:29–32)

In Chapter Four, we considered the call of Levi as he sat at his post in the customs house. It is a startling illustration of Jesus' originality, his breaking the mould, his openness to those on the periphery, dubbed "sinners". Having "left everything", Levi throws a party as a joy-filled expression of gratitude to Jesus for inviting him to be a follower, opening up an entirely new and unexpected chapter of his life.[7] It was also an opportunity to introduce him to his friends and acquaintances. Jesus is criticised to his disciples, probably on a later occasion, by some Pharisees and scribes for dining in such company; they are the ones who introduce the label "sinners". The Pharisees, "separated ones", were a lay movement, who were noted for their strict observance of the Law and its oral interpretations. Generally sincere and devout, they believed that, in obedience to God's will, they had to shun sinners so as not to be defiled. They would eat only in their own homes or with other Pharisees, extending to their family table the ritual purity required of the priests serving in the temple.[8] The scribes were the legal experts, powerful and privileged men, with close links to the temple.

In reply to their critique about his sharing table with tax collectors and sinners, people beyond the pale, Jesus states: "Those who are well have no need of a physician, but those who are sick; I have come to call not the righteous but sinners to repentance." The proverb he is quoting brings to mind the metaphor he used in the Nazareth synagogue. It emphasises, not without a touch of irony, that Jesus sees his mission as reaching out, being available and accessible, mainly to those considered "sinners". The whole point of being a doctor is to attend to the sick and bring them to health. Perhaps there is more than simply a proverb here, for in the Old Testament it was God who was considered to be the doctor or physician, and God's healing was understood as a restoration of a relationship, and therefore as entailing forgiveness.[9] The presence of the Healer, the Physician, was a sign that the messianic era had dawned.[10] For Jesus, sinners are the ones to whom, in a particular way, the offer of the gift of the Kingdom is made, and the invitation to adopt its values. This is Gladdening News indeed that, in Jesus, the merciful love and forgiveness of God seeks out and encounters those most in need, beyond all the barriers of status and class and occupation and education and religious practice and law-abiding observance.[11] Through these encounters, this crossing of boundaries,[12] people have the opportunity to see their need to be converted (*metanoia*, "repentance") and opt to change their lives. The prophet Ezekiel criticises the shepherds of Israel for their failure to care for the weak and sick, so Jesus' words here are also a challenge to his critics, questioning their "righteousness".

The story of the conflict that has emerged as a result of Jesus' style of table fellowship leads into a further conflict that has bearing on meals.[13]

> Then they said to him, "John's disciples, like the disciples of the Pharisees, frequently fast and pray, but your disciples eat and drink." Jesus said to them, "You cannot make wedding guests fast while the bridegroom is with them, can you? The days will come when the bridegroom will be taken away from them, and then they will fast in those days." (5:33–35)

The context remains Levi's party. The identity of those raising the next issue is unclear. "They" are probably the religious leaders.[14] They criticise Jesus because their own disciples and those of the Baptist fast and pray, two pillars of traditional Jewish piety, whereas Jesus' followers seem bent on having a good time with their eating and drinking. Fasting was a sign of contrition, penance, mourning or an expression of religious devotion, a way of begging God to bring in the messianic age.[15] All Jews fasted on the feast of Atonement (Lev 16:29; 23:27), and the Pharisees fasted on a voluntary basis twice a week, on Tuesdays and Thursdays; the disciples of John, as well as following his ascetic style, were coping with their master's imprisonment.[16] There seems to be no indication of repentance among the followers and new friends of Jesus!

Jesus' reply continues the banquet imagery, rich in Old Testament connotations,[17] pointing out that it is ridiculous to expect wedding guests to fast when the bridegroom remains with them. The time of salvation has dawned; it is a time for feasting; fasting represents a failure to recognise it. In that culture, wedding celebrations lasted for a week; there were dispensations from fasting and other religious duties;[18] killjoys were out of place.[19] The bridegroom will, however, be taken from them, and this will bring about a changed situation with different challenges, and his disciples will embrace fasting then.[20]

Jesus continues with a twofold parable or two mini-parables:

> No one tears a piece from a new garment and sews it on an old garment; otherwise the new will be torn, and the piece from the new will not match the old. And no one puts new wine into old wineskins; otherwise the new wine will burst the skins and will be spilled, and the skins will be destroyed. But new wine must be put into fresh wineskins. And no one after drinking old wine desires new wine, but says, "The old is good." (5:36–39)

No sensible person would do either of these things. Jesus' message and style are like a new garment and like new wine.[21] Any attempt to mix old and new will fail; there is a radical incompatibility between them. Jesus' openness to outcasts is fundamentally at variance with the basic Pharisee stance; other aspects of his teaching and style represent a very different spirituality. Compromise is not an option; it would be destructive of both. The final comment of Jesus, found only in Luke, seems to contradict the previous position. Perhaps it is ironic, explaining why people were slow to accept the teaching and the way of Jesus: "stubbornly clinging to the old, one fails to see the value of the new and therefore misses what God is doing."[22]

An alternative interpretation suggests that Luke consistently links Jesus' story with the story of God's dealings with Israel. The old garment needs repair; new cloth is not the solution, but the old need not be cast aside. The old wineskins are fine; for new wine, however, one needs new skins. Old wine is, in fact, good. "Jesus interprets his behaviours, which are questionable and innovative to some onlookers, as manifestations of God's ancient purpose coming to fruition, while the concerns of the Pharisees are rejected not only as innovative but also as quite inconsistent with God's programme."[23]

The Meal in Simon's House (7:36–50)

Luke records several occasions in which Jesus is invited to dine with the religious elite, invitations which he graciously accepts. The first of these meals takes place in the house of a Pharisee by the name of Simon. It is preceded by the contextualising comment that Jesus had a reputation for being a friend of tax gatherers and sinners.[24] It is a wonderful story, "a literary gem".[25]

> One of the Pharisees asked Jesus to eat with him, and he went into the Pharisee's house and took his place at the table. And a woman in the city, who was a sinner, having learned that he was eating in the Pharisee's house, brought an alabaster jar of ointment. She stood behind him at his feet, weeping, and began to bathe his feet with her tears and to dry them with her hair. Then she continued kissing his feet and anointing them with the ointment. Now when the Pharisee who had invited him saw it, he said to himself, "If this man were a prophet, he would have known who and what kind of woman this is who is touching him—that she is a sinner." Jesus spoke up and said to him, "Simon, I have something to say to you." "Teacher," he replied, "speak." "A certain creditor had two debtors; one owed five hundred denarii, and the other fifty. When they could not pay, he cancelled the debts for both of them. Now which of them will love him more?" Simon answered, "I suppose the one for whom he cancelled the greater debt." And Jesus said to him, "You have judged rightly." Then turning towards the woman, he said to Simon, "Do you see this woman? I entered your house; you gave me no water for my feet, but she has bathed my feet with her tears and dried them with her hair. You gave me no kiss, but from the time I came in she has not stopped kissing my feet. You did not anoint my head with oil, but she has anointed my feet with ointment. Therefore, I tell you, her sins, which were many, have been forgiven; hence she has shown great love. But the one to whom little is forgiven, loves little." Then he said to her, "Your sins are forgiven." But those who were at the table with him began to say among themselves, "Who is this who even forgives sins?" And he said to the woman, "Your faith has saved you; go in peace."

This story is found only in Luke. Mark and Matthew include a story in which an unnamed woman anoints the head of Jesus, prior to his passion, while he is dining in Bethany at the house of Simon the leper. In John, while Jesus is at table with his friends after the raising of Lazarus to life, Mary of Bethany anoints his feet and wipes them with her hair.[26] It is generally agreed that Mark and John are describing the same incident, with some variations. Luke's story has no connection with the passion, has a clearly alternative focus and is a different episode in the ministry of Jesus, though some cross influence has probably occurred during the oral transmission.[27] As it stands, the story unfolds with great artistry in dramatic form, sweeping between the three central characters "with passion and power".[28]

To make sense of the story, it has to be assumed that the woman has already either had some indirect knowledge of Jesus and his message, which led her to repentance,[29] or has heard him proclaiming his message of God's love for sinners. Perhaps "she had seen and heard him from the fringe of the crowd, and that had been enough to soften the hardness of her heart and to set her back on the road to self-respect."[30] Maybe there had been some direct contact between them previously. In some way, she has been moved by his message, has believed, repented and now wishes to thank Jesus.[31] We are not told or provided with any further details.[32]

A Pharisee named Simon invites Jesus to dine with him, probably after the synagogue service on the Sabbath. Perhaps this invitation stems from his respect for Jesus as a rabbi, a prophet even; it could be that he even finds aspects of his teaching interesting and attractive.[33] Jesus is open to the religious elite as well; they, too, need to hear his message; Jesus does not give up on them. However, since Jesus' presentation of God's love for sinners was at variance with the normal Pharisee viewpoint, the invitation to the meal may have been an excuse to cross-examine, advise, correct or challenge him.[34] It was customary to extend the welcoming greeting of a kiss. When the guests had taken their places, olive oil and water were brought so that they could wash their hands and feet. The thanksgiving prayer would then be said. We learn later that the basic gestures of welcome and hospitality were not offered, an omission the other guests would have observed. This was a public insult, especially as Jesus was a teacher, as Simon himself acknowledges. Jesus would be well aware of this.[35]

Having left his sandals at the door on entering, Jesus reclines on a divan.[36] Normally, the eldest or most senior guest would recline first, then the others. Usually the door was left open, and sometimes beggars would come in to pick up the scraps, or admirers to relish the conversation.[37] No doubt the presence of Jesus would attract onlookers, genuinely interested or simply curious. On this occasion, the person who enters is a woman who has been living an immoral life in the town, a prostitute, who has come to hear that Jesus is at table in the

Pharisee's house.[38] Jesus later gives the impression that she was already there when he arrived and, therefore, had seen the way in which he was publicly humiliated.[39] The reason for her presence is her desire to thank Jesus for setting her free.

The guests would be reclining on couches facing the table with their feet sticking out; she approaches from behind. She brings with her an alabaster jar or flask of perfume. Her initial intention was probably to use the perfume to anoint his hands and head as a sign of gratitude.[40] Now her intention is also to compensate for the host's rudeness to him.[41] Her emotions get the better of her, and she breaks down in floods of tears, which wet Jesus' feet.[42] Without thinking, in an attempt to remedy the situation, she lets down her hair, which is quite unacceptable in public, to wipe his feet dry.[43] She repeatedly kisses his feet, a sign of reverence, and anoints them. In that context, and given that he was reclining, she could not anoint his face. By unloosing her hair, she was making some form of an ultimate pledge of loyalty to him. With this dramatic act, she also entered into Jesus' pain of rejection and public humiliation.[44] The onlookers would have expected Jesus to be as embarrassed and shocked as they were, and to have rejected her, but he calmly allows all this to happen and accepts her intimate gestures. It is Simon who is shocked, embarrassed, offended and confused!

"Through all this," writes Caird, "Jesus did not turn; for he had no need; all that he needed to know about the uninvited guest he could read in the mirror of Simon's shocked face, and all he needed to do for the woman he could do by accepting motionless the homage of her penitent love."[45] What Jesus in fact read was: "If this man were a real prophet, he would know who this woman is who is touching him, and what a bad character she is."

The words presuppose that prophets have extraordinary knowledge,[46] and imply that Jesus did not know and that, had he been aware, he would have withdrawn from contact with her, as Simon himself would have done. It is becoming apparent that Jesus cannot be a true prophet. He ought to have told the woman to follow the accepted procedures and go to the temple and offer sacrifice in God's presence. The genuineness of his prophet status is questioned. Simon's attitude to the woman is negative and dismissive. In fact, however, Jesus shows that he does know who she is; she is a sinner but a repentant and pardoned sinner. Her reputation has not changed but she herself has.[47] Jesus knows what is going on in Simon's mind, so he turns to him, and states: "I have something to say to you."[48] Politely addressing Jesus as "teacher", Simon invites him to speak up.

Jesus responds by recounting a brief, straightforward parable in which a creditor has two debtors, one who owes him a little amount (50 *denarii*), the other a considerable sum (500 *denarii*), and, given that neither can repay him, unexpectedly he cancels both debts.[49] In Aramaic the same word is used for debts and for sins; the Greek verb can be used both financially and theologically: to cancel and to forgive. Initially the creditor is assumed to be God; the debtors cannot pay God, and God freely and generously forgives them both. This is another beautiful description of God's mercy. For the reader, there is also a sense in which the creditor then begins to look like Jesus, who forgives the woman and also forgives Simon for his rudeness and insult. Through the parable, Jesus shifts the focus of attention from the woman's sin to her response, her acceptance of the gift of forgiveness.[50]

Jesus then poses the question as to which of the two would respond with the greater love. Simon rightly supposes that it would be the one for whom the greater debt was freely cancelled. His reply is cautious and wary; maybe he anticipates what follows.[51] Jesus agrees with his verdict; love is the product of forgiveness. The woman has incurred the anger of Simon and his guests by her behaviour and possibly by thwarting their plan to some extent. But Jesus defends her as he brings out the significance of her actions and the contrasting dispositions of his host. He invites Simon to look at her.[52] He has, of course, observed her already with a negative, jaundiced, judgemental eye. Jesus is drawing him to see her in a different light as a person of quality. Then, gently or accusingly, he points out to Simon his economical love, his lack of hospitality, his failure to do his duty as host.[53] In Simon's own home Jesus publicly lists his 'oversights'. There was no foot bath, no kiss of friendship, no oil of respect. These the woman has substituted abundantly, effusively, extravagantly, with great love and unrestrained, spontaneous affection, generosity and gratitude, which reveal the pardon she has come to acknowledge. The text is beautifully balanced.[54] The woman "sees Jesus defending her, confirming her and in the process carving out a space for her in the community of his followers."[55] But in the long run, there will be a price to pay for Jesus' defending her and criticising his host.[56]

Jesus explicitly and publicly confirms God's forgiveness, which she has already experienced.[57] There is some discussion among scholars as to whether the sense of the text is that the woman's manifestation of love towards Jesus brings her (or merits, earns) forgiveness, or that her love is a consequence of her having been already forgiven, though this has not been described in the story. The original Greek is open to both positions. Some of the early Fathers of the Church, like

Augustine, Clement of Alexandria, Peter Chrysologus, took the former view, and this is adopted in the KJV and RSV versions. The latter position, in which the parable is integrated into the narrative, is the view of Ambrose, Origen and Cassian, and adopted by the JB, NRSV, NIV versions. This is the view which, along with most modern scholars, I have followed.[58] Jesus then finally speaks to the woman, something a rabbi should not do. His words are similarly un-rabbinic: "Your sins have been forgiven."[59] His confirming comment is reassuring, liberating and transforming.

As those at table wonder who this man can be who forgives sins, Jesus again addresses her: "Your faith has saved you; go in peace." This is the first time in the account of the ministry that these two terms have been clearly joined.[60] The guests' question, focusing on the identity of Jesus,[61] is answered implicitly: precisely because Jesus is a prophet with divine authority, he receives and forgives sinners.[62] The woman has not uttered a word, but her actions in risking rejection and insult in entering the house, in expressing her gratitude and in compassionately and daringly entering into Jesus' suffering, have manifested a deep and generous faith. Prior to this encounter, she must have shown trust in God despite her sinful past, and this facilitated the restoring of their relationship. As we saw in Chapters One and Two, when examining Luke's Infancy Narrative, Jesus comes to bring salvation and peace on earth. "Simon can also learn about the depth of God's forgiveness and its powerful effect through the experience of the woman," [63] and this can revitalise his understanding of God. But we do not know how he responds; the story is open-ended; he is on the threshold of a decision.

Reflections

This is a moving narrative of two-way love. The woman courageously breaks through the exclusion barrier and shows so many signs of a love, which is far from 'economical'. There is a self-forgetfulness about her, a spontaneity and genuineness. She is deeply grateful. Jesus accepts her with great respect, allowing her to express her feelings, and even to touch him. He welcomes the service she renders and allows her to remain close to him, refusing to send her away even though the cultural and religious expectations warrant it, even though the atmosphere is pulsating with shock and disapproval. Her love and faith clash with the cold, self-righteous, closed and withdrawn attitude of the male, religious elite present at the meal.

In contrast with Simon, who invites Jesus but violates the rules of hospitality, the woman, who is a member of the outcast poor, rejected by the religious elite as an untouchable, shows by her acts of hospitality that she does accept the prophet Jesus.[64] With a touch of genius, Luke's story highlights the contrast between these two very different people.[65] Jesus has made it clear that both law keepers, the legal purists, and lawbreakers are sinners and equally in need of forgiveness. That forgiveness is freely offered to both kinds. The woman has accepted the gift; her past now lies behind her, and she can move on into a new future. Simon's final response is unknown.[66]

Whether we have been forgiven much or little, God's forgiveness has frequently been offered to us. Perhaps we sometimes take this gift for granted. Perhaps our sense of wonder and appreciation has become dull and muted. The story invites us to recapture the dreamlike, scandalous magic of God's unfathomable compassion and forgiveness. And Simon challenges us, too, about genuine hospitality, about judging and about openness to what is different and new. Jesus turns his religious world upside down, presenting a very different image of God and a new way of assessing and of relating. Maybe there is still a Simon lurking within us and present in our Church.

The Multiplication of The Loaves and Fishes (9:11–17)

Perhaps the most dramatic meal scene in Luke is the feeding of the multitudes with bread and fishes. Matthew and Mark have two versions of the story, Luke and John only one. In Luke's overall narrative, after the meal at Simon's house, there are two parables (the sower and the lamp under the jar) and several miracle stories (the calming of the storm, the healing of the Gerasene demoniac, the restoring to life of a young girl and the healing of a woman with a problem of a gynaecological nature).[67] In the immediate context, the disciples, referred to as "the apostles" by Luke, have been sent on mission with the authority of Jesus; it is an experience of apprenticeship.[68] In their absence, the reader is informed of Herod's perplexity about the identity of Jesus.[69]

On their return the apostles told Jesus all they had done. He took them with him and withdrew privately to a city called Bethsaida. When the crowds found out about it, they followed him; and he welcomed them, and spoke to them about the kingdom of God, and healed those who needed to be cured. The day was drawing to a close, and the twelve came to him and said, "Send the crowd away, so that they may go into the surrounding villages and countryside, to lodge and get provisions; for we are here in a deserted place." But he said to them, "You give them something to eat." They said, "We have no more than five loaves and two fish—unless we are to go and buy food for all these people." For there were about five thousand men. And he said to his disciples, "Make them sit down in groups of about fifty each." They did so and made them all sit down. And taking the five loaves and the two fish, he looked up to heaven, and blessed and broke them, and gave them to the disciples to set before the crowd. And all ate and were filled. What was left over was gathered up, twelve baskets of broken pieces.

On their return, the disciples report back about what they have done, and Jesus withdraws with them to Bethsaida, outside Herod Antipas' territory, looking for some space and privacy. But the crowds find out and follow.[70] Jesus, adjusting to the thwarting of his plans, welcomes them graciously, proclaims the Good News of the Kingdom to them and makes that Kingdom real by curing those in need. Mark and Matthew, in their versions, emphasise that it is the compassion of Jesus that leads to his response (in Mark teaching, in Matthew healing, before the multiplication).[71]

The storyline is familiar; it highlights the hospitality of Jesus, a broader form of table fellowship, this time in a setting of rocks and grass.[72] The introductory phrase, "the day was drawing to a close," perhaps foreshadows the Emmaus story. The disciples, practical folk, explicitly referred to as "the twelve", are aware of the situation and want Jesus to send the crowd away to find food and lodging for themselves elsewhere in the local villages. On their recent journeys, however, they have themselves depended on the hospitality of local people, a sign of God's providential care, but they wish to move the goalposts now.[73] They do not entertain the possibility that Jesus could provide for the people's needs.[74] Jesus won't accept their solution and challenges their weak faith. He tells them to address the problem and set about offering hospitality to the people from their own meagre resources.[75] With some reluctance, they get the folk to sit down in groups of fifty.

Jesus then provides the banquet, fulfilling messianic expectations. Everyone who comes is welcome at the meal; some would doubtless be unclean and less than faithful to the Law. Jesus ignores issues concerning washing regulations, the cleanliness of the food and its correct preparation and whether it has been tithed. He ignores the social boundaries so characteristic of Jewish life.[76] As Luke tells the story, the gestures and language have clear eucharistic tones as Jesus takes the loaves and fish, looks up to heaven, blesses and breaks them and gives them to the disciples, who then set the food before the crowds and later gather up the fragments that are left over, a basketful each. Remarkable superabundance![77] There is no reference to the response of the crowd, which is unusual for Luke.

The original event was clearly symbolic, an indication that the messianic times were here, and an anticipation of the final, eschatological banquet. In the story, the care and concern of Jesus for the people is evident, his inclusion of everyone; he is the one through whom God's generous mercy is made present. For Luke, this event, which is a narrative fulfilment of the hunger beatitude[78] and Mary's *Magnificat* prediction,[79] is an educative experience for "the twelve", preparing them for their later servant role of offering to people the hospitality of God. Here they discover that what seems impossible can happen when Jesus is around and with the power he bestows.[80] It is surprising what Jesus can still do with the little we have, if we offer it to him.

A Healing and Subsequent Comments (14:1–14)

Soon after this episode, the journey to Jerusalem begins. Early in that journey Jesus visits the home of Martha and Mary, and a meal is prepared for him. We have already discussed this occasion. The next two occasions in which we find Jesus dining take place in the company of the religious elite. In the first, as Jesus takes his place at table, the Pharisee who has invited him is amazed because he does not wash first before dining. Jesus launches into a lengthy tirade against various aspects of Pharisee behaviour, which he then extends to the lawyers too (11:37–52). The episode closes on an ominous note: "When he went outside, the scribes and the Pharisees began to be very hostile towards him and to cross-examine him about many things, lying in wait for him, to catch him in something he might say."

The second occasion comprises a meal, a parable about places at table and teaching concerning guest lists. This section is a carefully crafted unit; it takes place on the Sabbath at the house of a leading Pharisee, in the context of a meal, in an atmosphere of hostility.[81]

> On one occasion when Jesus was going to the house of a leader of the Pharisees to eat a meal on the sabbath, they were watching him closely. Just then, in front of him, there was a man who had dropsy. And Jesus asked the lawyers and Pharisees, "Is it lawful to cure people on the sabbath, or not?" But they were silent. So, Jesus took him and healed him, and sent him away. Then he said to them, "If one of you has a child or an ox that has fallen into a well, will you not immediately pull it out on a sabbath day?" And they could not reply to this.

The last two occasions on which Jesus dined in Pharisee company proved difficult for him and challenging for his table companions. The current episode follows that trend. This time the invitation has come from "a leader of the Pharisees", "one of the socio-economic elite".[82] It is the Sabbath, a day of special celebration and an expression of faithfulness to the Law and Jewish identity.[83] Presumably, the meal at his house will follow the synagogue service. Other Pharisees and some scribes are also guests; it is unlikely that people other than Pharisees will be present; issues of ritual purity and status are in the background.[84] There is antagonism in the air, for these people are on the watch in a monitoring role to see if Jesus fails in any way to meet their standards and expectations. With typical sensitivity to atmosphere, Jesus is aware of the emerging scenario. He sees before him a man suffering from dropsy (modern edema). The man happens to be there; he is not the bait in a Pharisee trap.[85] He makes no request for healing; it is Jesus who makes the first move. His presence poses a threat to the ritual purity of the meal and the honour of the gathering.[86]

Jesus had found himself in a similar situation earlier when teaching in a synagogue on the Sabbath, when he took the initiative in healing a man with a withered hand. The scribes and Pharisees were on the watch so as to find grounds to accuse him. Inviting the man to stand before him, he asked his adversaries whether it is lawful to do good or to do harm on the Sabbath, to save life or destroy it. In the ensuing silence, he told the man to stretch out his hand, and it was restored. The response of the religious elite was one of intense anger (6:6–11). Likewise, some time later, while preaching in a synagogue on the Sabbath, he noticed a woman who was disabled, bent double for eighteen years. Calling her over, he laid his hands on her, saying: "Woman, you are set free from your ailment." The leader of the synagogue took umbrage at this Sabbath breach, and was not shy in letting those present know his view. Jesus put him firmly in his place, to the satisfaction of the crowd (13:10–17).[87]

On this occasion at the meal, Jesus puts a question to the company: "Is it lawful to cure people on the Sabbath, or not?" The issue concerns the interpretation of the Law.[88] The rabbis permitted Sabbath healing only when human life was in danger. A positive response would indicate laxity, a negative rejoinder would be an indication of lack of sympathy for a sufferer. Jesus' adversaries are silent; they refuse to be drawn into discussion. So, Jesus heals the man on the spot, releasing him from his malady and sends him away.

Turning back to them, Jesus does not refer to the Law but to their humanity, asking how they would react if a child or ox were to fall into a well on the Sabbath and risk drowning. Surely, they would immediately pull it out and save life.[89] "Compassion took precedence over the requirements of the Law."[90] Again there is stony silence. They know he is right; it is permitted to heal on the Sabbath; Jesus is an authoritative teacher.[91] What a way to start a meal!

Despite the inauspicious beginning, it seems that the meal continued, and Jesus entertained the guests with a parable and further comments about table etiquette:[92]

> When he noticed how the guests chose the places of honour, he told them a parable. "When you are invited by someone to a wedding banquet, do not sit down at the place of honour, in case someone more distinguished than you has been invited by your host; and the host who invited both of you may come and say to you, 'Give this person your place', and then in disgrace you would start to take the lowest place. But when you are invited, go and sit down at the lowest place, so that when your host comes, he may say to you, 'Friend, move up higher'; then you will be honoured in the presence of all who sit at the table with you. For all who exalt themselves will be humbled, and those who humble themselves will be exalted."

> He said also to the one who had invited him, "When you give a luncheon or a dinner, do not invite your friends or your brothers or your relatives or rich neighbours, in case they may invite you in return, and you would be repaid. But when you give a banquet, invite the poor, the crippled, the lame, and the blind. And you will be blessed, because they cannot repay you, for you will be repaid at the resurrection of the righteous."

In that culture, people of the same status, with similar ideas and values, would eat together, reclining on couches or mats on their left side, their right hands reaching out to the low central table. The host would be in the centre, his family on his right, the guests on the left, arranged in order of rank.[93] Part of the experience was table talk ('*symposium*'). On this occasion, it is Jesus who does the talking. As is so often the case with his parables, Jesus reflects with his audience about aspects of nature or life with which they are familiar. He has observed the jockeying for position around the Pharisee's table, he is aware of the importance of status and esteem in that culture, the desire for recognition. In parable, he extrapolates to wedding banquet imagery, though what he says applies to other celebrations.[94] In an honour/shame culture, rather than take the best place and then suffer the humiliation of having to step down, he suggests it is wiser to take the opposite tack and sit in the lowest place. The host may then seek you out and upgrade you to a more prestigious position at table, and the guests will note well how you have been honoured.

Jesus is not simply giving sound practical advice concerning blatant or cunning one-upmanship (Prov 25:6–7). In the parable, his words point to something deeper, the different mindset and values of the Kingdom, with its pattern of reversal, and a different way of defining social relations. "As in social etiquette, so in the spiritual realm, recognition eludes those who demand it and accrues to those who think more highly of others than of themselves."[95] In the world of Jesus it is the humble who are honoured, and it is God who bestows such honour. The final comment, a statement of divine reversal, which probably comes from another context, is apposite here: "For all who exalt themselves will be humbled, and those who humble themselves will be exalted."[96] This has been the pattern earlier in Luke's story of Jesus, with Elizabeth (1:7, 24–26) and Mary (1:47–48). Genuine value and honour comes as God's gift.

Jesus then shifts his attention from guests to host, and turns the normally accepted mores upside-down.[97] He is aware of the common culture of his day, the consciousness of status and rank, the seeking of advantage, connections and self-promotion, the practice of reciprocity.[98] He was aware, too, that, as part of their spirituality, the Pharisees refused to share table with those who did not share their values and their views on religious purity.[99] Given the importance of the guest list for formal dinners, Jesus provides his host with two alternative lists, each featuring four groups in carefully structured parallel. The first, the socially acceptable 'insider' list, is to be avoided: you do not invite your friends or your brothers or your relatives or your rich neighbours, with the expectation of reciprocity and repayment.[100] Jesus advocates the opposite, that they should reach out and offer hospitality to those who are poor, lame, disabled, blind.[101] This, of course, was absolutely unthinkable. It could entail loss of personal honour and status, deep upset for family and friends, the severing of social and economic links.[102]

Yet the list is in keeping with Jesus' own practice, as announced in his mission statement and his reply to the Baptist (4:18–19; 7:22), for these are the people who are hungry, isolated, sad and needy; the outcasts become included, which is the message of salvation.[103] Jesus insists on being subversive and countercultural in his vision of the Kingdom. Jesus is not saying that parties with friends are unacceptable, nor advocating the performing of good deeds for a heavenly reward.[104] The fact that there is no way that these categories of folk can repay the favour of being invited is in fact a blessing;[105] it means it is left to God to reciprocate, and God will do so in the end time in the resurrection of the just.[106]

The message of Jesus serves both as a warning and an invitation to his host and fellow guests; Jesus is still prepared to proclaim his message to them and offer them the opportunity to change and embrace the Kingdom. It is also a challenge to his disciples then and now. An inclusive and generous understanding of hospitality is required, being merciful like the Father (6:36).

The Parable of The Great Dinner (14:15–24)

The meal in the Pharisee's home continues with a comment from one of the guests, to which Jesus replies with another parable:

> One of the dinner guests, on hearing this, said to him, "Blessed is anyone who will eat bread in the kingdom of God!" Then Jesus said to him, "Someone gave a great dinner and invited many. At the time for the dinner he sent his slave to say to those who had been invited, 'Come; for everything is ready now.' But they all alike began to make excuses. The first said to him, 'I have bought a piece of land, and I must go out and see it; please accept my apologies.' Another said, 'I have bought five yoke of oxen, and I am going to try them out; please accept my apologies.' Another said, 'I have just been married, and therefore I cannot come.' So, the slave returned and reported this to his master. Then the owner of the house became angry and said to his slave, 'Go out at once into the streets and lanes of the town and bring in the poor, the crippled, the blind, and the lame.' And the slave said, 'Sir, what you ordered has been done, and there is still room.' Then the master said to the slave, 'Go out into the roads and lanes, and compel people to come in, so that my house may be filled. For I tell you, none of those who were invited will taste my dinner.'"

Jesus has just pronounced blessed those who invite the poor to their banquet, and guaranteed them a reward in the end time, the resurrection of the dead. One of the other guests takes a cue from this and pronounces blessed those who eat bread in the Kingdom of God. Perhaps he feels confident that he will have a place at that eschatological banquet.[107] With the word "Kingdom" ringing in his ears, Jesus offers further instruction, launching into another parable, which transfers the focus from the future Kingdom to the present; it is happening already.[108] In the parable, an unnamed individual decided to give an impressive dinner party and was lavish with his invitations, presumably offered to his social peers.[109] The presumption is that we are dealing with a small town community. When the meal was ready in the late afternoon, he sent his slave to inform them: "Come; for everything is now ready."[110]

The response proves to be other than expected, for all the invitees, having initially committed themselves to attend, now decline to participate, turning down the invitation and putting forward a variety of blatantly false excuses. Three are highlighted as representative (according to the rule of three in parables). One, probably an absentee landlord, has bought a piece of land and needs to go and inspect it. Another has bought five yoke of oxen, a not inconsiderable investment, and needs to try them out; this suggests that he is a successful landowner.[111] The phrasing is in parallel. A third uses his recent marriage as the reason why he cannot come. Unlike the others, who ask for their apology to be accepted, he simply states that he won't be there. The first two excuses are flimsy: one would conduct a detailed check of the field or test out the oxen prior to purchase.[112] The third excuse is rude for a man in that culture; besides he would be away for only a few hours.[113] It appears that there is a conspiracy, calculated to insult and dishonour the host.[114] The slave returns to his master ("lord") and informs him of the unexpected situation which has emerged.

Naturally, the host's initial reaction is one of anger; he has been embarrassed, snubbed and shamed by his peers. Rather than cancel the banquet, he creatively settles on an alternative scenario,[115] sending his slave out into the streets and narrow alleyways of the town with instructions to bring in the poor, the disabled, the blind and the lame, a list of invitees rather like that proposed by Jesus earlier in the meal, all of them unable to reciprocate the invitation (14:13; see 7:18–23). This kind of table fellowship will be a surprise to peer and poor alike, and will not enhance his social prestige.[116] The slave obeys instructions but has to inform his master that there is still room at the banquet table.

The next stage for the host (found only in Luke's version of the parable) is to order his slave to make a third trawl, going outside the confines of the town to the paths and byways where persons of low status, beggars, marginalised individuals, who need to be near the town to find a way of keeping alive, can be found.[117] His reason for this move is to make sure that the house will be full of guests, the banquet a success without the original invitees, for whom there will now be no room. The language of compulsion used in the text mirrors the social gap between host and invitees; the latter would be suspicious and wary.[118] Status boundaries are being breached. "The slave will need to use forceful persuasion to override that fundamental suspicion."[119]

The host's final statement can be taken in two ways. It can be part of the parable. The "I" is the host, the "you" (plural in the text) refers to the third group, who are presumed to have arrived.[120] The host's comment is not a judgement but a statement that his social relations will no longer be governed by the old system. He addresses the elite of Jesus' audience and Luke's audience too, with the challenge that they embrace social identity with the poor, those who cannot participate in the social games of reciprocity and status augmentation.[121] Or, the "I" is Jesus, the "you" his fellow guests at table.[122] Those who look forward to eating bread in the Kingdom need to accept his invitation ("my banquet") rather than continuing their opposition, otherwise they will exclude themselves.

In this parable once again, conventional ideas are radically challenged. In the upside-down world of Jesus, the Kingdom he is proclaiming, the sick and poor, the outsiders and people of low status, the marginalised are all included; they are offered a free place at table, with no strings attached. His own style of table fellowship makes this apparent. On the other hand, the religious elite are refusing the invitation to embrace the Kingdom. The excuses put forward are typical of the obstacles to entering the Kingdom, highlighted elsewhere by Jesus, posed by riches, possessions and family ties; but they are excuses covering deeper levels of rejection. The parable challenges them and all self-righteous and status-oriented people about their unwillingness to accept the current invitation of Jesus, and warns them of the future consequences. But, unlike the man in the parable, the invitation that Jesus extends to the poor is not an expression of anger, a reaction to being snubbed; it is right at the heart of his ministry, as his statement in Nazareth made clear.[123]

Some scholars maintain that the third group of invitees are to be understood as Jewish too: "the parable takes place entirely within the Jewish world."[124] Others are of the opinion that the third invitation symbolically represents an outreach to the gentiles.[125] Some believe that such outreach was not in Jesus' mind and that this element is an expansion by the early Church. Certainly, as Luke's church community listened to the story, they probably interpreted the first group as the Jewish religious elite, the second group as the marginalised in Israel and the third group as the gentiles.[126] It is true that Jesus seems to have understood his mission as directed primarily to the people of Israel (Matt 10:5; 15:23). However, he would have been aware of Isaiah 25:6–9, which speaks of God offering a banquet to "all the peoples", and Isaiah 49:6, which speaks of the Servant's being "a light to the nations so that God's salvation might reach to the ends of the earth." In his ministry, he did reach out to heal the centurion's servant (Luke 7:1–10) and the Syro-Phoenician woman's daughter (Mark 7:24–30). Shortly before the occasion of the meal in the Pharisee's house, which is still the setting for this parable, Jesus asked about those who would be saved, speaks about the narrow door and suggests the possibility of Jewish people being excluded and "thrown out", while "people will come from east and west, from north and south, and will eat in the kingdom of God" (13:28–29). Jesus possibly did intend a conscious allusion to the gentile mission; the feature may have been developed more fully in the course of the tradition, so that the parable was seen as giving a summons to the gentile mission.[127]

The parable continues to lay down a radical challenge for the way in which Christians understand and live out their discipleship. Our normal daily practice is challenged, and our eucharistic practice too.

Jesus Dines with Sinners (15:1–2)

Following Luke's narrative, it is not long before we find Jesus again sharing table. This time he is dining with his favourite people, and his practice again proves a source of contention:

> Now all the tax collectors and sinners were coming near to listen to him. And the Pharisees and the scribes were grumbling and saying, "This fellow welcomes sinners and eats with them."

We have already in the last chapter examined this beautiful section of Luke's story of Jesus, in which Jesus responds to criticism by telling three parables: the parables of the lost sheep, the lost coin and the two lost sons. Jesus explains in this way why it is that he seeks out those on the margins and enables them to experience the dawning Kingdom and come to realise the generosity and love of God. For his adversaries to understand where Jesus is coming from, a fundamental shift of mindset will be required. For those open to him, Jesus' words are revelation. God's invitation in Jesus is free and for all.

The Last Supper (22:14–38)

As we have reflected on Luke's story of Jesus, we have several times been made aware of that structural framework normally referred to as the journey narrative. We now pick up the story again when Jesus and his disciples have, in fact, reached Jerusalem, the theatre of his "exodus". After descending the Mount of Olives with his disciples, he weeps over the city because of the people's failure to recognise the time of their visitation from God (20:41–44). He then enters the temple and drives out those engaged in business there, for they have turned a house of prayer into a den of robbers. Each day he teaches there, leaving his hearers spellbound and the religious leaders more determined than ever on his destruction (20:45–48). Luke provides examples of this teaching, as Jesus responds to questions, tells parables, makes exhortations and prophesies about the future.

Inevitably things come to a head. The religious leaders desperately want rid of Jesus, but their fear of the people holds them back. Then Judas comes along clandestinely and offers to betray Jesus. After some discussion and a financial arrangement, he "began to look for an opportunity to betray him to them when no crowd was present."[128] Luke then tells the story of the final meal that Jesus shares with his disciples in the context of Passover.[129] The significant "hour" has now come, the "exodus" time has dawned.[130]

> When the hour came, he took his place at the table, and the apostles with him. He said to them, "I have eagerly desired to eat this Passover with you before I suffer; for I tell you, I will not eat it until it is fulfilled in the kingdom of God." Then he took a cup, and after giving thanks he said, "Take this and divide it among yourselves; for I tell you that from now on I will not drink of the fruit of the vine until the kingdom of God comes." Then he took a loaf of bread, and when he had given thanks, he broke it and gave it to them, saying, "This is my body, which is given for you. Do this in remembrance of me." And he did the same with the cup after supper, saying, "This cup that is poured out for you is the new covenant in my blood. But see, the one who betrays me is with me, and his hand is on the table. For the Son of Man is going as it has been determined, but woe to that one by whom he is betrayed!" Then they began to ask one another which one of them it could be who would do this.[131]

Jesus is aware of his impending death as he and "the apostles with him" gather, reclining as custom demanded for the solemn meal at which he is the host.[132] "Being with" is a designation of discipleship; the group has scarcely been mentioned during Jesus' time in Jerusalem. Jesus tells them with emotion in his voice that he has eagerly longed to eat this Passover with them before he suffers unto death,[133] stating that he would not eat it again until the Kingdom of God, already present in his ministry, not least in his table fellowship, finally reaches its consummation in the eschatological banquet.[134] Jesus is confident that death, predicted several times previously but now clearly imminent, will not be the last word.[135] He then shared a cup, perhaps to strengthen their fellowship, with the words:[136] "Take this and divide it among yourselves; for I tell you that from now on I will not drink of the fruit of the vine until the kingdom of God comes." "Fruit of the vine" is an expression found in the Old Testament (Deut 22:9; Isa 32:12), and echoes the blessing used with the cup. The two statements by Jesus are in parallel. This twofold reference to the Kingdom situates what follows clearly in that context, also suggesting that before that final fulfilment there will be a time gap.[137]

Jesus follows the ritual of the Passover meal, but there is no reference to the lamb. He gives his attention to the bread and cup, providing a new interpretation. He takes a loaf of bread, gives thanks to the Father, breaks it and gives it to them, saying: "This is my body which is given for you. Do this in remembrance of me."[138] The broken bread is a symbol of the body broken in the torture death of crucifixion, which will be for his followers a source of liberation and new life.[139] They are instructed to keep doing this in his memory. Remembering (*anamnēsis*) was central to the Passover meal; its purpose was to recall God's liberating the people from Egypt's slavery (Exod 12:14; Deut 16:3) and to look to the future with hope. But such remembering is more than a mental recalling; it creates a form of presence, a making present again. When his followers "remember" him by "breaking bread" (Acts 2:46; 20:7), he will be present among them.[140] The fellowship meals of his followers will recall the significance of his death on behalf of others, and should ensure that features of his life—his openness to outsiders, his comportment as servant, his indifference to status honour—remain central to the life of his community.[141] After these words, the meal itself continues.

When the meal is finished, Jesus takes the cup, with the words: "This cup that is poured out for you is the new covenant in my blood."[142] The imagery of blood poured out suggests violence and has a sacrificial ring. The emphasis seems to be on the idea of covenant, recalling Jeremiah's prophecy of a new covenant for the house of Israel, which concludes with the words "I will forgive their iniquity, and remember their sin no more" (31:31–34).[143] Covenants were usually sealed with sacrificial blood, and the phrasing suggests a sacrificial offering. The blood is poured out "for you", which can mean both "in place of you" and "on your behalf".[144] Jesus gives a new significance to the bread and the wine of that meal; both point to his death—body broken, blood poured out—which he accepts as the price he has to pay for the life he has led (his mission, his values, his message, his claims).[145] Those sharing this meal will benefit, but they are representative of all who will come to follow Jesus.

After this profoundly moving and symbolic gesture, Jesus, without a break, moves on to give some warnings and instructions to his disciples.[146] First, he speaks about his proximate betrayal by one whose hand is on the table where they are dining together, fracturing that fellowship.[147] The contrast is dramatic and quite breathtaking. While human tactical scheming and diabolical manoeuvring are certainly involved, what is happening is part of Jesus' destiny, God's overarching and providential plan.[148] Jesus does not reveal Judas' identity to the others, but intimates the tragic consequences of his culpable action. The disciples discuss with one another the possible identity of the culprit.

At this juncture, paradoxically, their focus switches, as a dispute erupts between them, not for the first time, about which of them is to be regarded as the greatest in the group, the top man.[149] There is clearly more than one way to let Jesus down. The disciples still fail to grasp the radically new values of Jesus and have not understood his very recent words of self-giving. Jesus addresses the situation with a statement and a brief parable:

> But he said to them, "The kings of the Gentiles lord it over them; and those in authority over them are called benefactors.[150] But not so with you; rather the greatest among you must become like the youngest, and the leader like one who serves."

The image of leadership in the Greco-Roman world is not flattering; those with power and wealth tended to seek to enhance their status and consolidate their power through generous acts that benefit their subjects or fellow citizens, who would then praise and support them; it was a system of patronage, and quite normal.[151] This is not the way Jesus understands human relationships or the way he himself operates, and it must not be the style of his followers. His words turn upside-down the normal expectations, hopes and social practice of our world, to which the disciples themselves obviously subscribe.

Jesus presses his point home with the parabolic saying: "For who is greater, the one who is at the table or the one who serves? Is it not the one at the table? But I am among you as one who serves." Jesus is the Master, the host at the table, where he has served the bread and wine; his habitual style throughout his ministry in his words and his actions has been to attend to the needs of others; he has been a servant. He sees himself as servant. This is the meaning of his body "given for you" and his blood "poured out for you". The gesture sums up the meaning of his life, just as it captures the meaning of his coming death. His way must be the model for theirs. "The form of leadership appropriate to Jesus' community, then, is one that is unconcerned with the accrual of status honour but itself reflects the humility of table servants and of those who occupy the bottom rung of social power and privilege, the young."[152]

The disciples at this stage seem incapable of understanding and accepting this. Central to the conversion Jesus demanded from the beginning of the ministry, the paradigm shift, the U-turn in mindset, outlook and living style, is the switch from a mentality of domination and control to one of self-giving, self-emptying and service. In spite of everything Jesus has said and done, his efforts to teach them, the disciples still have not got the message; they still have not understood what his mission and style are about.

Jesus then acknowledges that they have shown commitment to him, standing by him faithfully in times of trial and difficulty, and he rewards them for it. "I confer on you, just as my Father has conferred on me, a kingdom, so that you may eat and drink at my table in my kingdom, and you will sit on thrones judging the twelve tribes of Israel." The word translated here as "kingdom" can also be translated as "royal power". They will share in the royal power of Jesus by eating and drinking at the same table as he, and by exercising authority and governance.[153] But that authority, which is now conferred by Jesus, comes from God; it will be exercised in the future through their leadership and governance in the community of Jesus, for which they are now commissioned, with further fulfilment in the eschatological age beyond.

In the immediate future, however, a serious problem is created by Satan's onslaught on these disciples. Having successfully co-opted Judas, Satan will turn his attention on the others as the passion story unfolds.[154] The faith of the disciples will soon be severely tested. So Jesus, in the first place, prays for Peter, addressing him as "Simon, Simon", as when they first met.[155] His prayer of intercession is that his faithfulness may not be undermined during this time of trial. He then gives him the role of strengthening the others, when once he has recovered and repented.[156] Peter, confident as ever, claims that he is ready to go with Jesus to prison and even to death. He seems to have realised the seriousness of Jesus' intimations of coming death.[157] Jesus replies: "I tell you, Peter, the cock will not crow this day, until you have denied three times that you know me." It is quite a devastating prophecy of failed discipleship, even if the wording is gentler than in Mark.[158]

The final recommendation of Jesus to his struggling band recognises the danger confronting them that threatens not only their faith and commitment but even their life.[159] Jesus now reverses the recommendations that he had given the seventy disciples when they were setting out on mission earlier in their adventure of discipleship; then they were dependent on and received the hospitality and generosity of others. Now they are to take with them purse, bag and, surprisingly, even a sword (which replaces "sandals" in the original list (10:4)), for the circumstances have changed and are now hostile and will continue to be so in the future. Jesus is speaking symbolically as a warning.[160] He rejected violence earlier in the Sermon on the Plain (6:20–38). Jesus himself has no intention of seeking to escape, nor will he countenance violence in the face of arrest. When a sword is used, he heals the person who has lost his ear in the fray (22:49–51).

He quotes a piece of scripture which must be fulfilled: "And he was counted among the lawless." This is taken from Isa 53:12, and refers to the vicarious suffering of God's Servant; here it emphasises that Jesus will be dishonoured by being numbered among the lawless, treated as a criminal. While this will be literally true in that he will be arrested as if he were a bandit (22:52), twinned with Barabbas (23:18), and two rogues will suffer with him (23:52), the death he will endure is that reserved for the criminal class. It may also refer to his constantly associating with sinners, considered lawless by the religious elite.[161] At this point the literalist disciples produce two swords. Jesus' final remark betrays his exasperation and disappointment: "It is enough", indicating that further conversation is pointless; they are not on the same wavelength still.[162] This has been called "the utterance of a broken heart."[163]

They leave for the Mount of Olives, Jesus leading the way.[164] We know the sequel: betrayal by Judas, the disciples' sleepfulness in the garden, Peter's denials, the distant presence of some of them on Calvary and at the burial.[165] The final meal of Jesus presents a bleak and disconcerting picture of inadequacy and failure. "The disciples share this meal as sinners and broken people. They are the last of a long group of broken and sinful people who have shared meals with Jesus during his life and ministry."[166] Nevertheless, they remain his legitimate successors.

Fortunately, that is not the end of the story. The God of faithfulness and mercy is still around. The Father is faithful to Jesus and raises him from death, and the risen Jesus remains faithful to his disciples, encountering them and transforming their lives anew. In the next chapter, we shall look at Luke's presentation of these transforming experiences: the Emmaus narrative and the subsequent meeting of Jesus with the group of disciples in the room in Jerusalem. Both feature table fellowship.

Reflections

This theme of table fellowship, which threads its way through Luke's presentation of the ministry of Jesus, is extremely rich and quite complex. It reveals a great deal about the fascinating personality of Jesus. We encounter a man of incredible freedom and courage, who is true to his understanding of God and to his mission, as articulated in the Nazareth synagogue. He is a man of deep compassion and care as he reaches out to the broken, the outsiders, those considered sinful people. He is generous in his unconditional forgiveness. His table fellowship, expressed in the different episodes that we have considered, is the Gospel in a nutshell, for it reveals Jesus' acceptance and inclusivity, his desire to be close to those in need, to enable them to experience God's loving presence in their lives, to become members of the Kingdom. Table fellowship reveals a God who reaches out to us in love, wishing to be with us and share our lives, offering us a share in his life, which is salvation.

The table fellowship of Jesus was a prophetic gesture. Prophets reveal something of the God in whose name they speak and act. They also offer a critique of the current situation when it is at variance with the mind and heart of God. Inevitably, the way in which Jesus shares table is a challenge for the religious leaders of his people. His is clearly a different mindset and value system, a different understanding of God and God's ways. His teaching when in their table company makes this explicit.[167]

For us today, Luke's presentation of the story of Jesus is an invitation to allow ourselves to be embraced by God's extravagant love. At the Eucharist you and I frequently, perhaps daily, share Jesus' table as his friends, accepted and welcomed. We do so as disciples who, like the Gospel Twelve, often fail; we know his ongoing forgiveness and patience. It is important that we do not allow our sense of wonder to fade. In the Eucharist, we are caught up by Jesus into the meaning of the universe, the deepest mystery of God's love. I often imagine Jesus with a broken loaf in his hands simply saying: "Michael, this is me—for you." Amazing! I link these words with the expression of the Father to the older son in the parable: "All I have is yours." Jesus could not give us more than he gives us.

In developing this theme, Luke is addressing his largely gentile Church about their practice of inclusive fellowship in their community and in their celebration of Eucharist, the "Lord's Supper". I believe Luke raises some challenging questions to our Church today in relation to our Church communities and our current eucharistic practice.[168] As followers of Jesus, we are called to find ways of enabling people to experience what the Galilean peasants experienced in the table fellowship of Jesus. This is not limited to sitting around a table with a cup of tea or a glass of wine. Words that I associate with table fellowship are: acceptance, inclusion, affirmation, friendship, hospitality, encouragement, belonging, challenge, forgiveness, meaning, hope, joy. How do we translate all this into our parish and religious communities and places of mission, and into our daily personal lives, our encounters with others? What are the normal contexts in which "table fellowship" equivalents are a possibility? How are we present with others: our family and community, our work or recreation colleagues, the poor and sick and marginalised around us? How do we enable them to experience the love of God touching their lives, bringing them hope and meaning and a sense of worth? How do we draw them into the experience of the Kingdom?

These are issues that are central to our lives of discipleship and our Christian mission. We need creativity and courage, freedom and generosity like Jesus. Our faithfulness will also be a prophetic challenge to both religious and secular society and will therefore be uncomfortable. But, for our integrity there is no other option.

Notes

1   Robert J. Karris, *Luke: Artist and Theologian* (New York: Paulist, 1985), 47. Neyrey, *Passion*, 8–10, observes that Luke mentions meals 19 times, 13 of which are distinctive to Luke's editorial hand. Meals are inclusive events (Jew and gentile; saints and sinners; clean and unclean); he is interested in table etiquette; meals are symbols of election, forgiveness and eschatological blessing; meals stress reversal of roles.

2   Carroll, *Luke*, 133.

3   Joachim Jeremias, *New Testament Theology* (London, SCM 1971), 116. Wilfrid Harrington, *Mark* (Dublin: Veritas, 1979), 32, notes that the basis of table fellowship is messianic forgiveness.

4   Levine, *Stories*, 14, writes: "What is infectiously appealing about Jesus is that he likes to celebrate … . He is indiscriminate in his dining companions."

5   Tournier, *Guilt and Grace*, 189.

6   Karris, *Luke*, 57, refers to the "together with" and "separation from" aspects of Jesus' meals.

7   Carroll, *Luke*, 133, notes that leaving everything does not necessarily rule out continuing connection to household and further expressions of generosity. Green, *Luke*, 246, understands it as reorienting his life around God's purpose as manifest in Jesus' mission.

8   Culpepper, *Mark*, 84; McBride, *Mark*, 54–55. See Green, *Luke*, 247. Caird, *Luke*, 96, refers to spiritual quarantine.

9   Green, *Luke*, 249; McBride, *Luke*, 77, comments that the Pharisees were not

concerned about the sick but about themselves, lest they be infected.

10   Hos 14:4; Jer 3:22; 17:4; 30:17. See Harrington, *Mark*, 32.

11   Green, *Luke*, 248, sees Jesus' call to Levi as a programmatic call to discipleship for sinners, and Levi's response as the embodiment of repentance, and the banquet as a representation of the new community being formed around Jesus. Repentance (*metanoia*) is a major theme in Luke/Acts. Carroll, *Luke*, 133, comments that the meal setting becomes a central symbol of this reversal of social position.

12   Resseguie, *Spiritual Landscape*, 70.

13   These conflicts follow the Markan conflict pattern, but Luke combines the two scenes into one. Two further conflicts follow concerning the disciples who pluck corn on the Sabbath, and Jesus who heals a man on the Sabbath in a synagogue (6:1–11), but these have no bearing on the theme of meals. See Mark 2:1–3:6.

14   Reid, *Parables*, 250; Tannehill, *Luke*, 107; Resseguie, *Spiritual Landscape*, 150, n. 82. Green, *Luke*, 248, believes that it is not the Pharisees who ask this question; the issue may have raised in general table talk. Marshall, *Luke*, 224, maintains that the subject is an indeterminate "they".

15   Resseguie, *Spiritual Landscape*, 82, understands fasting as "boundary-creating activity", identifying a group as different from others.

16   Caird, *Luke*, 97. Reid, *Parables*, 251, suggests that the unusual phrase "disciples of the Pharisees" was constructed as parallel with "disciples of John" and the disciples of Jesus.

17   In biblical imagery, God is sometimes represented as the bridegroom of Israel (Hos 2:19; Isa 54:3–6; 62:5; Jer 2:2; Ezek 16); and the end time will be characterised by a great (messianic) banquet. Parties are not without deep religious significance.

18   Evans, *Luke*, 311.

19   McBride, *Luke*, 79. Marshall, *Luke*, 225, holds that Jesus, aware of his mission to bring in the age of salvation, could have seen himself as the bridegroom; it is purely metaphorical; it need not be messianic.

20   Caird, *Luke*, 97, suggests that the final comment about disciples fasting is out of kilter with the imagery because the celebration of the Kingdom had come to stay. It is part of later Church allegorisation. Similarly, Evans, *Luke*, 311. Reid, *Parables*, 253, maintains that most scholars doubt whether Jesus uttered this saying so early in his ministry; it reflects the post-resurrection experience of the early Church.

21   Tannehill, *Luke*, 109, sees the newness as referring to the various aspects of this controversy section: forgiveness, table fellowship, fasting, the Sabbath (6:1–11). In the experience of Luke's community, opposition continues because of the tendency to stick with the old. Caird, *Luke*, 98, comments that those satisfied with the old ways are not likely to be enthusiastic supporters of revolutionary change.

22   Carroll, *Luke*, 136; Reid, *Parables*, 254; Resseguie, *Spiritual Landscape*, 83. Marshall, *Luke*, 222, agrees; the new way of life must not be fettered by old ways. On p. 228 he states that the verse expresses the view of those who are content with the old, and make no effort to try the new. Evans, *Luke*, 312, sees the verse as an ironical comment on the religious perversity of Pharasaic conservatism in refusing Jesus and his message; it may be a piece of proverbial wisdom.

23   Green, *Luke*, 250. Reid, *Parables*, 254, acknowledges that more often Luke emphasises the continuity between Christianity and Judaism. Here, however, the message is that Jesus' teaching is something radically new, demanding a new response.

24   7:34. The other occasions are 11:37–52; 14:1–24; all are conflict situations.

25   Bailey, *Jesus Through Middle Eastern Eyes*, 239 and 241; Fitzmyer, *Luke*, 1:687, calls it one of the great episodes in the Lukan Gospel. Evans, *Luke*, 360, believes that style and language suggest that Luke was largely responsible for its present form. Bailey believes that it was written before the composition of the Gospels, and most likely given to Luke in written form during his Jerusalem sojourn in 56–58 CE; it records eyewitness testimony. Fitzmyer, *Luke*, 1:684, describes the story as conflated, but believes that it came to Luke in that way.

26   See Michael T. Winstanley, *Symbols and Spirituality*, (Bolton: Don Bosco Publications, 2007), 111–122.

27   Johnson, *Luke*, 128–29, argues strongly in favour of there being two separate incidents; Marshall, *Luke*, 304–306, is of the same view; likewise, Culpepper, *Mark*, 482. Reid, *Parables*, 91, notes the tendency in the Western Church to confuse the identities of Mary Magdalene, Mary of Bethany, the woman who anoints Jesus before his passion, the woman of this story and the woman taken in adultery. Each has her own identity. Brown, *John*, 1:449–50, maintains that there were two incidents, with some passing over of details in the oral stage. Fitzmyer, *Luke*, 1:687, however, seems open to there being one original incident of an anointing during a meal, which took different forms as the tradition developed.

28   Wright, *Luke*, 90. Bailey, *Jesus Through Middle Eastern Eyes*, 239, suggests a structure based on the typical prophetic template of seven inverted stanzas with a climax at the centre: introduction (the Pharisee, Jesus, the woman), the outpouring of the woman's love (in action), a dialogue (Simon judges wrongly), a parable (at the centre), a dialogue (Simon judges rightly), the outpouring of the woman's love (in retrospect), conclusion (the Pharisee, Jesus, the woman).

29   Marshall, *Luke*, 314 and 306.

30   Caird, *Luke*, 114.

31   Bailey, *Jesus Through Middle Eastern Eyes*, 242; Fitzmyer, *Luke*, 1:686–7, holds that the sinful woman comes to Jesus as one already forgiven by God and is seeking to pour out signs of love and gratitude; love is the consequence of her forgiveness.

32   Evans, *Luke*, 362, observes that it has to be presumed that she knew herself to be one of the company with whom Jesus associates, that he had already declared her sins forgiven, and that her actions were expressions of gratitude for this. Her actions can only be accounted for by something the story does not itself contain. Carroll, *Luke*, 177, suggests that previous contact motivates her action; this is not their first encounter.

33   Fitzmyer, *Luke*, 1:688, thinks the invitation stemmed from the Pharisee's desire to honour an important person.

34   This is Bailey's opinion, *Jesus Through Middle Eastern Eyes*, 242. Michael Fallon, *Gospel according to St Luke: An Introductory Commentary* (Bangalore: Asian Trading Corporation, 1997), 153, adopts a similar negative line. Carroll, *Luke*, 176, observes that the critical part played so far in Jesus' ministry by the Pharisees places a question mark

beside this meal invitation.

35   Fallon, *Luke*, 153, considers it a studied insult, and sees it as an expression of Simon's desire to humiliate him. McBride, *Luke*, 102, thinks that Simon has been polite according to the book, but has made no effort to make Jesus feel especially welcome. This is the view of Marshall also, *Luke*, 311.

36   Pagola, *Jesus*, 151, states that this way of dining was reserved for special occasions. He believes that the banquet was held in front of the house, where bystanders could listen to the conversation of the diners. The woman was probably a prostitute, not to be confused with Mary of Magdala or Mary of Bethany. Byrne, *Hospitality*, 74, makes the same point. Fitzmyer, *Luke*, 1:688, thinks the meal was a festive banquet, possibly a Sabbath meal after synagogue; also, Marshall, *Luke*, 308.

37   See Caird, *Luke*, 114.

38   Reid, *Parables*, 97, bucks the trend, claiming that nothing in the text says she was a prostitute; the nature of her sins is not mentioned; she could have been ill, disabled, a midwife or dyer, or have frequent contact with gentiles for the whole city to consider her sinful from association with the unclean.

39   "From the time I came in she has not ceased to kiss my feet." Bailey, *Jesus*, 244.

40   Johnson, *Luke*, 127, notes that *myron* is an oil with a pungent scent; but there is in this story no connection with the burial of Jesus nor any suggestion that the oil is particularly expensive.

41   Bailey, *Jesus*, 246.

42   Marshall, *Luke*, 308. Bailey, *Jesus Through Middle Eastern Eyes*, 247, suggests that her tears are not because of her sins, but because of his humiliation. "She is in anguish because, before her eyes, this beautiful person who set her free with his message of the love of God for sinners, is being publicly humiliated." Fitzmyer, *Luke*, 1:689, notes that traditionally the tears have been understood as tears of repentance; but she could have been weeping for joy at the realisation of the forgiveness she has already experienced.

43   Women were obliged to cover their hair in public. For a married woman failure to do so merited divorce. McBride, *Luke*, 103, notes that this was usually taken as a public signal that the woman was willing to negotiate a certain transaction. Reid, *Parables*, 97, suggests that a woman did not bind up her hair until married. Had she been a prostitute, she would have had carefully groomed and elaborately styled hair.

44   Bailey, *Jesus Through Middle Eastern Eyes*, 247. Tannehill, *Luke*, 135, says she publicly behaves with improper intimacy.

45   Caird, *Luke*, 114.

46   Johnson, *Luke*, 127, notes that it is "axiomatic" that a prophet can see the heart; Jesus knows her heart and also Simon's. Fitzmyer, *Luke*, 1:689; also, Evans, *Luke*, 362: Jesus shows prophetic discernment in knowing the Pharisee's inner thoughts. See 5:22; 6:8; 9:47; 11:17; 20:23.

47   Caird, *Luke*, 114. Mosetto, *Luca*, 165, suggests that Jesus' openness is itself profoundly prophetic.

48   Bailey, *Jesus Through Middle Eastern Eyes*, 251, points out that this is a classical Middle Eastern idiom that introduces blunt speech which the listener may not want to hear. Carroll, *Luke*, 178, notes that, addressed as a teacher, Jesus will respond as one:

with the woman's actions as an object lesson, he will seek to draw his host into a deeper understanding of God's mercy towards human beings, and what it means for life in community.

49   Pagola, *Jesus,* 151, notes that the creditor in the parable knows the suffering of those who cannot pay what they owe. 500 *denarii* is a large debt, the equivalent of a farm worker's wages for two years.

50   Bailey, *Jesus Through Middle Eastern Eyes,* 254. Reid, *Parables,* 94, maintains that the parable has one point: that one who has been forgiven much loves greatly the one who remitted the debt.

51   Marshall, *Luke,* 311.

52   Reid, *Parables,* 93, maintains that the story hinges on this question of Jesus. What Simon sees in the woman and her interaction with Jesus determines how Simon sees Jesus: she is a sinner, and Jesus is not a prophet. If Simon can see her as a forgiven woman who shows great love, he may perceive Jesus aright: not only as a prophet, but also as the agent of God's forgiveness.

53   Fitzmyer, *Luke,* 1:691, states that the application of the parable is not so much to contrast their deeds, as to stress the love manifested in them. Carroll, *Luke,* 178, Jesus defends the woman's honour and shames Simon with a stinging rebuke.

54   Carroll, *Luke,* 178–179, notes that each clause describing what Simon failed to give begins with the thing withheld. Each clause describing the woman's acts begins "But she."

55   Bailey, *Jesus Through Middle Eastern Eyes,* 257.

56   Carroll, *Luke,* 179: Simon has failed to act as a hospitable host; the unwelcome guest has provided the hospitality that Jesus should have received from him. The story gives the most dramatic enactment so far of the inside out reversal that attends Jesus' ministry.

57   Johnson, *Luke,* 128, notes the use of the perfect passive, indicating what has been done for her. Her expression of love "is not the basis for forgiveness, but the demonstration of it." Also, Byrne, *Hospitality,* 75; Fitzmyer, *Luke,* 1:692; Marshall, *Luke,* 304, 314. Reid, *Parables,* 95, notes that the perfect passive connotes a past action whose effects endure into the present. The "was" of v. 37, meaning "used to be", indicates that her sins had been forgiven before she came to Simon's home.

58   Byrne, *Hospitality,* 75; Caird, *Luke,* 114–5, Marshall, *Luke,* 313, take this view also. Similarly, Pagola, *Jesus,* 152, who states that Simon sees in her the suggestive gestures of her profession; Jesus sees the tangible sign of God's forgiveness. Carroll, *Luke,* 180, notes that the perfect tense intimates that mercy has preceded her demonstration of love. A previous encounter with Jesus evidently resulted in the offer and grateful acceptance of forgiveness. He translates: "I am able to tell you this—that her sins have been forgiven because, as we can all plainly see, she has, (like the forgiven debtor) loved much." Reid, *Parables,* 95, n. 14; in the parable love follows forgiveness.

59   As with the paralysed man in Luke's version, 5:20.

60   Johnson, *Luke,* 128; see 8:12, 48; 17:19; 18:41; Acts 15:11.

61   It picks up the Baptist's issue in 7:20, anticipates Herod's question in 9:9, and recalls 5:21.

62   Marshall, *Luke*, 304. Carroll, *Luke*, 180, states that behind the passive voice "have been forgiven" is the action of the merciful God. Forgiveness mediated by Jesus has its source in God.

63   Tannehill, *Luke*, 136–137. Reid, *Parables*, 96, n. 15, notes how most commentators and translators entitle the episode "The Woman who was a Sinner" (with slight variations), rather than "The Woman who showed great love."

64   Johnson, *Luke*, 129.

65   Byrne, *Hospitality*, 76; McBride, *Luke*, 101, also stresses the contrasts.

66   Bailey, *Jesus Through Middle Eastern Eyes*, 258. Fallon, *Luke*, 153, comments that Simon is exposed as the real sinner, too self-opinionated to realise it. But he has been offered the insight that would enable him to change.

67   The section in Mark's Gospel that follows these "mighty works" of Jesus (6:44–8:27) has been excised by Luke; scholars call it "the great omission".

68   Byrne, *Hospitality*, 84, speaks of "apprenticing the Twelve for leadership and service in the renewed People of God."

69   The feeding miracle will partly provide a response to his question. See Francis J. Moloney, *A Body Broken for a Broken People* (Mulgrave: Garratt, 2015), 132.

70   Byrne, *Hospitality*, 84, observes that whereas Mark has Jesus take the disciples to a deserted place, Luke prefers a city. Green, *Luke*, 363, refers to the rural environs of Bethsaida; the people should therefore be close to the possibility of food and lodging.

71   Mark 6:34; Matt 14:13. Carroll, *Luke*, 207, notes that Luke also omits reference to the shepherdless sheep, because Jesus is their shepherd.

72   Carroll, *Luke*, 208.

73   Carroll, *Luke*, 206.

74   Green, *Luke*, 363, recalls the big catch of fish when Peter became a disciple; there are echoes of Elijah and of the desert manna. On their earlier mission, they were told to take no bread and no money; yet they have a few loaves and think of buying food!

75   Carroll, *Luke*, 208. He also highlights the difference between the disciples and the generous women who have provided for the group from their own resources (8:2–3).

76   Green, *Luke*, 365.

77   McBride, *Luke*, 119, points out that the language is heavy with the symbolism of the Eucharist. Johnson, *Luke*, 147, notes that the sequence of verbs anticipates the eucharistic gestures at the Last Supper. Green, *Luke*, 364, denies any eucharistic significance for Luke; these are commonplace gestures at any Jewish meal. Carroll, *Luke*, 208, accepts the ritual of the meal and sacredness of the occasion, but makes no reference to Eucharist.

78   Johnson, *Luke*, 147.

79   6:21; 1:53.

80   Byrne, *Hospitality*, 85; Carroll, *Luke*, 208; McBride, *Luke*, 119; Moloney, *Body Broken*, 133. In Luke, the multiplication is followed by Jesus' questioning The Twelve about his identity, his passion prediction, and the transfiguration (all of which provide the answer to Herod's earlier question). The whole section has to do with the instruction and formation of the apostles. Johnson, *Luke*, 144, entitles the section "Preparing a Leadership for the People", and, p. 147, points out that the leadership of Israel are

rejecting Jesus, so now Jesus begins to prepare a new leadership for the restored Israel; Luke fixes our attention on the relationship between Jesus and The Twelve. Carroll, *Luke*, 208, refers to the education of the disciples for their role as leaders of the community.

81   Green, *Luke*, 540.

82   Carroll, *Luke*, 296; Green, *Luke*, 545. Carroll comments that these meals among the social elite regularly featured excessive eating and drinking, use of hospitality to increase one's social prestige, and animated conversation. Johnson, *Luke*, 226, believes that the invitation to the meal was hypocritical. Marshall, *Luke*, 578, suggests the Pharisee may have been a member of the Sanhedrin.

83   Reid, *Parables*, 160, notes the escalating opposition between the Pharisees and Jesus as the Gospel story develops. However, they are absent from the passion narrative. In Acts their antagonism ceases and some become believers. There were many different Jewish sects in Jesus' day, and differences between Pharisee groups. Nor were they the prevailing force at the time of Jesus; that became the case after the destruction of Jerusalem. This is the fourth Sabbath controversy (6:1–5, 6–11; 13:10–17). This story is unique to Luke. Green, 547, *Luke*, notes that when appearing in the company of the legal experts, the Pharisees have been consistently portrayed as adversaries of Jesus and the plan of God.

84   Green, *Luke*, 545.

85   Caird, *Luke*, 175. Marshall, *Luke*, 578, suggests the possibility that the man's presence was arranged. Also, McBride, *Luke*, 188; or perhaps the man was aware that Jesus was going to attend the party and just turned up, seeking a cure.

86   Green, *Luke*, 544.

87   This story has many points of contact with the current episode; for details see Green, *Luke*, 543.

88   Green, *Luke*, 547, maintains that Jesus is not seeking to subvert the Law, but to query conventional wisdom regarding its interpretation.

89   Carroll, *Luke*, 297, notes the link made by Cynic and Stoic authors between dropsy (with its symptom of a desperate need for water) and greed or avarice. This Jesus picks up explicitly later (16:14, 19–31), but acquisitive striving—seeking status and honour and the leveraging of reciprocity to gain social advantage—receive immediate critique in the rest of this episode. Tannehill, *Luke*, 228, makes the same link; dropsy was a metaphor for insatiable desire.

90   McBride, *Luke*, 189.

91   Green, *Luke*, 548.

92   Caird, *Luke*, 175, suggests that many sayings of Jesus came to Luke without any indication of the original context, and he provides a narrative setting for three discourses on feasting. Green, *Luke*, 549, notes the similar structure of the two sections 7–11 and 12–14.

93   Reid, *Parables*, 161; Tannehill, *Luke*, 229. Green, *Luke*, 550, notes that where one sat (was assigned or allowed to sit) at a meal *vis-à-vis* the host was a public advertisement of one's status; the matter of seating arrangements was carefully attended.

94   In Matt 23:6, Jesus criticises the lawyers and Pharisees for seeking the first places at banquets.

95   Caird, *Luke*, 175.

96   See the *Magnificat* (1:46–55), 6:20–26; 9:46–48; 10:15; 22:24–30. This passage (14:12–14) is found only in Luke.

97   Green, *Luke*, 550, comments that because meals were used to publicise and reinforce social hierarchy, invitations to meals were carefully considered so as to allow to one's table only one's inner circle or only those persons whose presence at one's table would either enhance or at least preserve one's social position.

98   Green, *Luke*, 552, notes that invitations served as currency in the marketplace of prestige and power; reciprocity was expected.

99   Green, *Luke*, 553, observes that here the Pharisees are portrayed as persons who exploit hospitality for a self-serving agenda; their patterns of hospitality secure their positions of dominance in their communities and insulate them from the needy.

100   Green, *Luke*, 550, notes that the ethics of reciprocity, the gift and obligation system; gifts were never "free".

101   Carroll, *Luke*, 300, refers to the careful structure, pointing out that the first list is more ornate, the second staccato-like; Evans also, *Luke*, 571.

102   Green, *Luke*, 550, comments that privileged people would not invite the poor to their meals because this would possibly endanger social status, be a wasted invitation because it could not be reciprocated and embarrass the poor because they would be obliged to decline, being unable to reciprocate. On p. 553, he states that this would be the death knell for the ethics of patronage.

103   Green, *Luke*, 542, indicates that Jesus has a distinctive view of the world, shaped by his experience of the Spirit, his understanding of the merciful God, and his awareness of the presence of the Kingdom in his ministry.

104   Marshall, *Luke*, 583; the Semitic idiom is "not so much X … as rather Y."

105   Resseguie, *Spiritual Landscape*, 78, concludes that a spiritual life characterised by selfless generosity replaces self-seeking ambition for present rewards.

106   The Pharisees believed in resurrection. Carroll, *Luke*, 301, thinks that here Jesus is speaking of a resurrection only for the just. In 16:19–31, there is the threat of punishment for the rich who are not generous to the poor. Similarly, Green, *Luke*, 554: the "righteous" are those whose worldview is transformed along the lines Jesus promulgates. In Acts 24:15, the resurrection is for all.

107   Caird, *Luke*, 177; Carroll, *Luke*, 302; Johnson, *Luke*, 228; Green, *Luke*, 558; who also notes that their presumption was based on being children of Abraham and their noble status. Bailey, *Through Peasant Eyes*, 89–93, discusses at length the idea of the final banquet, the symbol for salvation (Ps 23:5; Isa 25:6–9, "for all the peoples"). In the intertestamental period, the banquet was linked with the coming of the messiah, but Gentiles and imperfect Jews would be excluded. Bailey, *Through Peasant Eyes*, 93, divides the parable into an introduction and seven stanzas.

108   McBride, *Luke*, 194; Marshall, *Luke*, 588, for whom the meal stands for salvation as a present experience and future consummation. Matthew has a version of this parable after Jesus has reached Jerusalem (22:1–14); there the meal is a wedding feast for the king's son.

109   Green, *Luke*, 555, notes the cultural use of invitations to promote one's status

in the community; meals signal demarcation lines.

110   This procedure of a double invitation was common custom. It was helpful for potential guests to assess the social propriety of the situation, and for the host to determine the amount of food (especially meat) required. (Marshall, *Luke*, 588; Bailey, *Through Peasant Eyes*, 94; Green, *Luke*, 558; McBride, *Parables*, 60). Evans, *Luke*, 573, suggests the idea that the first invitation was already present in God's election of Israel, now further implemented by Jesus' message: "Come ... ."

111   Reid, *Parables*, 313, n. 14, suggests 100 acres of land; similarly, Green, *Luke*, 560, adding that peasant families might have three to six acres per adult.

112   Bailey, "Through Peasant Eyes", 96–98, provides cultural details. The land excuse is "paper thin", the ploughman's "a transparent fabrication".

113   Bailey, "Through Peasant Eyes", 99. Reid, *Parables*, 314, suggests that perhaps the bridegroom had accumulated too many social obligations.

114   Carroll, *Luke*, 303; Bailey, "Through Peasant Eyes", 95. Tannehill, *Luke*, 234, speaks of "a co-ordinated act of ostracism"; Green, *Luke*, 559, refers to closing ranks, shaming him publically, a social strategy the effect of which is the host's defamation. Donahue, *Gospel*, 141, refers to 1 Macc 3:56, where the exemptions from joining up for war are for building houses, betrothal and planting vineyards. But in Luke there is no war scenario. Johnson, *Luke*, 231, refers to Deut 20:5–7, adding that there can be no exemptions when it is a question of the Kingdom.

115   Green, *Luke*, 561, comments that his anger does not lead to reprisal but to a dramatic switch from the system of reciprocity and status preservation; he acts in a way that despises the social order in which he had previously demonstrated his deftness.

116   Reid, *Parables*, 314, calls it "social suicide". In the view of the Qumran community, people such as these would be excluded from the messianic banquet. Bailey, "Through Peasant Eyes", 100, sees this as an "unexpected, visible demonstration of love in humiliation"; it is "costly grace", for the original invitees will be angry and taunt the host. Green, *Luke*, 562, refers to the host as stepping outside the patronal ethics of the Mediterranean world; he creates a new social order in which normal boundaries are inconsequential, and initiates a new community grounded in gracious and uncalculating hospitality.

117   Reid, *Parables*, 315, lists tanners, traders, beggars, prostitutes as the inhabitants of these areas; they were extremely vulnerable. Green, *Luke*, 562, sees these as the utterly destitute and impure not allowed to live within the city walls. Bailey, "Through Peasant Eyes", 101, does not see these as outcasts, but as people outside the host's community.

118   Bailey, "Through Peasant Eyes", 108, notes that in the Middle East an unexpected invitation must be refused, especially if the guest is of lower rank than the host. "Grace is unbelievable". Also, Marshall, *Luke*, 590.

119   Carroll, *Luke*, 305. Luke omits the violent treatment of the servants and the punishment of the guests who refuse, and the burning of their city, as in Matt 22:5–6.

120   Green, *Luke*, 562, believes that this is the more natural option; the second person plural is addressed to a servant; but the plural can be a narrative device whereby the master speaks to those outside his own story.

121   Green, *Luke*, 563.

122 Bailey, "Through Peasant Eyes", 109, argues for this option. Green, *Luke*, 555.

123 Tannehill, *Luke*, 234; Reid, *Parables*, 317.

124 Reid, *Parables*, 317.

125 For example, Caird, *Luke*, 177.

126 Caird, *Luke*, 177; Bailey, "Through Peasant Eyes", 101, 110; he discusses this issue from 101–109. He notes (101) that the third command to the servant is given but not carried out; it remains an unfulfilled future task as the parable closes. Jesus did reach out to outcasts but did not formally conduct a gentile mission. That came later. Carroll, *Luke*, 306, notes that it is a mistaken interpretation that the gentiles supplant the Jews.

127 Marshall, *Luke*, 587.

128 The word translated "betray" (*paradidōmi*) means to "hand over"; the verb is later used of Pilate and the religious authorities (23:25; 24:20).

129 Moloney, *Body Broken*, 135, notes that scholars believe that Luke is probably not following Mark, but "is working creatively with other sources." As well as the meal theme, there is the literary element of a farewell speech. On p. 141, he maintains that the passage is not primarily concerned with the words of institution; it is about his last testimony to the disciples within the context of the meal. The centre of gravity is the four dialogues. He recalls the main features of the traditional farewell discourse: prediction of death (22:15, 22); prediction of attacks on the dying leader's disciples (22:31–34); an exhortation to ideal behaviour (22:24, 25–26); a final commission (22:31–32). This discourse element establishes the disciples as his legitimate successors. See also Neyrey, *Passion*, 6–8; he deals with the whole supper under that rubric. Karris, *Luke*, 65, agrees that the centre of the supper is the discourse, not the words of institution; also, Matera, *Passion Narratives*, 160–61. Carroll, *Luke*, 428, refers to a "poignant farewell discourse", and 431, "an extended farewell speech"; Tannehill, *Luke*, 316–17; Johnson, *Luke*, 348. Green, *Luke*, 75, heads the section "Teaching at the Passover Table"; the literary form is a farewell address set within a Passover meal along the lines of a Greco-Roman symposium. Luke is the only Synoptist to do so; John has five chapters of discourse and little interest in the meal. In Acts 20:17–38, Paul delivers a similar farewell speech.

130 While "hour" could simply be factual, the term is probably intended to refer to the appointed hour of Jesus' destiny. For a description of a Passover meal, see Evans, *Luke*, 783.

131 Moloney, *Body Broken*, 139, suggests the following alternating structure: a) 14–18: the sharing of the first cup and the promise of fulfilment of the Kingdom; b) 19–23: the account of the meal and the prediction of betrayal by Judas; a) the part which the disciples will play in the Kingdom; b) 31–34: the prayer of Jesus for Peter, but the prophecy of denial; a) 35–38: the difficulties that will confront the disciples in their future mission.

132 Carroll, *Luke*, 431, notes that The Twelve are here not as individuals but in their representative role as commissioned leaders of the community that Jesus is gathering, the nucleus of an Israel undergoing restoration. Evans, *Luke*, 783, comments that Jesus is with the future leaders of the Church. Green, *Luke*, 757, notes that Luke does not usually employ the term "apostles"; here it refers to their representative function. Johnson, *Luke*, 336–37, observes three small but significant changes from Mark: the more solemn "hour",

"apostles" rather than "the twelve", and the disciples recline "with him", emphasising the central role of Jesus as host. Tannehill, *Luke*, 312, raises the question as to whether others were present; Luke is focusing on The Twelve.

133   Carroll, *Luke*, 432, asserts that for Luke this meal *is* a Passover meal; Fitzmyer, *Luke*, 2:1378–82. "With desire I have desired" (see Gen 31:30; Num 11:4; Ps 105:13; Acts 5:28; 23:14) accents the deep emotion.

134   Passover was always celebrated in thanksgiving for the past and with hope for final deliverance by God. Tannehill, *Luke*, 312–13, discusses the minority view, which he seems to favour, that Jesus did not partake of this meal. This could be an expression of determination to fulfil his destiny; it could also be a prayer for the coming of the Kingdom. Evans, *Luke*, 784, discounts this view. Johnson, *Luke*, 337, sees fulfilment as referring either to the eschatological banquet or the eucharistic celebrations of the Christian community. Green, *Luke*, 759, maintains that the eagerness with which Jesus wishes to share this meal indicates that Jesus does partake. On p. 760 he acknowledges the importance of the post-resurrection meals with Jesus and the community meals in Acts; but these are not the final consummation; it remains a future reality. Marshall, *Luke*, 796–97, maintains that Jesus does share the meal with his disciples. He believes that Luke sees a hint of the fellowship between Jesus and his disciples at the Lord's Supper.

135   Green, *Luke*, 759. Neyrey, *Passion*, 13, sees these words as a prediction of death and also of future vindication and triumph; reference to Kingdom has an imminent aspect (resurrection) and an eschatological one (parousia). Matera, *Passion Narratives*, 162, maintains that the prophecy of death already carries a note of victory.

136   Tannehill, *Luke*,314, notes that to share this cup was unusual; he detects a eucharistic aspect here, even if the words of interpretation are reserved for the second cup. Johnson, *Luke*,337, notes that there were four cups of wine at the Passover meal, each with its own blessing. Green, *Luke*,761, states that this may be the first cup taken at the beginning of the meal, but thinks it is the second because of Jesus' interpretive words, which move the focus away from exodus to his own death and the coming of God's reign. Such a sharing of the cup is unconventional, but would underscore the solidarity of those gathered. For Marshall, *Luke*,799, the act of drinking together unites the participants into a table fellowship with one another.

137   Byrne, *Hospitality*, 172–173.

138   There is a difficult textual problem here. The widest extant attestation is accepted by the majority of modern scholars (like Byrne *Hospitality*, 172, n. 2; Tannehill, *Luke*, 314; Green, *Luke*, 761). Some important manuscripts omit the phrases "which is given for you. Do this in remembrance of me." Carroll, *Luke*, 432–33, argues for the shorter version because it coheres thematically with the rest of Luke's narrative; Luke does not envisage Jesus' death as a vicarious, atoning sacrifice. He suggests that early in the second century, under the influence of widely dispersed liturgical traditions (particularly 1 Cor 11:23–25), Luke 22:19b–20 was inserted to fill out the seemingly incomplete words of institution of the Lord's Supper. Marshall, *Luke*, 799–801, rehearses the arguments for and against the longer text, as does Evans, *Luke*, 786–88, the latter opting for the shorter version. Mark (14:22) reads "he took a loaf of bread, and after blessing it he broke it, gave it to them, and said, 'Take; this is my body.'" Luke omits "take" and adds "which is

given for you", and "do this in remembrance of me."

139   The gestures of Jesus recall the multiplication scene (9:16). Luke's form of words is close to Mark 14:22 and Matt 26:66, except that he uses *eucharisteō;* it is closer still to Paul (1 Cor 11:23–25). Green, *Luke*, 761, maintains that the breaking of the bread is not metaphorical (indicating a broken body); it has no symbolic significance; it is the giving which suggests giving one's life for others. Jesus is interpreting his death through his words, not his actions. Marshall, *Luke*, 803, sees both sacrificial and martyrological motifs here.

140   Johnson, *Luke*, 344.

141   Green, *Luke*, 762.

142   Mark (14:24) reads: "This is my blood of the covenant, which is poured out for many." Marshall, *Luke*, 805–806, sees this as a covenant inaugurating sacrifice. In Luke, it is the cup (with its contents) that is the symbol of the new covenant brought about by the blood of Jesus shed for the disciples.

143   Green, *Luke*, 763, emphasises that this is not a covenant discontinuous with that of old; there is continuity between God's ancient purpose and its fulfilment in the coming of Jesus.

144   Carroll, *Luke*, 436; Johnson, *Luke*, 339; Tannehill, *Luke*,315. He points out that grammatically it is the cup that is poured out, rather than the blood, and maintains that the sacrifice may be a covenant-founding sacrifice (Exod 24:6–8) rather than an atoning sacrifice. Green, *Luke*, 763–34, believes that in the light of Exod 24:8, Jesus' death atones for the sins of the people, and thus enables them to participate in the renewed eschatological covenant with God. This idea is missing in Acts (except for 20:28); elsewhere Luke emphasis the saving role of Jesus' exaltation.

145   McBride, *Luke*, 286. Johnson, *Luke*, 342, says "it is by the giving of his life in sacrifice—donation to God for the sake of others—that a regeneration of the people can take place." For Neyrey, *Passion*, 17, the Eucharist is a Passover, a covenant sacrifice, an atonement sacrifice. But Luke's emphasis is on the meal, not the sacrifice.

146   Moloney, *Body Broken*, 141. This element of the discourse establishes the disciples as his legitimate successors. See also Neyrey, *Passion*, 6–8.

147   Carroll, *Luke*, 437, notes that the "hand" receives bread and cup but is also a metonym for the enemy's power, that, allied with the power of darkness (22:53) is strong enough to effect Jesus' death. The term has been used in reference to Jesus' opponents (9:44; 20:19; 21:12; 24:7). In Mark, reference to the betrayer comes earlier in the meal. Neyrey, *Passion*, 18, notes that prophecies about the future are characteristic of farewell speeches; from now on the focus of Jesus' speech falls on his followers.

148   Luke uses *dei* ("must") in 9:22; 17:25; 24:26. He refers to scriptural fulfilment in 18:31; 22:37; 24:27, 46; both aspects come together in 24:44. The last reference to the Son of Man states: "they will see the Son of Man coming in a cloud with power and great glory" (21:27), words which intimate vindication to follow suffering.

149   See after the second passion prediction: "Jesus, aware of their inner thoughts, took a little child and put it by his side, and said to them, 'Whoever welcomes this child in my name welcomes me, and whoever welcomes me the one who sent me; for the least among all of you is the greatest'" (9:46–48). He has also criticised the religious leaders

324

for status seeking (14:7; 20:46), and warned his followers about imitating them (12:1).

150   McBride, *Luke*, 288, observes that "Benefactor" was an honorific title used by the kings of Egypt and Syria. Powell, *The Gospels*, 103, notes that in the Roman world emperors and other public figures were sometimes referred to as Benefactors; their existence was thought to be a blessing to society. Tannehill, *Luke*, 317, refers to the prevalent patron-client system.

151   For a good description of this situation see Green, *Luke*, 768. The issue is not abuse, but the system itself.

152   Green, *Luke*, 769.

153   Tannehill, *Luke*, 319; Byrne, *Hospitality*, 174. It is not a question of judging. Johnson, *Luke*, 345, notes that this recalls Exod 24:11, and anticipates the post-resurrection meals. Green, *Luke*, 770, points out that the transfer of leadership is a typical function of farewell discourses; Neyrey, *Passion*, 25, refers to leadership succession. On p. 27–28 he locates these meals after the resurrection (24:30–35, 41–43; Acts 1:3–4; 10:41–42) and notes their exercise of leadership and governance in Acts (2–3; 4–5; 8:20–23; 11:2–18; 15:7–14). Matera, *Passion Narratives*, 165, recalls 12:32: "Fear not, little flock, for it is your Father's good pleasure to give you the kingdom."

154   Green, *Luke*, 771, notes that this exchange is an element in the typical farewell discourse format.

155   Green, *Luke*, 772, suggests that the doubling of Peter's name may suggest that his vocation as apostle is at stake, that his faithfulness may be endangered. Evans, *Luke*, 802, refers to "intensification of feeling". The image is that of sifting wheat from chaff; this was Satan's role in Job 1–2. Evans, *Luke*, 802, suggests that the emphasis may be on "shaking"; Neyrey, *Passion*, 33, on being separated and scattered.

156   Johnson, *Luke*, 346, points out that Jesus implicitly predicts Peter's rehabilitation; his strengthening role is seen in Acts 1:15–26. Green, *Luke*, 773, n. 112, points out that this is one of the rare occasions when the content of Jesus' prayer is provided. Neyrey, *Passion*, 31, 34, interprets Peter's strengthening role as a commission to be the shepherd leader. The "turning" takes place in 22:32, evidenced by his weeping, the strengthening begins with 24:34, after he sees the risen Lord.

157   Green, *Luke*, 774.

158   For Luke, Peter's denial of Jesus is not viewed as a failure of faith, but as an act of cowardice.

159   Carroll, *Luke*, 442.

160   Marshall, *Luke*, 823, suggests that the saying is "grimly ironical", expressing the intensity of the opposition that Jesus and the disciples will experience, endangering their very lives. On p. 825 he suggests that the saying may refer to an attitude of mind rather than outward equipment. Matera, *Passion Narratives*, 166, concludes that a time of persecution is about to begin.

161   Green, *Luke*, 776. Jesus' enemies reckon that his activities lie outside the boundaries of Torah. Karris, *Luke*, 70, suggests that his own disciples are the transgressors because they jockey for position; Neyrey, *Passion*, 44, because they misunderstand and are in possession of swords.

162   Commentators struggle to explain these words. Byrne, *Hospitality*, 174,

understands Jesus' expression as exasperation, because the apostles take his words literally; also, Johnson, *Luke*, 347. Tannehill, *Luke*, 323, suggests an expression of disgust, or that two swords are sufficient to fulfil the prophecy; possibly the apostles are to be considered "lawless" because of their fear and attempted violence. Carroll, *Luke*, 443. Karris, *Luke*, 69, notes that to understand swords literally is to misunderstand the peaceful Jesus.

163   Manson, *Sayings*, 341.

164   We have considered Jesus' prayer in Gethsemane earlier, and will explore aspect of the Calvary scene in the next chapter.

165   Having excused the disciples' sleepfulness in the garden as induced by grief, Luke omits Mark's reference to their deserting Jesus and taking flight to a man. Whereas in Mark none of the male disciples are present on Calvary, Luke includes "all his acquaintances including the women ... ." Thus, his presentation of the disciples is much less negative than Mark's.

166   Moloney, *Body Broken*, 137.

167   Karris, *Luke*, 70, maintains that Jesus was crucified because of the way he ate. Through his meals with the poor, he criticised the way of life of the religious elite; he proclaimed a different God; he was leading the people astray.

168   For an excellent discussion of this, see Moloney, *Body Broken*, 205–237.

Chapter Thirteen
Calvary

Since that Passover-season Friday on Jerusalem's Calvary, the cross has been the defining sign or symbol of Christianity. Despite attempts to have it removed from public places, it remains the icon of the world's transformation.[1] The early Christians were obliged to seek to explain how an instrument of torture, humiliation and disgrace was, in fact, an indication of liberation and new life, a revelation of God's love. This was a daunting task, given that Jesus was condemned by imperial Rome and rejected by the religious leadership of his people. Perhaps for us today, accustomed to seeing a cross in our churches, schools, in most rooms in our houses, on a chain around our neck, it's worth pondering its significance afresh. This is a huge task, so in this chapter I propose that we reflect on the death of Jesus as Luke presents it.

There are, as you well know, four Gospel passion narratives. The versions of Mark and Matthew are very similar. John has the same basic events but treats them in his own unique way, with much symbolism and theological development. Luke has much in common with Mark, but there are a number of differences, to which we will refer as the story unfolds.[2] We are all familiar with the story of the passion and death of Jesus, but in my experience most people have their own version of events, which is like a cocktail, a mixture and harmonisation of items selected from the different evangelists, usually without realising that this is the case. This *mélange* approach probably entails that we are not sensitive to the theology of each evangelist, his particular themes, emphases and message. This is an impoverishment, I feel.

I intend to omit the arrest of Jesus, Peter's denials and the trials before the Sanhedrin, Herod and Pilate, and to concentrate on the Calvary scene.[3] It is good to remember that, although there are solid factual details and a chronicle-like sequence, Luke is more interested in bringing out the theological significance of the events he is describing. It is also important to view the passion in the context of the whole Gospel. The main themes that we have encountered as the Gospel story unfolds reach their climax and conclusion here, in Jerusalem, the place of Jesus' "exodus".

The Crucifixion (23:33–34)

> When they came to the place that is called The Skull, they crucified Jesus there with the criminals, one on his right and one on his left.

Jesus, the rejected prophet, has reached the place of execution. Luke follows the tradition in naming it "The Skull" (*Calvaria*), a name derived from the shape of the hill and the presence of some caves there, or because it was a place of executions where skulls could be found near the surface.[4] The Aramaic term is omitted, since it would have meant little for his readers (Mark 15:22). No details are given of the actual crucifixion; only three words are used in the Greek; the horrible process was well known to Luke's readership.[5] The Romans preferred executions to be located in public places; this would serve as a deterrent. The crucifixion of two others with him is also a factor of the basic tradition. Luke describes them with a different term than Mark, preferring the generic "malefactor" to "revolutionary bandit".[6] Luke omits mention of the offering of a drink of wine and myrrh. Earlier, on the way to Gethsemane, Jesus had quoted scripture: "he was counted among the lawless" (22:37, quoting Isa 53:12).[7]

> Then Jesus said: "Father, forgive them; for they do not know what they are doing."[8]

Only Luke includes these words of Jesus.[9] Earlier in the ministry, during the Sermon on the Plain, Jesus has spoken about loving one's enemies and praying for those who abuse us (6:27–36), urging his hearers to be merciful like the Father (6:36; 15:11–32). And one of the items in the prayer that he taught his disciples, "the Lord's Prayer" as we call it, is "forgive us our sins, for we ourselves forgive everyone indebted to us" (11:4). In Isaiah 53:12, the Servant intercedes for transgressors. So Jesus, in extreme circumstances, is practising what he has preached.[10] In his ministry he has sought to restore and reconcile sinful people (5:20, 24, 32; 7:34, 47–50; 11:4; 15:1–32; 17:3–4), so there is consistency. In the midst of his suffering, Jesus has not lost sight of the Father.

Some think that Jesus is praying here primarily for the Romans, his executioners. Others include the Jews who are responsible for his death.[11] If so, the prayer would suggest that the Jews acted out of ignorance. This runs contrary to the general view of the New Testament, with its indications of deliberate blindness and malevolence, and is a more humane understanding of the complex responsibilities for Jesus' death.

> And they cast lots to divide his clothing.

The executioners divide his clothes among them, as was the custom, casting lots for them, not using dice but guessing the number of outstretched fingers behind one's back. There may be an allusion to Psalm 22:18, but this is not explicit as in John, nor is the symbolism developed.[12] Herod, as part of his mockery of Jesus, dressed him in "an elegant robe", probably a white mantle, before sending him back to Pilate; this is probably not intended here.[13] Jesus is stripped naked, a great humiliation and indignity; he is deprived of his identity; he is a nobody.[14]

The Mockery (23:35–43)

The next main scene is devoted to the mocking of Jesus as he hangs in pain on the cross; it unfolds in three phases.

> And the people stood by, watching; but the leaders scoffed at him, saying, "He saved others; let him save himself if he is the Messiah of God, his chosen one!" The soldiers also mocked him, coming up and offering him sour wine, and saying, "If you are the King of the Jews, save yourself!" There was also an inscription over him, 'This is the King of the Jews.'
>
> One of the criminals who were hanged there kept deriding him and saying, "Are you not the Messiah? Save yourself and us!" But the other rebuked him, saying, "Do you not fear God, since you are under the same sentence of condemnation? And we indeed have been condemned justly, for we are getting what we deserve for our deeds, but this man has done nothing wrong." Then he said, "Jesus, remember me when you come into your kingdom." He replied, "Truly I tell you, today you will be with me in Paradise."

In Luke's version of the Calvary scene, those who are responsible for the mockery of Jesus are the Jewish leaders, the Roman soldiers and one of those crucified with him. The mockery focuses on Jesus' messianic claims and his ability to save.[15] Any mocking by the bystanders, the ordinary people passing by, as in Mark (15:29), is omitted. They simply stand by and "watch"; they are present throughout. This, located at the beginning of the mockery section, along with the 'good thief' at the end, provides a more sympathetic framework. Luke has already mentioned a large number of people following Jesus on the way to Calvary, possibly suggesting that their attitude is not one of curiosity or negativity. "For Luke, ... observing Jesus on the cross could harden the hostility of some and soften the hearts of others."[16]

The mockery by the leaders (*archontes*, probably including the chief priests: 23:13; 24:20) is probably intended as another example of Israel's formal rejection of the Messiah (as 23:13, 18–25), the innocently suffering righteous one.[17] Scoffing repeatedly,[18] they invite Jesus to save himself, as he had in the past saved others, if he really is the "Messiah of God, the Chosen One". The conditional, "if", is a slight alteration of Mark and accurately conveys their lack of faith.[19] Their words pick up the affirmation of Jesus earlier in the trial (22:67–71; 23:2; see also 9:20; 9:35). Psalm 22:7–8 reads: "All who see me mock at me; they make mouths at me, they shake their heads; 'Commit your cause to the Lord; let him deliver—let him rescue the one in whom he delights'."[20] The irony is that Jesus in fact is Messiah and Chosen One, but he becomes the Saviour and Christ not by saving himself (and showing the power these titles imply), but by committing himself into God's hands and by then being vindicated in the resurrection.

Next it is the turn of the Roman soldiers, hitherto referred to as "they" (23:26, 33, 34). Luke has omitted mention of the soldiers ill-treating Jesus after the sentencing. Again, the conditional is used, as they mockingly shout: "If you are the King of the Jews, save yourself." This was the term used by Pilate in the trial (23:3). As they mock him verbally, they offer him vinegary wine (an echo of Ps 69:21), which shows how they evaluate him.[21] In Mark's Gospel, this takes place later just before Jesus dies. John, too, records it at that point in his narrative, but it is an act of kindness.

Their mockery of Jesus as "King of the Jews" is more appropriate on gentile lips than "King of Israel", which is part of the Jewish mockery in Mark. This seems to be linked with the inscription fixed to the cross over Jesus' head, which reads "This is the King of the Jews". This item of information, the normal procedure with both an informative and a deterrent aspect, mentioned now rather than earlier, is common to all of the evangelists. This was part of the agenda in his trial before Pilate, but both Pilate and Herod were aware that Jesus was not making a claim that would threaten the emperor's sovereignty. The "this" is derisive, but, ironically, the placard is true.[22]

The mockery continues. In Mark, both of the men crucified with Jesus join in. In Luke, only one gets involved in this way. This victim picks up the theme of the previous mockery, the messiahship of Jesus, which he clearly does not accept. He suggests that Jesus should save not only himself but the two of them as well! If this man were a zealot, he would have only scorn for Jesus, who was not interested in armed resistance or nationalist/political messiahship.

The verb used for his abuse of Jesus is "blasphemed", which reflects a later Christian view. This man receives no answer from Jesus.

The other criminal is of a different mind and rebukes the first. He urges his companion to fear God's coming judgement and admits that he and his companion are justly suffering punishment because they are guilty. Jesus, however, he acknowledges to have done nothing wrong. He is innocent. This man joins Herod and Pilate in affirming Jesus' innocence. Addressing Jesus, he then makes that beautiful petition: "Jesus, remember me when you come into your kingdom."[23] Only the blind beggar and the ten lepers address Jesus by name in this way (17:13; 18:38), and the meaning of this name is "saviour". In contrast to the soldiers and religious leaders, he acknowledges Jesus' kingship and is "its first willing subject."[24] He manifests insight into Jesus' identity; he seems to realise that this kind of kingship is different from the normal Jewish messianic expectation and may transcend death.[25] Several scholars take the words as they stand to refer to the parousia (when you come again as king), a future event that would be the inauguration of the messianic era and which, for Jews, would include the raising of the dead.[26]

Jesus' reply is emphatic and goes further, promising him salvation that very day. "Today you will be with me in paradise." The focus thus shifts from future hope, from the end of the world, to the immediate present.[27] The era of salvation has become a present reality (2:11; 4:21; 5:26; 19:11). This has been seen in many of the Gospel stories. "Paradise" was the Persian word for a park or garden and was used of the garden of Eden (Gen 2:8–15). It had come to mean the future abode of the righteous beyond death, an image of the new creation, and had acquired a technical sense (Isa 51:3).[28] While not eliminating future eschatology, when God's reign will be fully realised, Luke has emphasised its present realisation during the ministry of Jesus. Jesus' kingly power is operative from that moment. "God's plan comes to fruition through, not in spite of, the crucifixion of Jesus, so that Jesus is able to exercise his regal power of salvation in death as in life."[29] The meaning of death assumes a new significance: it leads his people straight into his presence.

In this incident, Jesus is again seen as the saviour of the outcast who turns to him; Jesus is seeking and saving to the end. Appropriately, Jesus' last words to a human being in the story are addressed to an outcast.

The Death of Jesus (23:44–46)

We now come to the scene in which Luke describes the death of Jesus and provides his interpretation.

> It was now about noon, and darkness came over the whole land until three in the afternoon, while the sun's light failed; and the curtain of the temple was torn in two. Then Jesus, crying with a loud voice, said, "Father, into your hands I commend my spirit." Having said this, he breathed his last.

Luke's version is again different from that of Mark. Dereliction is entirely lacking. Instead of Psalm 22, Psalm 31:5 is quoted. There is an air of calm, restfulness and peaceful surrender. There is a reference to darkness at noon, but the reference to the temple veil comes before Jesus' death rather than after.[30] The centurion's response is different. There are male disciples as well as women present at the scene.

Luke leads into his presentation of Jesus' death by describing two preparatory or anticipatory events. After Jesus has been crucified about noon, darkness covers the whole land for the next three hours.[31] Luke specifies that "the sun's light failed". This could not have been an eclipse, since this is astronomically impossible at the Passover full moon, and eclipses do not last more than about seven or eight minutes.[32] At that time in the Greco-Roman world, many believed that unusual portents took place at significant or tragic moments, like the death of an important person.[33] Perhaps Luke envisages nature affected by what is happening to Jesus; what is taking place has cosmic implications. In the prophetical books of the Bible, such darkness was linked with divine judgement and the awaited day of the Lord (Amos 8:9; Joel 2:10, 30–31; 3:15; Zeph 1:15).[34] Jesus referred to "the power of darkness" at the time of his arrest (22:53); this is Satan's time.

The evangelist then mentions that the curtain of the temple sanctuary (*naos*) was torn in two.[35] The passive verb implies that this is the action of God. In Mark, this is the first effect of Jesus' having breathed his last. Generally, Luke sees the temple in a positive light; for Jesus and later for the disciples, it is a place of prayer and teaching. However, on reaching Jerusalem and entering the temple, Jesus has driven out the merchants and recalled God's will that the temple should be a house of prayer, not a den of robbers; for this he incurred the opposition of the leadership (19:45–48). There were two curtains in the temple, one before the Holy Place, the other separating the Holy Place from the Holy of Holies. Most commentators take this event as applying to the inner curtain to the Holy of Holies, entered only by the high priest once a year to pray for the atonement of the nation's sins. The significance of the incident for Luke would probably be that it is an omen of the temple's future destruction, a symbol of God's judgement on the temple, and his readers would probably understand it that way. It may also suggest that the temple has served its purpose; its rites are no longer necessary or meaningful.[36] It could also be a symbol that access to the presence of God is now open even for gentiles, a positive sign;[37] God is no longer remote.

There is no mention of Jesus' desolation nor of any activity around the cross. It is now the ninth hour, which was the time for evening prayer in the temple, and Psalm 31:5 formed part of that prayer. It also formed part of night prayer for the pious Jew.[38] In Luke, Jesus cries out only once, with a loud voice,[39] using this psalm: "Father, into your hands I entrust my spirit." The introductory "Father" is added to the psalm, and the tense of the verb adapted from future to present.[40] It is the psalm of the suffering righteous one, who places in God's hands all he is and has. The psalm on the lips of Jesus is an expression of inner poverty, of dependence and confidence in God, and of surrender to the will of the Father. It also conveys a firm trust in the God who is faithful to his promises; it expresses the hope of vindication, the conviction that there will be a victory. In this final act of conscious commitment, Jesus entrusts his whole life to the Father's care. Jesus is convinced that "the hands into which he commits his life are gracious."[41] "When Jesus 'places over' his spirit to the Father, he is bringing round to its place of origin his life and mission."[42]

The term that Jesus uses to address God in prayer itself communicates a profound sense of trust and surrender. The core of Jesus' relationship to God is revealed in his addressing him as "Abba, my Father", as we have seen in an earlier chapter. It was almost without precedent for a Jew to pray to God in such a way, whereas for Jesus it appears to have been the norm. "Abba" was the word used by little children when chattering to dad; by the time of Jesus it had come to be used by older children too. It was part of the day-to-day language of family intimacy and denoted courtesy, warmth, trust, confidence and readiness to obey. The basic Hebrew concept suggests a relationship of tenderness, care and authority on the one hand, and trusting obedience on the other. Jesus takes the highly unusual step of adopting this familiar term as his regular and characteristic manner of approaching God in prayer. He encouraged his disciples to address God in the same way. "Abba" seems to have captured Jesus' understanding and intimate experience of God. Luke has Jesus refer to his Father's house as an adolescent (2:49); he prays to the Father on the Mount of Olives (22:42), when crucified (23:34) and now as he dies. It is not surprising that Luke places the term on the lips of the dying Jesus.[43] According to Neyrey,[44] in the overall context of the Gospel and Acts, the words "Father, into thy hands I commit my spirit" imply Jesus' conviction that his imminent death is not final; there will be a future victory. Clearly, there is a similar implication in his earlier words to the 'good thief', also peculiar to Luke: "Today you shall be with me in Paradise." The final words of Jesus are essentially a statement of faith (or trust) in the God-who-raises-from-the-dead.

For Luke, then, Jesus dies (the verb is "expired", *exepneusen)* with this prayer on his lips, a prayer of trust in God. "With these words, he breathed his last." Jesus dies peacefully in trust.[45] "Jesus dies as he has lived, connected to God through prayer, fully entrusting his life and his future to the One he knows as Father."[46] But the spirit Jesus hands over to the Father in breathing his last is the spirit empowered and commissioned to prophetic-messianic vocation by the Spirit.[47] He is also "entrusting to God the future of his Spirit-empowered, Spirit-directed, Spirit-authorised mission", leaving that work to others.[48]

Reactions to The Death of Jesus (23:47–49)

When the centurion saw what had taken place, he praised God and said, "Certainly this man was innocent." And when all the crowds who had gathered there for this spectacle saw what had taken place, they returned home, beating their breasts. But all his acquaintances, including the women who had followed him from Galilee, stood at a distance, watching these things.

Luke is not interested in apocalyptic signs but in the changes that take place in people's hearts, the responses given to the event of Jesus' death. Previous to Jesus' death, all is negative, now the responses are positive. Luke provides four: that of the centurion, the people, his friends and a member of the supreme council of the Jewish people.

The centurion, who was responsible for the crucifixion, seeing what had taken place, "gave praise to God", a typically Lukan reaction (2:20; 5:25–26; 7:16; 13:13; 17:15; 18:43). His glorifying God is linked with his further comment: "Truly, this was an upright man." The word can mean juridically innocent. This theme has run through the passion account; the centurion is confirming the view of Pilate, Herod and the 'good thief'.[49] Before and after Jesus' death, a Roman has proclaimed him to be innocent of any crime. But the word signals more than innocence; it also means righteous. Taunted as the "chosen one", Jesus is now proclaimed as God's righteous one, the suffering servant: "the righteous one, my servant" (Isa 53:11); it is a Christological title.[50] The fact that the centurion is a gentile looks to the future.

The crowds, who with their leaders earlier demanded Jesus' death, have been present on Calvary, simply watching (23:27, 31);[51] the Greek suggests a spectacle or entertainment. Now they beat their breasts/chests as an expression of grief as they head back to the city. While probably not repentance in the full sense, their returning may spatially suggest a movement in the direction of genuine repentance, at least a preparation for what will happen in Acts.[52] This balances the intensely negative reaction of the rulers and soldiers.

Luke next makes mention of Jesus' acquaintances, who stood "at a distance". Undoubtedly, they would not have been allowed to go closer. This refers to male disciples, probably including the apostles, who, Luke suggests, had not been totally faithless.[53] There were women too, "who had accompanied him from Galilee" (8:1–3). The verb actually means "followed with", and is the language of discipleship. Luke does not name them here, as do Mark and Matthew. They are part of the nucleus of the Galilean community that will be the first Church in Jerusalem.[54] The comment that the women "saw all this happen" is important for their later role at the tomb after the Sabbath rest. However, the acquaintances of Jesus are standing "at a distance" (see Ps 38:11), perhaps "indicating a weakened discipleship that is as yet unwilling to identify too closely with Jesus in his humiliation and death."[55]

The Burial (23:50–56)

> Now there was a good and righteous man named Joseph, who, though a member of the council, had not agreed to their plan and action. He came from the Jewish town of Arimathea, and he was waiting expectantly for the kingdom of God. This man went to Pilate and asked for the body of Jesus. Then he took it down, wrapped it in a linen cloth, and laid it in a rock-hewn tomb where no one had ever been laid. It was the day of Preparation, and the sabbath was beginning. The women who had come with him from Galilee followed, and they saw the tomb and how his body was laid. Then they returned, and prepared spices and ointments. On the sabbath they rested according to the commandment.

In other parts of the empire, the Romans usually left the corpses on the cross for wild animals and birds to feed on, but the Jewish Law required burial before nightfall (Deut.22:23), so they permitted this. A Jew named Joseph from

Arimathaea comes forward to bury Jesus. He is described as "a good and upright man", who "lived in the hope of seeing the kingdom of God", a phrase which numbers him among the genuinely pious members of the people.[56] Surprisingly, he is a member of the Council, but Luke states that he had not consented to what the others had planned, decided and carried out. Out of respect for the Law, he asks for, and seemingly obtains, permission to take down the body of Jesus and bury it.[57] There is no reference to the centurion being questioned by Pilate about Jesus' death, as in Mark. Joseph wraps the corpse of Jesus in a shroud and places it in a new tomb in which no one had previously been laid.[58] There is no mention of a stone being placed at the entrance. In Luke's account, the burial of Jesus is not dishonourable, as it is in Mark.[59]

The women, who had been eyewitnesses of the ministry in Galilee, now follow. Having been present for what happened on Calvary, they take note of the place of the tomb and then go back to prepare spices and ointments. There is no reference to them buying them, as in Mark. They are not named.[60] On the Sabbath, they rest, faithfully observing the Law. They will ensure continuity in the story, for they will be the first witnesses to the empty tomb, and the first to proclaim the resurrection and will be in the group which receives the Spirit.

Reflections

There is, I believe, much for us to reflect upon in Luke's presentation of Calvary. Clearly, he intends Jesus' death to be the pattern for Christian death, since he later describes the death of Stephen in a similar way: "Lord Jesus, receive my spirit", and "Lord, do not hold this sin against them" (Acts 7:59–60). The prayer of forgiveness and the prayer of surrender are important throughout our lives but particularly as we face our death. The frequency with which Jesus' exhortations that we be forgiving people occur in the Gospel story is an indication both of our ongoing need to forgive and of the difficult challenge this can sometimes be. "Forgive, and you will be forgiven" (6:37); "Forgive us our sins, for we ourselves forgive everyone indebted to us" (11:4). When Peter asks Jesus how many times he should forgive someone who offends him, and generously suggests seven times, Jesus indicates that it should be seventy times seven times, which indicates that there is no limit (Matt 18:21–22). To die with forgiveness in our hearts, with no one unforgiven, is the way of Jesus.

The phrase from the psalm that Jesus quotes as he dies, entrusting himself to the Father's love, is one which we use in the night prayer of the Church. Before we retire for the night, we commit into the Father's hands the day that is coming to a close: the things that we have tried to do for the Kingdom, the love we have given and received, the mistakes that we have made, the opportunities grasped or missed, the difficulties that have arisen, the problems still unsolved, the anxieties which trouble us, the graced/gifted situations that we have recognised. All this we confidently place into God's safe and gracious hands. And our prayer can stretch back beyond any single day to the various stages of our life's journey so far: significant moments, significant events and relationships, significant failures and mistakes. Often, we neglect to commit our past into God's safe keeping. It can be at once a prayer of thanks, a prayer of sorrow, a prayer for healing but above all a prayer of trust. If necessary, God can still put things right; God can also turn water into wine.

But obviously this is a prayer that we can use at any time. There are always so many people and situations that we may wish to commit to God's faithful love— people whom we love, people whom we serve, people with whom we share life and ministry, in sickness and separation, in journeying, struggle and change, in all our coming and our going. In doing so, we place our trust in God's merciful love and providential care.

This phrase of the psalm is particularly appropriate, I believe, for our future, be that our personal future, especially in time of uncertainty and change, or our future as parish and religious communities or as wider Church, as we struggle with the challenges which confront us locally and worldwide. Naturally, there can be fear around, and anxiety, and the urge to cling to what is known and secure. It is difficult to let go and to move on. There are also issues and problems and tragedies far greater than we seem able to cope with. There are dreams and hopes and expectations that we hold dear. We do believe that our God is gracious; we believe that God is worthy of our total trust.

And we return to the context in which Jesus uttered this prayer as we think of our death. It will come one day, though we know not when or where or how. Death is the supreme letting go, the culmination of those many acts of letting go that punctuate our lives. Death is the moment of our utter poverty, when we are completely dependent on God's sustaining love for our ongoing existence, and when we are invited to surrender all we are into God's hands, trusting that death is not the end but a beginning. That trust is strengthened by our belief that God vindicated Jesus' trusting surrender through the resurrection. And it is a full sharing in his risen life that awaits us beyond the grave, a place in the Father's house or "paradise" forever.[61]

Notes

1   Rowan Williams, *God with Us: The Meaning of The Cross and Resurrection—Then and Now* (London: SPCK, 2017), 3-7.

2   Johnson, *Luke*, 380, states that Luke shapes the tradition in a distinctive fashion, and exercises more freedom than Matthew with his Markan source.

3   Byrne, *Hospitality*, 181, suggests a fourfold structure: the crucifixion; the response of onlookers before Jesus dies; Jesus' death; the response of onlookers after his death. Carroll, *Luke*, 464, speaks of a "vivid display of a righteous man facing death with equanimity, courage and integrity." Caird, *Luke*, 250, notes how belief in the fulfilment of the Old Testament prophecies concerning the righteous Servant of the Lord has coloured the form and language of the passion narrative. There are allusions to Psalms 22 and 69.

4   Brown, *Death*, 2:937. He mentions the Adam tradition, depicted in some pictures and carvings.

5   Tannehill, *Luke*, 340, sees the crucifixion as the climax of a "status degradation ritual", which has been in process since 22:63. "It is the final act of social rejection of one who is so dishonoured that all kinds of verbal and physical abuse are permitted."

6   He uses *kakourgoi* rather than *lēstai*. Their presence is repeated several times (vv. 32, 33, 39, 41, 47). Matera, *Passion Narratives*, 183, notes that the Greek order can be translated as "two other criminals were led away ... ." which recalls the scriptural quotation at the end of Supper (22:37).

7   Brown, *Death*, 2:970, notes that there is no vocabulary indication that Luke saw this passage fulfilled here.

8   There is a textual problem with Jesus' word of forgiveness, as some important manuscripts omit it. Most of the commentaries prefer to include it: Carroll, *Luke*, 466; Brown, 2:975–81; Caird, *Luke*, 251; McBride, *Luke*, 307; Marshall, *Luke*, 868. Johnson, *Luke*, 376, believes that on thematic grounds, there is every reason to consider it authentic; similarly, Tannehill, *Luke*, 341. Fitzmyer, *Luke*, 2:1503, disagrees.

9   For a discussion of the authenticity of this verse, see Brown, *Death*, 2:975–981. He concludes, p. 980, that "it is easier to posit that the passage was written by Luke and excised for theological reasons by a later copyist than that it was added to Luke by such a copyist who took trouble to cast it in Lukan style and thought." Tannehill, *Luke*, 340–341, notes that this prayer balances Jesus' final prayer; they bracket the death scene.

10   See Stephen in Acts 7:60; the ignorance motif is found also in Acts 3:17; 13:27; 14:16; 17:30; 26:9. Karris, *Luke*, 85, notes that the effects of Jesus' death are felt in advance through the reconciliation of Herod and Pilate (23:12).

11   Brown, *Death*, 2:973; Carroll, *Luke*, 466; Caird, *Luke*, 251; Tannehill, *Luke*, 341. McBride, *Luke*, 307, refers to "all those involved in his death"; Green, *Luke*, 820.

12   This psalm is often referred to as the psalm of the righteous sufferer; it played a large part in early Christian reflection on Jesus' passion.

13   Carroll, *Luke*, 466, wonders whether it includes the robe which Herod gave Jesus. Karris, *Luke*, 85–87, develops the theme of "clothing" in the passion narrative; he suggests that Herod decks Jesus in a white mantle, Roman style, preparing him for

selection for office by the religious leaders and people. They select Barabbas instead.

14   Karris, *Luke*, 86, quotes Haulotte, that "in biblical culture to be deprived of clothing was to lose one's identity." Also on p. 99; similarly, Green, *Luke*, 820. Brown, *Death*, 2:953, holds that the evidence favours complete despoliation, but the question is not settled.

15   Caird, *Luke*, 251, comments: "With restraint and economy he portrays the different attitudes of the spectators: the vulgar curiosity of the crowd, the contemptuous derisions of the rulers, the callous frivolity of the guard, the bitter invective of the criminal." The word "save" occurs several times, and forms part of each form of mockery. Brown, *Death*, 2:984, notes the pattern of threes, frequent in the passion. He also (n. 1) links the mockery (two "ifs") with the temptation story.

16   Brown, *Death*, 2:990.

17   "Rulers" is an umbrella term; Mark has the chief priests and scribes, to which Matthew adds the elders. The term contrasts with "the people"; for Luke, the people as a whole are not hostile to Jesus, but the rulers are (Brown, *Death*, 2:991).

18   Carroll, *Luke*, 467, suggests a "chorus of insult". Green, *Luke*, 820, believes that the verb "scoff" recalls Ps 22:7, which refers to a worm, scorned, despised and mocked. Brown, *Death*, 2:991, notes that Luke uses the same verb as Ps 22:8a (see also 16:14). It can mean to look down one's nose at.

19   The hope that God will rescue the righteous one from suffering and death (Wis 2:18) is fulfilled in a way other than the Jews expect. Wis 2:18 reads: "For if the righteous man is God's son, he will help him, and will deliver him from the hands of his adversaries." There are echoes of Isa 42:1: "the chosen one". This term occurs in 9:35, the transfiguration scene. Green, *Luke*, 821, notes that the leaders refer to Jesus correctly, employing language that draws together the identity of Jesus as the Servant of Yahweh and as the Messiah. The categories are there, but the leaders repudiate Jesus' salvific role. Neyrey, *Passion*,132, notes that Luke highlights the salvation theme; he sees Jesus as the "saved saviour".

20   Luke omits Mark's "he cannot save himself" and "come down from the cross".

21   Brown, *Death*, 2:997, refers to "a burlesque gift to the king"; similarly, Green, *Luke*, 821; Tannehill, *Luke*, 342, who also suggests a Jew/ gentile parallel with Jesus' condemnation.

22   Brown, *Death*, 2:998–999, believes that that the mockery by the soldiers is totally a Lukan formulation.

23   Green, *Luke*, 822, notes that "remember me" echoes words repeatedly addressed to God whose memory is a source of divine blessing in keeping with his covenant. Neyrey, *Passion*, 135, reminds us of those who petition Jesus during the ministry, and Jesus' promise that those who ask will receive (11:9).

24   Carroll, *Luke*, 468; his translation is "when you reign as king". 19:38 reads: "Blessed is the king who comes in the name of the Lord." Karris, *Luke*, 101, sees vv. 40–43 as the high point of the Gospel. On p. 102 he refers to the "repentant malefactor", a representative of all repentant evildoers. Tannehill, *Luke*, 343, suggests that in effect he is asking for royal clemency. Neyrey, *Passion*, 136, considers his statement as tantamount to a confession of faith in Jesus.

25   Carroll, *Luke*, 468. This is the longest speech in the Calvary scene. Caird, *Luke*, 252, suggests he may have wished to be kind to Jesus, and seized on the words of the placard on the cross to say something to offset the taunts of his companion—a cup of cold water, which received a reward out of all proportion to his request.

26   Marshall, *Luke*, 872. Some manuscripts read "come in your kingdom" rather than "come into your kingdom".

27   Byrne, *Hospitality*, 182, refers to the "great Lukan 'Today'." Johnson, *Luke*, 378, notes that the word signifies a special moment of revelation or salvation (2:11; 4:21; 5:26; 13:32–33; 19:9; 22:34, 61).

28   Caird, *Luke*, 252; Johnson, *Luke*, 379, notes that in the time of Jesus and later, the term had acquired a strong future reference. See also 2 Cor 12:4; Rev 2:7.

29   Green, *Luke*, 823; Neyrey, *Passion*, 137: Jesus assumes his kingly reign not at his parousia but ironically on the cross and in his resurrection.

30   Brown, *Death*, 2:1938, observes that in this way Luke concentrates the negative signs of God's wrath before Jesus' act of trust.

31   Green, *Luke*, 825, comments that an effect of mentioning time is to slow down the pace of the narrative.

32   Brown, *Death*, 2:1039–42, notes that, although many translators prefer "the sun's light failed", textually "the sun having been eclipsed" is more original, even if not scientifically accurate. There is no independent evidence for a longer eclipse. Luke does not seem to have other weather phenomena like a sirocco in mind. Brown suggests that Luke, "confusedly or by art" connected the memory of a solar eclipse months or years before Jesus' death with Mark's tradition of the darkness. Luke understands the darkness as an eschatological sign from God.

33   Caird, *Luke*, 253; Brown, *Death*, 2:1043, gives several examples.

34   Caird, *Luke*, 253, suggests symbolic descriptions of the significance of the cross.

35   Brown, *Death*, 2:1043, notes that if the Greek particle *de* is conjunctive, the eclipse and rending of the veil are yoked as negative signs; if adversative, the rending is linked with Jesus' cry. Resseguie, *Spiritual Landscape*, 98, sees darkness as a giant cloak and the temple veil as a garment. The garment of darkness that cloaks the entire land at midday represents the momentary triumph of the powers of darkness. The veil is a garment which clothes the temple.

36   Resseguie, *Spiritual Landscape*, 98–99, sees the rending of the veil as an act of disrobing the temple and removing its distinctiveness as sacred space at the moment before Jesus dies. This is the dissolution of the symbolic world surrounding the temple; God exposes the temple as inadequate to accomplish God's purposes; it is unable to provide for the spiritual needs of a nation. God's purposes are now fulfilled in Jesus. Fitzmyer, *Luke*, 2:1518, believes that the outer curtain is intended, rather than the inner.

37   Johnson, *Luke*, 379; Byrne, *Hospitality*, 183; Carroll, *Luke*, 469, notes that Jesus had used the temple court as a classroom, and the disciples later went to the temple to pray and teach. Green, *Luke*, 825–6, does not believe that the destruction of the temple is symbolised; rather, it is "God's turning away from the temple in order to accomplish his purposes by other means." Luke neutralises its centrality in preparation for the

centrifugal mission of the followers of Jesus.

38   McBride, *Luke*, 310. Brown, *Death*, 2:1069, doubts this, believing that the date when the psalm came to be used in evening prayer is uncertain, and that a loud cry does not suggest evening prayer.

39   Luke uses *phōnein*, a softening of Mark's more violent *boan*, "to scream". Neyrey, *Passion*, 146–147, notes that the evangelists have put different sets of words on the lips of the dying Jesus; he quotes from the psalms; we need to bracket consideration of his emotions or psychology.

40   Johnson, *Luke*, 379, notes that the psalm portrays the rejection of the righteous one by his adversaries, but expresses a quiet confidence in God's saving power. Chrupcala, *The Salvation of God*, 226, states that a brief cry of prayer, besides being spontaneous, in which the entire intimacy of the petitioner is assumed, is a sign of profound dependence of man on God and the faith in him (*sic*). For Luke, Jesus' dying words are transformed to a trustful supplication of unwavering faith and obedient acceptance of the will of God.

41   Karris, *Luke*, 108. Neyrey, *Passion*, 147, maintains that Luke has two things in mind, pastoral and theological. Jesus shows the community the proper way to die; Jesus expresses faith in the God who raises the dead.

42   Brown, *Death*, 2:1068. He notes the earlier use of the leaders seeking to lay "hands" on Jesus and his being given over into the "hands" of sinners; now Jesus places his spirit into the Father's "hands". Brown recalls the Spirit in 1:35; 3:22; 4:1; 4:14.

43   Brown, *Death*, 2:1068, notes that Luke wishes that Jesus' followers should imitate Jesus' sentiments when they face death (see Acts 7:59–60).

44   Neyrey, *Passion*, 147–155. He refers to Peter's inaugural sermon (Acts 2:14–36) and his use of Psalm 16:9–10: "You will not abandon my soul to Hades, or let your Holy One experience corruption." That trust in God has been vindicated through the resurrection; this verse contains the fuller content of Jesus' dying prayer. Throughout the Gospel, Luke consistently presents Jesus as knowing God's promises of salvation and believing in their fulfilment (9:22; 18:33; 22:69; 23:43; 23:46; 24:7; 24:26–27; 24:44–46). Tannehill, *Luke*, 345–346, also refers to this.

45   Byrne, *Hospitality*, 183, notes that this is not a literal description of a person dying from crucifixion. The narrative seeks to bring out the deeper meaning. Carroll, *Luke*, 470, suggests that Luke is presenting Jesus as a model for dying as also for living; he seeks to enlighten and inspire his readers. Matera, *Passion Narratives*, 186, believes that Jesus dies as the suffering righteous one who peacefully entrusts his soul to the Father.

46   Carroll, *Luke*, 470.

47   Carroll, *Luke*, 470.

48   Carroll, *Luke*, 470.

49   23:4,14, 15, 22, 41.

50   In Acts 3:13–14, alluding to Isa 52:13–53:12, the term "righteous" is linked with Jesus' death. Matera, *Passion Narratives*, 187, believes that this means that he stands in the correct covenant relationship with God. In Acts, it is a messianic title.

51   Johnson, *Luke*, 384, notes that Luke's view is against the weight of the tradition. Earlier, the people were involved in asking for Jesus' crucifixion. Now their eyes are

opened as they see what has taken place. Marshall, *Luke*, 877, considers it unjustified to read repentance into their reaction.

52   Johnson, *Luke*, 382, comments that the populace, only marginally involved in the death of the prophet, are now stunned and remorseful, ready to respond to the call to conversion in Acts 2:37–41. Also p. 385; the reader is being prepared for later developments; also, Carroll, *Luke*, 472; McBride, *Luke*, 310. Green, *Luke*, 828, recalls the Jerusalem women and the parable of the tax collector in the temple (18:9–14).

53   Johnson, *Luke*, 383, notes that Luke has omitted the scene of the disciples abandoning Jesus in the garden; so this group probably includes disciples; likewise Green, *Luke*, 828; Matera, *Passion Narratives*, 188.

54   Johnson, *Luke*, 383.

55   Green, *Luke*, 828. Tannehill, *Luke*, 346, considers this "a sign of their continuing weakness as followers."

56   See earlier Zechariah, Elizabeth, Simeon and Anna. Johnson, *Luke*, 383, believes that Luke is portraying him as a member of the "faithful people of God" like them; also, Tannehill, *Luke*, 348. In Mark, he is simply an upright Jew who wishes to keep the Law concerning burials before the Sabbath; in Matthew, he is a disciple (27:27); in John, a secret disciple for fear of the religious authorities (19:38).

57   Johnson, *Luke*, 385; the leadership were not unanimous, then, in rejecting Jesus the prophet. McBride, *Luke*, 311, suggests that he was absent from the Sanhedrin session.

58   Wright, *Luke*, 287, notes that since only the body of Jesus is in the tomb, there would be no danger of making a mistake, as could have happened if there were other bodies in the tomb, as was often the case. Matera, *Passion Narratives*, 189, links the tomb in which no one had been buried with the colt on which no one had ridden (19:30), and suspects a regal allusion.

59   See Winstanley, *Little People*, 163–166.

60   In the narrative at the empty tomb, the women are named as Mary of Magdala, Joanna, Mary the mother of James, and others (24:10).

61   See John 14:1–3.

Chapter Fourteen
The Resurrection

The strong hints, which we noticed at the Last Supper and Calvary, that the death of Jesus would not be the end of the story reach fulfilment "on the first day of the week."[1] The account of Jesus' burial concluded with the note that the Galilean women, who were present on Calvary, saw the tomb where Jesus' body was laid by Joseph of Arimathaea. They then went to prepare spices and ointments, minded to anoint the body of Jesus but only when the Sabbath was over, thus faithfully observing the Law. Now, at early dawn, they make their way to the tomb, carrying their spices.[2] Before we continue with Luke's description of the events of that "first day of the week"—the discovery of the empty tomb, the Emmaus story, the appearance of the risen Lord to the disciples at table and the ascension—perhaps we should pause and take a look at the wider picture.

A Historical Interlude

Our liturgical celebration of Easter Sunday, on "the third day",[3] suggests that the situation of desolation, utter crisis and emptiness, which the friends of Jesus must have felt after his death and burial, did not last long, less than 48 hours, in fact. Luke's Gospel supports this, as his account of Easter is compressed into that one day, the culmination of Jesus' "exodus".[4] However, that is probably not the case historically. The earliest tradition about that Sunday morning is probably found in John, where Magdalene goes to the tomb; she finds the stone removed but no Jesus.[5] She departs to find Peter and the Beloved Disciple, and informs them that the tomb is empty, suggesting that people have removed the body;[6] they go to the tomb to see.[7]

All four Gospels provide an account of the discovery of the empty tomb. A key factor in that scenario is the appearance of an angel or angelic young men,[8] who with different wording interpret the empty tomb and proclaim the Easter kerygma. While most Christian scholars accept the historicity of the discovery of the empty tomb,[9] they believe that the angelic visitor(s) and message are not factual but a later addition to the basic story, providing an explanation for the empty tomb tradition. This is a classic biblical technique. It transforms the tradition so as to create a vehicle for the proclamation of Easter faith. The reason for its emptiness becomes part of the narrative.[10]

It is the view of most scholars that, in all probability, the disciples fled Jerusalem and hotfooted it back to Galilee.[11] Some of them had probably done so as early as Thursday evening, the rest after the Passover Sabbath. In his wonderful Emmaus narrative, Luke captures, I think, their near despair, their shattered dreams, the empty void which was their future: "We had hoped that he was the one to redeem Israel." The disciples returned to Galilee as confused, broken and disillusioned people. It was also safer for them there. They may have resumed their former occupations.[12] Probably some followers and sympathisers remained in Jerusalem; perhaps they were residents.[13]

But soon, something decisive happened back in Galilee to change it all. There are unexpected, out of the blue encounters or meetings between Jesus and Magdalene, Jesus and Peter,[14] and a group of the others.[15] Fearful, disillusioned, heartbroken people were suddenly transformed; there was a complete turnaround. Maybe these meetings, these experiences, happened at a meal or by the lake, or both; but it is these meetings that gave birth to faith in the resurrection of Jesus.[16] The way the disciples later described what had happened was to claim that Jesus appeared to them (or "let himself be seen by them").[17] They recognised him. The initiative was with Jesus; the experiences were God's gift, God breaking into their lives again. Possibly the risen Lord poured out the Spirit on them. These encounters also explained why the tomb was empty, why it had been pointless and misguided to seek the living among the dead.[18]

It would seem that for the Feast of Pentecost, if not before, the disciples, family and friends of Jesus returned with other pilgrims to Jerusalem for the celebration. Their fear and confusion dissipated, they joined the disciples who had remained. While they were there, something else happened: the presence of the Spirit of God was charismatically manifested.[19] The first community came to be established and was centred in Jerusalem. Filled with the Spirit, the disciples began to go out with great courage and tell people with deep conviction that the Jesus whom their leaders had had killed by the Romans was alive; God had vindicated Jesus' trusting surrender, his self-giving in love, by raising him from death; therefore, God really was behind his message and values and lifestyle and Kingdom dream. With the resurrection of Jesus, the last days have arrived, the new age has been inaugurated, the final phase of God's interaction with the world.[20]

Initially, simple phrases were used to articulate their deep faith conviction: "Jesus is Lord."[21] There were short formulas like "Jesus died and rose again,"[22] and other formulas that stressed the contrast or antithesis between death and resurrection, or death and life.[23] Most expressions used the language of resurrection ("God raised Jesus from death", or "raised Jesus to life"); other expressions adopted the language of exaltation or glorification ("God exalted him to his right hand").[24] The earliest written statement is found in 1 Cor 15:3–5: "For I handed on to you as of first importance what I in turn had received: that Christ died for our sins in accordance with the scriptures, and that he was buried, and that he was raised on the third day in accordance with the scriptures, and that he appeared to Cephas, then to the twelve." Paul is quoting a very early tradition, probably from the mid-thirties CE. As well as in the letters of Paul, there are good examples of these early formulas in Peter's five early sermons in Acts.[25]

In the light of the resurrection, the disciples proclaimed Jesus as Messiah and Saviour and Lord. They invited their hearers to accept the forgiveness he brought, to share the life of God which he made available, to experience salvation, to become part of his new community, God's new people. This new community quickly developed; the word spread—and the rest we know. It is perhaps worth recalling that language of resurrection does not mean that Jesus came back to life as it was before (like Jairus' daughter or the son of the widow of Nain); it does not refer to the reanimation of a corpse. It means that Jesus moved forward into a radically new and very different kind of life, beyond the limitations of space and time. There is continuity—it is the same Jesus but there is immense difference and transformation, a completely new dimension.[26] Jesus has been freed from death and from all that holds back humanity's growth towards God, and is now actively present in the world.[27]

Fifty years later, Gospel writers (Matthew, Luke, John) composed narratives to proclaim this Good News.[28] Each evangelist used his own unique style, reworking early traditions according to his own theological vision and aims.[29] There are two basic traditions: in Matthew, Mark (by implication) and John 21, the main appearance of the risen Jesus to his disciples occurs in Galilee, whereas in Luke and John 20 it takes place in Jerusalem.[30] Some of these resurrection narratives perhaps overemphasise the physical side, corporeal continuity, and can give the wrong impression; but at the same time they also make it clear that Jesus is different. Paul, who alone can speak at first hand, tends to stress the element of otherness or difference, speaking of a spiritual body, a glorified body.[31] Our language of space/time breaks down when it is used to describe something beyond normal human experience; it is a pale approximation. The early disciples did not have the language needed to describe what they had experienced; it was beyond the scope of human categories. In their attempts, they are pushing human language to the limits; they have to use metaphor or analogy. One key element of the narratives is Jesus' commissioning of his disciples. The wording is different in each Gospel, reflecting the style of the individual evangelist. They articulate and put into the mouth of Jesus what over the years they have come to understand the mission entails.[32]

These narratives are not meant to provide biographical information, reconstructing the events. They are catechetical stories; they draw out and explore different aspects of the meaning of faith in the risen Christ: gift, surprise, conversion, forgiveness,[33] friendship and closeness, evangelising mission.[34] But they are based on the real experiences of the early disciples. Because of what God has done for his Son in raising him from death, new possibilities have been opened up for human beings; our understanding of God and our relationship with God have been changed.[35] With this background, we can now pursue our examination of Luke's presentation of the Easter events, all situated in and around Jerusalem.

The Tomb (24:1–12)

The text describing the discovery of the tomb reads as follows:

> But on the first day of the week, at early dawn, they came to the tomb, taking the spices that they had prepared. They found the stone rolled away from the tomb, but when they went in, they did not find the body. While they were perplexed about this, suddenly two men in dazzling clothes stood beside them. The women were terrified and bowed their faces to the ground, but the men said to them, "Why do you look for the living among the dead? He is not here, but has risen. Remember how he told you, while he was still in Galilee, that the Son of Man must be handed over to sinners, and be crucified, and on the third day rise again." Then they remembered his words, and returning from the tomb, they told all this to the eleven and to all the rest. Now it was Mary Magdalene, Joanna, Mary the mother of James, and the other women with them who told this to the apostles. But these words seemed to them an idle tale, and they did not believe them. But Peter got up and ran to the tomb; stooping and looking in, he saw the linen cloths by themselves; then he went home, amazed at what had happened.

The women come at first light to the tomb, carrying their spices with them in order to anoint the body of Jesus. They discover the stone rolled away,[36] and this must have been disturbing. On entering the tomb, straight away they find that the body of Jesus is not there, which causes them deep perplexity. As they stand there in bewilderment, two men in dazzling apparel, the clothes of heaven, appear beside them.[37] Naturally, the women are terrified; they fall prostrate on the ground, realising their heavenly origin.

The men reproach them, together asking why they are looking for the living among the dead, a question with strong and exciting implications. They then declare the amazing news: "He is not here, but has risen."[38] They go on to remind them of Jesus' words while in Galilee, words which they had heard when in his company there and ought to have remembered, namely, that he "must" be handed over to sinful people, be crucified, and on the third day rise again.[39] At this point the women do recall the words of Jesus and, coming to faith, leave the tomb and spontaneously go to find the eleven and the rest of the group, and relay to them what has happened—what they had seen, been told, and its significance.[40] Luke at this (late) point names the women: Mary Magdalene, Joanna, Mary the mother of James and their other female companions.[41] These are the first witnesses to the resurrection of Jesus. The response of the male disciples to their witness is incredulity and rejection, for their words seem utter nonsense, "an idle tale".[42] However, Peter runs off to the tomb to check it out. He stoops and looks in; he sees the linen cloths lying there.[43] He then goes home, amazed at what has happened, and possibly a little more open-minded, but not yet a believer. An empty tomb is simply an empty tomb; it does not of itself lead to resurrection faith.

Emmaus (24:13–35)

The Emmaus story is one of the most beautiful narratives in the New Testament. It is an exquisite masterpiece in which Luke's theological and artistic talents are seen at their finest, "a gem of literary art".[44] Dominating Luke's Easter narrative,[45] it takes up again the themes of the journey, the meal and mercy, themes prominent in Luke's telling of the Gospel story, as we have seen.[46]

In the various Gospels, there are several resurrection appearance narratives, and they tend to have a number of common features, rather like a basic template or pattern. A situation is described in which the disciples, bereft of the Master, are despondent, disappointed and fearful. Then Jesus suddenly becomes present.

Sometimes there is a form of greeting by Jesus; initially there is some hesitancy or doubt or non-recognition on the part of the disciples. There follows the climactic moment of recognition. Finally, Jesus sends them forth on mission. This scheme provides a useful framework for our reflections.[47]

Now on that same day two of them were going to a village called Emmaus, about seven miles from Jerusalem, and talking with each other about all these things that had happened. While they were talking and discussing, Jesus himself came near and went with them, but their eyes were kept from recognizing him. And he said to them, "What are you discussing with each other while you walk along?" They stood still, looking sad. Then one of them, whose name was Cleopas, answered him, "Are you the only stranger in Jerusalem who does not know the things that have taken place there in these days?" He asked them, "What things?" They replied, "The things about Jesus of Nazareth, who was a prophet mighty in deed and word before God and all the people, and how our chief priests and leaders handed him over to be condemned to death and crucified him. But we had hoped that he was the one to redeem Israel. Yes, and besides all this, it is now the third day since these things took place. Moreover, some women of our group astounded us. They were at the tomb early this morning, and when they did not find his body there, they came back and told us that they had indeed seen a vision of angels who said that he was alive. Some of those who were with us went to the tomb and found it just as the women had said; but they did not see him." Then he said to them, "Oh, how foolish you are, and how slow of heart to believe all that the prophets have declared! Was it not necessary that the Messiah should suffer these things and then enter into his glory?" Then beginning with Moses and all the prophets, he interpreted to them the things about himself in all the scriptures.

As they came near the village to which they were going, he walked ahead as if he were going on. But they urged him strongly, saying, "Stay with us, because it is almost evening and the day is now nearly over." So he went in to stay with them. When he was at the table with them, he took bread, blessed and broke it, and gave it to them. Then their eyes were opened, and they recognized him; and he vanished from their sight. They said to each other, "Were not our hearts burning within us while he was talking to us on the road, while he was opening the scriptures to us?" That same hour they got up and returned to Jerusalem; and they found the eleven and their companions gathered together. They were saying, "The Lord has risen indeed, and he has appeared to Simon!" Then they told what had happened on the road, and how he had been made known to them in the breaking of the bread.

The story begins on the first day of the week. In fact, in Luke's Gospel everything takes place on that "day". The two disciples are making their way home after the Passover festival to the village of Emmaus, about seven miles (11 km) from Jerusalem; the location of this village is uncertain.[48] Some scholars suggest that they may be man and wife, if Cleopas is the same person as the Clopas mentioned in John's version of the Calvary scene as the mother of one of the Mary's present (John 19:25).[49] As they walk along leaden-footed, they share the depths of their distress and disappointment. As so often happens in situations of grief and bereavement, they recall what has taken place, retrace familiar contours in an attempt to keep the person alive, clinging in tight-gripped desperation to a past that had meaning and which brought joy and love. We sense the tragedy and poignancy of their situation, the pained brokenness of shattered dreams, articulated later in the story: "Our hope had been that he would be the one to set Israel free." We detect the tones of anguish, bitterness and near despair, and glimpse the empty void that is their future.

A significant factor in the setting for the story is that the two disciples are travelling away from Jerusalem. A salient feature of Luke's presentation of the ministry of Jesus is, as we have seen, his structural emphasis on Jesus' journey up to Jerusalem, clearly inaugurated in 9:51, and continuing until the solemn entry into the city. It is there that the events called in the transfiguration scene Jesus' "departure" or "exodus" (9:31) take place. It is in Jerusalem that the gift of the Spirit will be bestowed. It is from that city that the apostles will set forth on another journey in mission to the nations. Yet these disciples are walking away; they have turned their backs; they have thrown in the towel; they have abandoned their friends and God's sacred story.[50] As we learn later, they have even heard the women's tale of the empty tomb and angelic vision with its Easter proclamation—but they are walking away in grief and unbelief, hopes shattered, expectations in pieces.

As they walk, the two disciples are engaged in deep conversation, a spirited debate.[51] Then, suddenly, a stranger is walking with them, as the risen Jesus takes the initiative and breaks through, unannounced and unexpected, into the shredded web of their lives and into the midst of their tragedy. When he asks about the topic of their discussion,[52] they stand still, their sadness obvious. Then they avidly seize on his ignorance as simply a visitor to the city,[53] and capitalise on the opportunity to tell their story all over again. He listens to their words and to their angst, listens with compassion and understanding, lives with them their questioning bewilderment. He is content to wait, prompting them with a question or two to enable them to bring out their problem, not forcing the pace, not rushing in with instant solutions. He walks their way with them along the twisting, dusty road, stopping and starting with their halting rhythm.

But the two disciples fail to recognise him, and their failure is protracted. "Something kept them from seeing who it was."[54] This motif of non-recognition is one of the devices by which the evangelists underline the 'otherness' of Jesus, the radical transformation which has taken place. Its persistence in this story adds considerably to the dramatic effect and suspense. It also serves to illustrate the truth that vision of the risen One is not a human achievement; it is gift, God's free gift.[55]

At this point in the unfolding of the story, Luke very skilfully, and not without considerable irony,[56] puts on the lips of Cleopas a summary of the early Christian kerygma and catechesis (similar to the preaching of Peter and Paul in Acts 2:22–24 and 13:26f.).[57] Jesus is described in terms of the popular estimate of him as "a prophet powerful in action and speech before God and the whole people."[58] A brief résumé of the passion follows, with emphasis on the responsibility of the Jewish leaders.[59] Luke's Cleopas goes on to express the hopes that Jesus had aroused in their own hearts that he was, in fact, the prophet, the prophet-like-Moses, the liberator of his people—hopes dashed by his untimely death.[60] Finally, he mentions the empty tomb tradition: the women's visit, the absence of the body, the astounding angelic vision and proclamation, the journey to the tomb made by some of the group of disciples[61] in search of corroboration as hope was rekindled and as suddenly snuffed out in scepticism, a scepticism which they apparently shared. They are very much aware of all the events, the facts, but they fail to understand their significance.[62]

Jesus then responds, jolting them initially with a reproach for their obtuse failure to understand God's ways, their slowness of heart.[63] From the Jewish scriptures, he provides the key to the recent events: "Was it not necessary that the Christ should suffer before entering into his glory?" Jesus leads them through the Bible (Moses, the prophets and the psalms), highlighting the evidence of God's purpose, the links between the scriptures and his vocation and destiny, detecting an underlying common pattern in God's ways that was a foreshadowing of the pattern of his own messianic mission: rejection leading to acceptance, suffering leading to glory.[64] No specific texts are mentioned. Jesus had himself explicitly spoken of this in what we call the passion predictions (9:22, 44; 18:31–33). Jesus shows them that not only is suffering not incompatible with messianic kingship, it is necessary, for it is God's providential pathway to glory.

So enthralled and taken up are they by the conversation, that the miles imperceptibly slip by, and suddenly Jesus and the two disciples find themselves on the outskirts of Emmaus village, probably the couple's home. There is a heightening of suspense. The two are no longer so self-absorbed; they respond to the stranger, concerned for his need. Jesus makes as if to go on,[65] a gesture which evokes that beautiful invitation, almost a demand:[66] "Stay with us, for evening draws on and the day is almost over" (24:29 NEB).

The disciples thus take the initiative in response to Jesus and his words. It is not without significance that Jesus waits to be asked, for he never imposes himself, never forces his friendship; with remarkable sensitivity, he reverences our freedom. But once the offer of hospitality is extended, he accepts promptly (see also Rev 3:20; John 14:23). Later they sit at table together.[67] Again, Jesus is sharing table with people who have failed, but this time they are his failed disciples.[68] Jesus, though the guest, assumes the role of host: "He took the bread, said the blessing; then he broke it and handed it to them." As has happened so often in the ministry, as Luke tells the story, we find Jesus eating with broken people. He reaches out and touches them in their failure and disloyalty, their fragility and inadequacy, and breaks with them the bread of reconciliation and friendship.[69] That outreach and acceptance in table fellowship transforms their understanding and opens their eyes, and, no doubt recalling earlier meals they had shared, at last they recognise him. At this, he vanishes from their midst.

The Emmaus narrative does not conform precisely to the normal pattern of appearance stories in its conclusion, for there is no explicit commissioning. Nevertheless, the sense of mission is strongly in evidence, for the effect of the encounter with the Lord is that the two disciples depart without delay, in spite of impending darkness, and retrace their route to Jerusalem in order to reach out and share with the others of their band this Gladdening News so filled with promise. Having abandoned Jerusalem in disappointment and scepticism, they now return in faith, with a spring in their step and a smile in their eyes, their hearts on fire, to begin afresh and to bear witness to the resurrection. "Where before they were ex-followers of a dead prophet, now they are followers of the Risen Lord." [70]

On their arrival, the two disciples find the eleven and the rest of the company assembled, and their news is confirmed: "The Lord has been raised and has appeared to Simon." The risen Jesus has in the meantime reached out to Simon in a similar way, extending to him, too, his forgiveness and fellowship, his reconciliation. Simon, the first official witness to the resurrection of Jesus, can now strengthen the faith of the other disciples (22:32). Easter faith has already been born in Jerusalem.[71]

The Appearance to The Group of Disciples (24:36–49)

As the whole company of his followers talk together excitedly about these extraordinary occurrences, Jesus interrupts them as he suddenly appears in their midst, wishing them peace.[72] Their immediate reaction is one of intense fear, panic and doubt ("emotional turmoil and cognitive confusion"); they think they are seeing a ghost.[73] Jesus asks why they are afraid and doubting, inviting them to look at his hands and feet, even to touch him. The bodily reality of the risen Jesus is emphasised, though not subject to the normal limitations of our humanity in terms of time, space and movement.[74] He is clearly not a disembodied spirit or a ghost! It really is the same Jesus. Joy invades their wonder and disbelief as they struggle to come to terms with what is happening, which seems too good to be true.[75] Jesus asks whether there is anything to eat and partakes of the grilled fish they provide, a clear indication of his bodily reality; one presumes that the customary bread was also available. Table fellowship is again experienced.[76]

Jesus uses this opportunity at the meal table, in what amounts to a farewell speech, to open the scriptures to them: the Law, the prophets and the psalms. What he shared with the Emmaus couple he now expounds to the whole group. Recalling his teaching during the ministry, he reiterates the message that whatever scripture had said about him had to be fulfilled.[77] He opens their minds to a new level of understanding. He specifies two things. First, the scriptures make it clear that the Messiah must suffer and rise from the dead on the third day. Secondly, the Good News of repentance and forgiveness must be proclaimed in his name to all the nations, starting from Jerusalem.[78] Their role or mission, now formalised, is to bear witness to all that has occurred and all that Jesus has explained. Throughout his ministry they have heard his teaching, been present for his acts of mercy and healing, have encountered him in his risen state and have now been led to understand the scriptures and grasp God's saving plan. They have themselves experienced this transforming forgiveness so profoundly in table fellowship with him.[79] Finally, he reveals his intention to send upon them what the Father promised, commanding them to stay in Jerusalem until they are clothed with power from on high, the Holy Spirit. Empowered by the Spirit, they will be enabled to carry out faithfully their mission of witness and proclamation to the world.[80]

The Ascension (24:50–53)

Then he led them out as far as Bethany, and, lifting up his hands, he blessed them. While he was blessing them, he withdrew from them and was carried up into heaven. And they worshipped him, and returned to Jerusalem with great joy; and they were continually in the temple blessing God.

Luke's Gospel closes with another journey, as Jesus leads the group out across the Kidron, as he had done before, and up the hill to Bethany.[81] He does not speak again but gives a final blessing and is carried up into heaven, completing his "exodus".[82] His movement is twofold, away from them and up into heaven. This "signifies the finality of Jesus' departure (until the parousia) and Jesus' glorified status."[83] At this the disciples worship him, which is a clear indication that they have finally recognised his true identity. Then they make their way back to the city, as instructed, but do so replete with joy. They are people transformed. From that moment on, they were continually in the temple blessing God and waiting for the fulfilment of Jesus' final promise. The Gospel ends in the place, setting and atmosphere where it began. The next phase, the phase of mission, will begin there too. Its Spirit-directed unfolding and expanding will be described in Luke's second book, the Acts.[84]

Reflections

This final section of Luke's Gospel is a rich source for our reflection. The women, who approach the tomb of Jesus in order to perform a final act of love for the Master, have their sorrow turned to joy at the message conveyed by the two angelic figures. It is a classic Lukan reversal, a transformation beyond their wildest dreams and expectations. They listen to the angels' word and remember what Jesus had told them in Galilee. Spontaneously, they rush to tell the eleven and the other members of the group this amazing news. It just has to be shared. Remembering and sharing must be twin aspects of our mission.

In the Emmaus story, Luke is less concerned with the resurrection of Jesus as a past event than with the active presence of the risen Lord in the life of the community. He is interested in highlighting those aspects and areas of our living where Jesus continues to encounter us today.[85]

First, it is so easy for us to empathise with the Emmaus couple in their loss and bereavement experience, and in their need to talk about their dreams and their pain and disillusionment. We have ourselves been there too. We, also, "had hoped". At times, our schemes and dreams and plans fall apart. It is a struggle to see meaning in failure or change, oppression or injustice, in loss of any kind. We can feel let down by friends and family, by people in leadership roles, by those we seek to serve and to whom we minister, by the Church, by God. There can be much anger and frustration and hurt within us.

Luke is assuring us that Jesus is present with us in these situations, in our stumbling and groping, when we feel 'let down'; he is walking our way alongside us as faithful companion and friend. It is so important to acknowledge our pain and to share our feelings with him in our prayer, to allow him into our messiness and shadows. His strengthening and liberating presence is frequently mediated by others, fellow travellers, who, through their own suffering and journeying, have learned how to 'be with', have learned how to listen, empathise, offer a healing space, the gift of hospitality. It is important to be able to trust and share about our disappointments. Some people carry this kind of pain for years and years, and it can affect and infect relationships, decisions, attitudes, ministry.

Secondly, the failure of the disciples to recognise Jesus can stimulate us to ask what it is in ourselves that can hinder the realisation of his presence with us. The disciples seem too depressed, too caught up in their problems and grief. Perhaps their God is too small, their expectations too limited and narrow. They are not open to what is new and unexpected and freely given, to a God of such unfathomable love, a God of surprises. We, too, can at times be bogged down in the rut of routine or the heavy sands of our problems and preoccupations; or we can be just too busy. We can be blinded by our self-centredness or introspection, deafened by the strident sounds inside and around us. Perhaps we are looking for a God fashioned to our own sketchy design; perhaps we are pining for what is tried and comfortable, afraid of letting go, of losing our control and security. Like the Emmaus couple, we can thus be closed to the divine stranger, and he goes unrecognised.

Thirdly, one of the points that the evangelist wishes to teach us, through this narrative and also the later appearance of Jesus to the larger group of disciples, is that in the study and prayerful pondering of scripture, the risen Lord is to be encountered, is reassuringly present, deepening our insight and understanding, widening our perspectives, firming up our commitment, disturbing and challenging our lives, "setting our hearts on fire". The risen Jesus is present whenever his life-giving word, the Good News of God's forgiveness, acceptance and faithful love, is proclaimed. It is a word which also summons us to model our lives on the messianic pattern of his and to surrender in trust to the mystery of God's loving plan. Today there is much greater interest in reflecting on scripture, in *lectio divina*. Perhaps we need to ask ourselves whether we are indeed people of the word.

In addition, one of the details of the narrative which fascinates me is the change that takes place in the disciples as they listen to Jesus' words. As long as they are concerned exclusively with their own problems and grief and disappointment, their horizons are shrouded in thick cloud. But their focus changes; they begin to look beyond themselves; they see the stranger's need for food and shelter and rest; they open their hearts to the other. The clouds then begin to lift and the sun filters through. In this, I believe that the evangelist is reminding us that the risen Lord is present and can be encountered wherever there is care and service of others, however ordinary and prosaic its mode of expression might be. Selflessness can open our eyes so that we may catch a glimpse of him. I think that it is also true that our love, hospitality and acceptance of others can be the occasion for them to perceive that he is touching their lives too.

Furthermore, for the two disciples, recognition finally takes place at table in the breaking of bread, and the larger group seem to be dining, too, when Jesus appears to them. Luke is reminding us that it is in the Eucharist that the presence of the risen Lord continues in the Christian community; in the eucharistic celebration he can be encountered most powerfully in our midst. Like those original disciples, we celebrate the Eucharist repeatedly as fragile and imperfect people. Eucharist is a reconciling event. It is an encounter with the risen Jesus which has the potential to transform and reshape our lives.[86]

Finally, like the women from the tomb, the two disciples are on fire to share their Good News, reaching out in mission to the others. And the following episode highlights this element, as Jesus sends them out, "preaching repentance for the forgiveness of sins to all nations." Failed disciples have been forgiven and restored; they have experienced the compassionate mercy of God; they can vouch for the truth of the message that they proclaim. This surely gives us courage as we reach out to others in mission and ministry.

Thinking of mission, we can, I believe, find in these narratives an exciting model for our ministry, as we journey with people entrusted to our care. We are called to walk alongside them, even when they are travelling in the wrong direction! We are to be present with them, accepting them where they are, listening to their story, feeling their hopes and their disappointments. We move at their pace, respecting their dignity and freedom. There is a time to ask a question, a time to suggest an explanation, a time to offer a challenge, a time to share our experience too. We can accept and offer hospitality, and share 'table fellowship'. We may break together the bread of Word and Sacrament, and forge together new ways of responding to the Gospel of Jesus. Together we may experience new Emmaus moments, and, our hearts burning within us, find our way to a new Jerusalem, a place where we have never been before.

Notes

1   Tannehill, *Luke*, 349, maintains that Luke's resurrection chapter is basically the story of the risen Messiah's revelation of God's redemptive plan to his followers, in preparation for their mission. Reginald H. Fuller, *The Formation of the Resurrection Narratives* (London: SPCK, 1972), 95, believes that Luke has introduced considerable changes to Mark, or is following an independent tradition, with an eye on Mark as well. Francis J. Moloney, *The Resurrection of the Messiah: A Narrative Commentary on the Resurrection Accounts in the Four Gospels* (New York: Paulist, 2013), 99, n. 80, notes that almost all scholars accept that Luke had Mark before him; he alternates between a creative use of Mark and an equally creative use of his own source.

2   The oldest account of the empty tomb is probably that reflected in John, Magdalene's first visit (20:1–3). The emptiness of the tomb did not give rise to resurrection faith (though the Beloved Disciple is said to have come to belief). It was the appearances of Jesus to his disciples which gave rise to faith, as well as providing the explanation why the tomb was empty. In passing on the tradition it was necessary to insert an explanation. See Raymond E. Brown, *The Virginal Conception and Bodily Resurrection of Jesus* (London: Geoffrey Chapman, 1974), 122–23.

3   "The third day" means the decisive day; in Hosea, it denotes "soon". For some, the Jewish view was that a person was really dead after the third day, so it means God raised Jesus from real death; see Pagola, *Jesus*, 390. For Lohfink, *Jesus of Nazareth*, 299, the dating stems from events which took place at the tomb.

4   In Luke, Jesus ascends on Easter Sunday night after the appearance to the group (24:50–51); he later describes an ascension in Acts. In John, after the Thomas appearance, the Gospel ends. There is no room in these accounts for Galilee appearances. (Brown, *Bodily Resurrection*, 102).

5   Moloney, *Resurrection*, 145, sees this as the oldest tradition. In the other Gospels, other women accompany Magdalene; the purpose of the visit is to anoint the body of Jesus; their presence would improve credibility, though the witness of women was valueless in the Jewish world. Mark 16:9 relates an appearance to Magdalene; she told the others, who would not believe her message. Lohfink, *Jesus of Nazareth*, 299, notes elements that suggest a real event. Female witnesses argue in favour of plausibility;

polemical opposition presupposes that the tomb was empty. Pagola, *Jesus*, 403, observes that the earliest confessions and hymns, and also Paul, do not mention the empty tomb; it did not play a significant role in the birth of faith.

6   Brown, *Bodily Resurrection*, 120, comments that the presence of the stone was not mentioned in the Johannine burial account, and so could have been original (besides, the risen Jesus can pass through obstacles!).

7   The Beloved Disciple perceives the action of God in this, but remains silent about it. There are traces of this sequence in Luke 24:10–12, 24.

8   A young man in Mark, sitting inside the tomb on the right; an angel in Matthew seated outside on the rolled-back stone; two men in Luke, standing inside; two angels in John, seated inside. For other variants in the four traditions, see Brown, *Bodily Resurrection*, 118. On p. 122, he observes that angelic interpreters were no more than mouthpieces of revelation, without any personality. Marshall, *Luke*, 883, considers the angelic message "a literary device" to bring out the significance of the discovery of the empty tomb.

9   Moloney, *Resurrection*, 144; Lohfink, *Jesus of Nazareth*, 299.

10   Brown, *Bodily Resurrection*, 124, notes that the pre-Pauline formula includes the reference to the third day (which was the first day of the week); this reference probably reflects the events surrounding the empty tomb. Moloney, *Resurrection*, 143, maintains that that there is a pre-Gospel tradition before Mark and John "with roots in solid historical memory".

11   See Pagola, *Jesus*, 387. Jesus mentions this on the way to Gethsemane (Mark 14:28); see also John 16:32. The Markan man at the tomb says: "Go, tell his disciples and Peter that he is going ahead of you to Galilee; there you will see him just as he told you" (16:7). Likewise, the angel at the tomb in Matthew, and then Jesus himself (28:7; 28:10). Lohfink, *Jesus of Nazareth*, 289, maintains that lived history lies behind these words.

12   Lohfink, *Jesus of Nazareth*, 290.

13   Lohfink, *Jesus of Nazareth*, 298.

14   1 Cor 15:3–5; Luke 24:34 (a formulaic reference); John 21:1–14. Brown, *Bodily Resurrection*, 109, suggests that Jesus appeared to Peter at the lakeside, and later to The Twelve at a meal. The glorified Lord poured out his Spirit on them and commissioned them. John 21 is a composite narrative. The implications of Jesus' resurrection gradually became evident and came to be incorporated in the narratives.

15   Brown, *Bodily Resurrection*, 106–08, suggests that the various evangelists are describing the same basic appearance to The Twelve, through which they are commissioned for their future task. The words of commissioning are different in each of the Gospels; they reflect the style of the individual evangelist. Probably the risen Jesus did not use words.

16   The appearances, not the empty tomb, give rise to resurrection faith. Lohfink, *Jesus of Nazareth*, 290–91, states clearly that the appearances to Peter and the inner group of disciples took place in Galilee. Luke and John locate the appearances in Jerusalem for theological reasons.

17   "Let himself be seen" or "made himself visible" is probably a better translation than "appeared".

18   Moloney, *Resurrection*, 144, asserts that most Christian scholars adhere to the

historicity of the empty tomb.

19   Brown, *Bodily Resurrection*, 110, refers to a charismatic manifestation of the Spirit they had already received. Lohfink, *Jesus of Nazareth*, 303, stresses the eschatological dimension of this outpouring; an outpouring of the Spirit was an element of end time expectation (Joel 2:28; 3:1–5). Earlier, he stresses the link between the resurrection of Jesus and the expectations of end time general resurrection; eschatology was strong in that first group; that is why they returned to Jerusalem, which would be the centre for end time events.

20   Williams, *God with* Us, 62.

21   Phil 2:10–11; Rom 10:9; 1 Cor 12:3. For this see Brown, *Bodily Resurrection*, 78–80. He suggests one, two or four-member formulas; he believes the antithetical formulas are probably earlier. The emphasis is on the activity of the Father (the divine passive is often used). See also Joseph Ratzinger, Benedict XVI, *Jesus of Nazareth: Part 2: Holy Week—From the Entrance into Jerusalem to the Resurrection*, trans. Philip J. Whitmore (San Francisco: Ignatius Press, 2011), 2:248–251.

22   1 Thess 4:14.

23   Rom 8:34; 4:24; 14:9; 2 Cor 13:4.

24   Pagola, *Jesus*, 3 88–90: *egeirein, anistanai*. The language of exaltation and glorification is found in early hymns (Phil 2:6–11; 1 Tim 3:16; Eph 4:7–10; Rom 10:5–8); resurrection and exaltation are used interchangeably. There is also the language of being alive (maybe more acceptable for gentiles). But there is no "immortality of the soul" language. Bodily resurrection indicates the whole person; but it is a glorified body. The early disciples did not have the language to describe what they had experienced.

25   Acts 2:14–41; 3:12–26; 4:9–12; 5:29–32; 10:34–43; and Paul in 13:16–47. Luke is the author of these speeches, taking up earlier material; it gives an idea of how the first Christians proclaimed their faith, the sort of thing they were saying.

26   See Rom 6:9–10. Brown, *Bodily Resurrection*. 87, speaks of the continuity of the corporeal element of personal existence. Lohfink, *Jesus of Nazareth*, 295–97, notes that ideas of exaltation, rapture/translation, resurrection, were already available in Jewish thought (Isa 52:13–15 and Ps 110; 2 Kgs 2:1–18; Isa 26:19 and Dan 12:2). All three are used in the early Church for Jesus; see also Brown, *Bodily Resurrection*, 76. Resurrection was understood as an eschatological event and was for many (or all). Probably, the disciples understood Jesus' resurrection (as an individual) as introducing the general resurrection as a kind of prelude, and expected this rather soon ("firstborn": 1 Cor 15:20; Col 1:18; Rev 1:5). Brown, *Bodily Resurrection*, 76, notes that the choice of resurrection language was not inevitable; there was no expectation of the raising of a single individual.

27   Williams, *God with Us*, 65. Ratzinger, *Jesus of Nazareth*, 2:244–246, comments that Jesus breaks into an entirely new form of life, a life which opens up a new dimension of human existence; it is an evolutionary leap. On p. 266, he refers to the dialectic of identity and otherness, of real physicality and freedom from the constraints of the body.

28   Ratzinger, *Jesus of Nazareth*, 2:248, distinguishes the confessional tradition and the narrative tradition.

29   N. Tom Wright, *The Resurrection of the Son of God* (London: SPCK, 2003), 660, affirms that the individual evangelists have clearly felt free to shape and retell their stories

in such a way as to bring out their own particular emphases and theological intentions. Williams, *God with Us*, 76, describes the resurrection stories as "abrupt, confused, vivid and unpolished"; their untidiness is one of the main reasons for taking them seriously as historical reportage. He notes the lack of Old Testament echoes. The Gospel accounts are pressed into existence by facts; they do not fit into any pre-existing pattern. Nothing like it had happened previously; it is an event which inaugurates something completely new. (pp. 77–80)

30   Gerald O'Collins, *The Easter Jesus* (London: Darton, Longman and Todd, 1973), 23, 36–38, notes that in Paul's list of recipients of resurrection appearances (1 Cor 15:3–8), he provides no geographical details. The important thing is that Jesus was raised and appeared; *where* Jesus met his disciples matters little. Peter and the disciples are the primary witnesses to the resurrection: that is the historical truth, wherever the evangelists place them.

31   1 Cor 15:8–11; 9:1; Gal 1:13–23; Phil 3:5–14. Brown, *Bodily Resurrection*, 87, notes that Paul does not agree with Luke! On p. 89, he refers to "the artistry of effective narration."

32   Gerald O'Collins, *Easter Faith: Believing in the Risen Jesus* (London: Darton, Longman and Todd, 2003), 25, holds that historical authenticity can hardly be claimed for any words attributed to the risen Christ. See also Wright, *The Resurrection*, 679.

33   Pagola, *Jesus*, 400, comments that Schillebeeckx sees forgiveness as the matrix in which faith in Jesus as the risen one is born. Rowan Williams, *Resurrection: Interpreting the Easter Gospel* (London: Darton, Longman, Todd, 2014 (3rd edition)), xii, sees the resurrection stories as having to do with a sense of the absolution by God, creating forgiven persons, whose relationship with God, and, derivatively with each other, is transformed.

34   Pagola, *Jesus*, 392, 399. The stories do have a basis in reality. They recall experiences of Jesus' unexpected presence; early uncertainties and doubts; process of conversion; reflection on scripture; sense of mission.

35   Moloney, *Resurrection*, 148, concludes: "There is no 'knock-down' objective historical proof for the resurrection events reported in the Gospel narratives. But there is objective evidence that the earliest Church came into existence because of the encounter with the Risen Jesus—whatever that means." He quotes E. P. Sanders, *The Historical Figure of Jesus*, (London: The Penguin Press, 1993), 280: "That Jesus' followers (and later Paul) had resurrection experiences is, in my judgement, a fact. What the reality was that gave rise to the experiences I do not know."

36   Luke did not mention the stone when describing the burial. It was the normal practice to locate one at the tomb entrance. While Mark is Luke's source for the empty tomb episode, he has reshaped it. For a study of Mark's version see Winstanley, *Little People*, 167–171.

37   Johnson, *Luke*, 387, suggests that mention of two men and their shining clothes may recall the transfiguration scene. Later the two are referred to as "angels" (24:23); similarly, Tannehill, *Luke*, 349 (also in Acts 1:10, the ascension, there are two interpretive angels); McBride, *Luke*, 314; Carroll, *Luke*, 476–77. In Mark, there is one man dressed in a white robe, already seated on the right. In Matthew, there is an earthquake and an angel

appears and rolls away the stone; while the women are on their way to give the message to the disciples, Jesus himself appears to them, and gives them the same message about Galilee (28:8). In John, Magdalene goes to the tomb alone, finds it empty, returns to tell Simon Peter and the disciple Jesus loved. They return to the tomb, and leave again. Magdalene has also returned to the tomb and sees two angels in white, sitting where the body of Jesus had been lying, one at the head, the other at the feet.

38   The Greek (*ēgerthē*) is better translated as "he has been raised" (by God). Green, *Luke*, 837, recalls Jesus words to the Sadducees in 20:38: "he is a God not of the dead but of the living."

39   9:22 (but no women present); 9:44 (women present but no mention of resurrection). The wording is slightly different ("sinners" and "crucifixion" are here included). Luke changes the message in Mark and Matthew that tells the women to inform the disciples that Jesus will meet them in Galilee; Jesus had also mentioned this after the Last Supper *en route* for the mount of Olives (14:28). Luke's focus is on Jerusalem. Fuller, *Resurrection Narratives*, 97, states that his changes are clearly motivated by his editorial requirements; he intends to record the appearances of the risen Jesus in Jerusalem, not Galilee. Johnson, *Luke*, 387, notes that it is typical of Luke's presentation of the resurrection tradition to recapitulate the earlier story and show how Jesus' words have been fulfilled. Carroll, *Luke*, 477, notes the importance of prophecy/promise and fulfilment in this chapter of Luke (also Fuller, *Resurrection Narratives*, 99). On p. 98, he points out that Luke uses "must" (*dei*) forty-one times, more frequently than the other evangelists.

40   Johnson, *Luke*, 391, maintains that their remembering indicates that they have come to faith and understanding; similarly, Moloney, *Resurrection*, 80. Green, *Luke*, 838, notes that to remember, as well as cognitive evocation, includes the nuance of understanding or insight. In Mark, the women are told to go and inform the disciples, but fail to do so (16:8). In Luke, they do so without there being any instruction. Moloney, *Resurrection*, 80, emphasises the importance for Luke of "remembering". The use of "apostles" prior to the resurrection is typically Lukan; Fuller, *Resurrection Narratives*, 99, notes that for Luke an apostle is a witness to the saving events from Jesus' baptism till his ascension.

41   Magdalene and Joanna were mentioned in 8:2–3, along with Susanna, who is not mentioned here; Mary, the mother of James is now included. Unlike Mark, Luke has not mentioned them by name on Calvary or at the burial; Mark's three lists are not entirely consistent.

42   Johnson, *Luke*, 388, comments that the term (*lēros*) (medically meaning "delirious") could hardly be more condescending; "there is a definite air of male superiority in this response." Green, *Luke*, 840, notes the cultural bias against women as reliable witnesses.

43   The Western manuscript tradition does not contain reference to Peter's visit, possibly because it was thought to be an interpolation from John, but most other manuscripts do include it, and most modern scholars accept it. See Green, *Luke*, 480; Johnson, *Luke*, 388; Fitzmyer, *Luke*, 2:1542, 1547. Carroll, *Luke*, 479–80; Evans, *Luke*, 899–900, are among those who do not.

44   Fuller, *Resurrection Narratives*, 104. Evans, *Luke*, 901, recognises its dramatic quality and its artistry. Fitzmyer, *Luke*, 2:1554–55, believes that there is a tradition behind the story (like Mark 16:12–13) upon which Luke has freely built; indications include Emmaus, Cleopas, and the kerygma of v. 34. Fuller, *Resurrection Narratives*, 106, provides a possible early form, which may stem from the Syrian community.

45   Carroll, *Luke*, 480.

46   Carroll, *Luke*, 482, observes that in rejoining his followers the risen Lord resumes his teaching role, feasts with them at table, and interprets the recent hope-deflating events in the light of the Jewish scriptures.

47   This scheme was first proposed by C.H. Dodd, *The Founder of Christianity* (London: Collins, 1971) 175; "The Appearances of the Risen Christ: An Essay in Form-Criticism of the Gospels," in *Studies in the Gospel: Essays in Memory of R.H. Lightfoot*, ed. Dennis E Nineham (Oxford: Blackwell, 1957), 9–35; also see Brown, *John*: 2:972–975. Green, *Luke*, 842, suggests a structure involving inverted parallelism, and Carroll, *Luke*, 482, a concentric structure.

48   For details of possibilities, see Marshall, *Luke*, 892–93; he concludes that certainty is impossible. Fitzmyer, *Luke*, 2:1562, observes that what matters for Luke is the place's proximity to Jerusalem; likewise, Johnson, *Luke*, 393. Moloney, *Resurrection*, 96, lists several authors who miss the importance of the fact that they are walking away from Jerusalem. Carroll, *Luke*, 483, notes that the village is near Jerusalem but not Jerusalem itself; the spatial movement away from the city bears symbolic meaning.

49   Caird, *Luke*, 259; McBride, *Luke*, 317. Fitzmyer, *Luke*, 2:1561, suggests that the unnamed disciple may be one of the eleven; 2:1563, he dismisses any link between Cleopas (Cleopatros) and Clopas. Fuller, however, *Resurrection Narratives*, 107, notes that Jews often took a similar sounding Greek name in addition to their Semitic name. On p. 108 he lists several names which have been proposed; similarly, Marshall, *Luke*, 894.

50   Francis J. Moloney, *Reading the New Testament in the Church: A Primer for Pastors, Religious Educators, and Believers* (Grand Rapids, MI: Baker Academic, 2015), 129; *Resurrection*, 81–82, they have made the wrong choice, abandoning God's saving story; McBride, *Luke*, 316.

51   Carroll, *Luke*, 483, notes the use of two verbs *homilein* and *syzētein*, suggesting a spirited exchange of differing opinions.

52   Here the verb is *antiballō*, which means to toss back and forth.

53   The Greek is *paroikein*. Johnson, *Luke*, 393, notes that the term is appropriate for someone staying in the city for the festival. Byrne, *Hospitality*, 187, considers the question sharp, cynical and ironic.

54   Moloney, *Resurrection*, 82, believes that the use of the divine passive indicates the action of God here. In *Reading*, 129, he comments that although God is not mentioned, God is responsible; God is not abandoning the disciples; likewise, Byrne, *Hospitality*, 187. Carroll, *Luke*, 483, refers to God's agency in the concealment and disclosure alike. Caird, *Luke*, 257, writes: "In retrospect their failure to recognise him seemed so odd that they could only suppose a supernatural restraint had been imposed on their vision and not removed until their minds were prepared for the staggering revelation" to come. Green, *Luke*, 845, disagrees with this view. Fitzmyer, *Luke*, 2:1558, sees it as a literary device to

advance the story and create suspense. They need to be instructed first. Evans, *Luke*, 905, holds that probably a supernatural action of God is denoted; this he sees as a theological narrative device.

55   Moloney, *Resurrection*, 96, n. 52, quotes with approval Tannehill's view that they are not without guilt in their inability to recognise Jesus. They are not ready to deal with Jesus' death, and this is a culpable failure. Johnson, *Luke*, 395, translates "reluctant to believe", implying moral failure.

56   Jesus is treated as an uninformed stranger, yet is the subject of all that has happened.

57   Moloney, *Reading*, 130, calls this "a catechetical-liturgical process."

58   Jesus refers to himself as a prophet in 4:24 and 13:33, both linked with rejection and death. In Acts, he is put forward as the expected prophet like Moses (3:22; 7:37), an alternative eschatological expectation. See Tannehill, *Luke*, 353; on p. 356, he writes that scripture and the story of Jesus are being read in the light of a presumed prophetic destiny that includes suffering, rejection and even death.

59   Fitzmyer, *Luke*, 2:1564, notes that the Jewish authorities are held responsible, not the Romans (see 23:13). Again, Luke substitutes "crucified" for "put to death".

60   Moses is described like this in Acts 7:22; see also Deut 34:10–12. See Green, *Luke*, 846; Fuller, *Resurrection Narratives*, 110. There is an echo of Anna's words in 2:38. Their expectations of national deliverance were misguided.

61   In Luke's empty tomb story, Peter went to the tomb alone.

62   Moloney, *Resurrection*, 83; *Reading*, 130. They have not remembered his words. Green, *Luke*, 848, notes the importance of "seeing" for Luke. Carroll, *Luke*, 484, too observes that the disciples cannot see; visual perception is a metaphor for understanding.

63   Carroll, *Luke*, 484, n. 11: "heart" in both cognitive and affective dimensions, as the locus of thinking, attitude, and life-orienting commitment.

64   Caird, *Luke*, 258. For Johnson, *Luke*, 396, "glory" means kingly rule and authority; similarly, Tannehill, *Luke*, 355. Evans, *Luke*, 910, understands "glory" as a heavenly mode of existence connected with the resurrection. Moloney, *Resurrection*, 84, calls this a liturgy of the Word. He notes the use of the passive to indicate Jesus' role in responding to God's design, and the mention of fulfilment and necessity (*dei*). No specific references are provided by the evangelist. For Fuller, *Resurrection Narratives*, 111, the fulfilment of scripture is the principal motif of the story. It is also part of the primitive formula in 1 Cor 15:3–4.

65   The Greek is *prospoieō*, meaning to pretend, to act as though.

66   The verb *parabiazō* means to force or urge; it denotes compulsion.

67   Fitzmyer, *Luke*, 2:1567, points out that according to Jewish reckoning, the Sunday is over; Luke seems to consider the time after sundown to be the same day.

68   Robert. J. Karris, "God's Boundary-Breaking Mercy", in *The Bible Today*, 24 (1986), 27–28.

69   Green, *Luke*, 849, links the gesture with 9:16, the miraculous feeding. Fitzmyer, *Luke*, 2:1568, recalls also 22:19, the multiplication and the Supper; also, Marshall, *Luke*, 898. Fitzmyer, *Luke*, 2:1559, states that the action of Jesus recalls the Supper, and becomes the classic Lukan way of referring to the Eucharist. Moloney, *Reading*, 131,

writes: "The memory of the many meals that Jesus has shared with them, and especially the meal he shared on the night before he died, opens their eyes and anticipates the many meals that will be celebrated in the future"; also, *Resurrection*, 84–85; similarly, Johnson, *Luke*, 396. Caird, *Luke*, 259, refers to other meals that Jesus had held with his friends, perhaps like the Last Supper, as anticipations of the messianic banquet of the Kingdom.

70   McBride, *Luke*, 320. Johnson, *Luke*, 397, notes that the same verb is used both for opening the scriptures and the opening of their eyes. "As they perceived the true, messianic meaning of the Scripture, they were also able to 'see' Jesus in the breaking of the bread." Also, Tannehill, *Luke*, 358; Evans, *Luke*, 914.

71   Moloney, *Resurrection*, 85. He notes that the name Simon is used here, as at his original call (4:38) and in foretelling the denials (22:31). He too is a failed disciple, a sinner who has been forgiven. Luke states the appearance to Peter, as does Paul in 1 Cor 15:5; there is no narrative.

72   Johnson, *Luke*, 398, sees the Emmaus story as providing an emotionally satisfying bridge between the shock of absence and the shock of full presence. Some manuscripts omit the greeting; Carroll, *Luke*, 489, 90, considers it an interpolation by a scribe wishing to conform Luke with John (20:19, 26). As Tannehill, *Luke*, 359, points out, mention of "peace" recalls 1:79; 2:14, 29; 10:5–6; 19:42; it is more than a conventional greeting. For Green, *Luke*, 854, peace for Luke means salvation. Carroll, *Luke*, 488, 491, notes the repetition of the pattern of divine activity through Jesus' revelatory presence and teaching in overcoming obstacles to the disciples' understanding and secure faith. Moloney, *Body Broken*, 151; *Resurrection*, *87*, lists the many parallels between the Emmaus story and the room scene: they are talking to one another; Jesus appears; he is not recognised; he asks a rhetorical question; there is scripture-based instruction; there are revealing actions with bread and fish; Jesus disappears; they return to Jerusalem.

73   Carroll, *Luke*, 490.

74   This is also the case in John 20: 19–29, which contains explicit mention of the nail marks. The emphasis in Luke is on Jesus' physical reality. In all appearance stories, Jesus is the same person, but different. There is continuity but transformation. Paul (1 Cor 15: 43–49) gives greater emphasis to the transformation; Luke and John perhaps overemphasise the physicality. Caird, *Luke*, 260–61, notes that for Jews, reality was always particular and concrete; it was inevitable that this concreteness should find expression in materialistic imagery. Ratzinger, *Jesus of Nazareth*, 2:269, refers to Luke exaggerating in his apostolic zeal.

75   McBride, *Luke*, 322; Green, *Luke*, 855, who also notes that incontrovertible evidence of Jesus' embodied existence is not capable of producing faith; scriptural illumination is required.

76   Moloney, *Resurrection*, 87, notes that the meal table is the place where he gives them his final instructions. The incident recalls the meal of 9:16. This and the Emmaus meal bring the many Gospel meals to a climax. Byrne, *Hospitality*, 191, also emphasises the meal context; also, Tannehill, *Luke*, 360. Green, *Luke*, 855, n. 9, believes that this should not be read into the text; Evans, *Luke*, 920, maintains that this is not a meal. Carroll, *Luke*, 492, sees Jesus as guest and recipient of the disciples' hospitality; in the future, they will be the providers of hospitality.

77   Carroll, *Luke*, 492, notes how the psalms (added here to Law and prophets) feature prominently in the Christological exegesis of scripture, especially in the speeches of Acts (2:25–28; 4:25–28; 13:33–37). Green, *Luke*, 856, adds that they play an important role in Luke's interpretation of the passion. He also stresses divine purpose and fulfilment.

78   Green, *Luke*, 857–58, notes the importance of Isa 49:6 for Luke (2:32; Acts 13:47). Instead of a centripetal orientation for the universal mission, it is now centrifugal. "Already the effects of the rending of the temple veil at Jesus' death are being felt." "Repentance" means the realignment of one's life (dispositions and behaviours) towards God's purpose. In Acts, the name of Jesus is an important motif.

79   Moloney, *Resurrection*, 88, observes that it is on the basis of their own experience of repentance and forgiveness that they are commissioned to bear witness to the nations. They are well qualified to do so. Tannehill, *Luke*, 361, notes that forgiveness was central to the mission of John the Baptist and Jesus; it is in Jesus' name, with his authority, that the message is to be proclaimed to all. Carroll, *Luke*, 492, speaks of Jesus' ministry of "release" (*aphesis*), (1:77; 3:3; 4:18–19).

80   Johnson, *Luke*, 403, suggests that this promise recalls that of 1:35 to Mary. On p. 406, he recalls that in the cases of both Moses and Elijah their spirit was transmitted to their successors at their departure (Deut 34:9; 2 Kgs 2:9). Green, *Luke*, 853, reminds us that the ministry of Jesus has been conducted in the power of the Spirit. Evans, *Luke*, 925–26, sees the exalted Jesus as the dispenser of the Spirit from heaven.

81   Green, *Luke*, 859, notes that this passage contains many textual problems; the NRSV text represents current scholarly consensus. Carroll, *Luke*, 495, notes that Bethany recalls the beginning of Jesus' triumphal entry into Jerusalem. The event now underway is a triumphal exit. Green, *Luke*, 860, observes that whereas Luke has hitherto marked chronology carefully and explicitly, he does not do so here. The impression is that the ascension too took place on the Sunday evening, but Luke leaves open other possibilities, which he exploits in Acts 1:1–11. The group present here is wider than the apostles. In Acts 1:12–15 those present number 120 persons.

82   See 2 Kgs 2:1–18 concerning Elijah and Elisha. Johnson, *Luke*, 403–404, recalls the blessings by Moses (Exod 17:11 LXX; Num 20:11; Exod 39:43) and Aaron (Lev 9:22); Carroll, *Luke*, 495, suggests Moses (Deut 33) and Jacob (Gen 49:28). Some scholars (like McBride, *Luke*, 323 and Evans, *Luke*, 928) refer to Lev 9:22 and Sir 50:20–22, which suggest reference to a priestly Jesus, operating outside the temple and city. But Luke has so far shown no interest in this idea. The leave-taking of Moses and Abraham is a more likely model. Carroll, *Luke*, 496, notes that after "he withdrew from them", not all manuscripts add "and was carried up into heaven"; he believes that this is a later addition, though this is not certain. For most readers, the ascension imagery completes the story, as Jesus is vindicated by God and is exalted to God's right hand as Messiah and Lord. Marshall, *Luke*, 909, considers evidence for omission to be weak.

83   Green, *Luke*, 861, understands this as a visible and concrete way of expressing the elevated status of Jesus, his glory and regal power. His way of suffering and humiliation is embraced by God. The ascension is a prelude to the outpouring of the Spirit and consequent mission of the Church.

84   There is an alternative and longer version of the ascension in Acts 1:1–11.

Johnson, *Luke,* 404, comments that ancient historians were less fastidious in such matters of overlap than are some contemporary scholars. See Byrne, *Hospitality,* 192.

85   Green, *Luke,* 843, notes the themes of journey, hospitality/table fellowship, and scriptural fulfilment. Fitzmyer, *Luke,* 2:1557–59, lists geographical, revelatory, Christological (as fulfilling Old Testament prophecy), eucharistic.

86   Fitzmyer, *Luke,* 2:1569, acknowledges a eucharistic reference in "the breaking of bread". Carroll, *Luke,* 487, sees the Emmaus meal as a proleptic anticipation of the bread-breaking meals of the community in Acts, and of the eschatological banquet.

Conclusion

We have now accomplished several excursions in Lukan terrain, exploring as we walked many of the themes in his presentation of the life and significance of Jesus of Nazareth. In doing so, we have probably come to appreciate better the great artistry of his narrative, the richness of his theology and spirituality and the strength of his challenge to our living.

Clearly, God is behind the story and behind our walking. It is God's saving plan and purpose that inexorably drives forward the events of Luke's narrative. Luke shows that the God of Jesus is the God of Israel, the God of mercy and faithful love. And it is God's merciful love and faithfulness that is behind the coming of Jesus into our world. For the developing and expanding Christian communities that he is addressing, Luke wishes to forge clear links of continuity with the story of Israel. He stresses the importance of fidelity to the Torah. His allusions to the Old Testament scriptures are myriad, some obvious, some subtle. He makes a point of showing that in Jesus, these scriptures reach their fulfilment, the dreams of the prophets come to realisation, their promises are honoured. This in turn indicates that God is faithful and can be trusted. God is also a God of surprises, who cannot be predicted or controlled, a God who seems to delight in turning situations on their head, reversing what seems negative in favour of something new and free and life-giving. His compassion and faithfulness take unexpected twists, often in favour of the poor and vulnerable. The most striking surprise and reversal is the resurrection of Jesus.

The Spirit is actively present from the outset: creative, inspiring, life-giving. Early characters in the story, whom we have encountered in the Infancy Narrative, are open to that presence. The beginning of Jesus' ministry is strongly influenced by the descent of the Spirit, anointing him for messianic mission. The Spirit remains with him throughout his journey and into his "exodus", and in his final message to his disciples, Jesus bids them wait for a fresh outpouring. The Acts describe the powerful and transforming action of the Spirit in the coming into being of the Christian community and its growth and development into the gentile world after the Pentecost event.[1]

Anointed by the Spirit as the Davidic Messiah, the life of Jesus is focused on the God, whom he calls "Abba", "Father" and who is utterly central to his life. Jesus is totally dedicated to his mission, the "must" of his life, the establishment of God's Kingdom. The nature of Jesus' mission, made clear in the Nazareth synagogue, is characterised by the word "release" (*aphesis*): liberation from all aspects of oppression, be this personal, social, cultural, institutional or physical, mental, spiritual. Such release is an experience of the salvation that Jesus brings in all dimensions of human experience.[2] Luke presents Jesus the Messiah as "a prophet mighty in deed and word before God and all the people."[3] As a prophet, Jesus claims to speak in God's name and reveals the God in whose name he speaks and acts. He brings healing and wholeness, forgiveness and freedom. He reaches out especially to those on the margins of religion and society, the outsiders (tax gatherers and prostitutes, lepers and the sick, sinners, women[4] and children), and does so with amazing openness, acceptance and a desire to include. He makes real and present the compassion and mercy of God, God's salvation. One significant prophetic gesture in this regard is his table fellowship, which graphically sums up what his ministry is about (seeking and finding and celebrating God's saving love). This openness is occasionally extended beyond the confines of Israel, to individuals from Samaria and the gentile world, and this sets the scene for the rapid development of the gentile and Samaritan mission later in Acts.

At the same time, as a prophet, his words, lifestyle and values are inevitably a critique of the world in which he lives, religious and secular. He seeks to challenge narrow-mindedness and prejudice and forms of exclusivity, discrimination and injustice. He is critical of misuse of the temple and of the common cultural mentality of power seeking, privilege, patronage and upward mobility. Jesus advocates status inversion, an alternative and countercultural way of relating to people and structuring society. He sees himself as a servant, and advocates self-giving and service as his way and the way of discipleship. All this, of course, invites hostility and opposition, particularly from the Pharisees, and we have caught a taste of this conflictual side of his ministry as we have walked. When Jesus finally reaches Jerusalem, the place of his "exodus", it is the priestly aristocracy who successfully orchestrate his shameful death at gentile hands. His death he accepts, placing himself, his mission and his future into the Father's hands. The faithful Father vindicates this trust and endorses his teaching, values and self-giving lifestyle by raising him from death and establishing him as "Lord".

The evangelist highlights that Jesus is a man of prayer and puts him forward as a model for his followers. Jesus himself offers a special prayer at his disciples' request, a prayer well known to all of us. His prayer in the garden and at his crucifixion, prayers of abandonment to God's will and forgiveness of enemies, are indications of Jesus' integrity. His dying prayer is placed before us as an illustration of how we should approach death, in trusting surrender to the God of life. In his teaching, Jesus advocates perseverance in our asking and trust in God's loving and providential care for us. An aspect of prayer that frequently occurs in Luke's narrative is praise; this is a response in the Infancy Narrative to the recognition of God's presence and action in the remarkable events that take place; later, it forms a frequent response to the realisation of God's presence and action in Jesus' healing activity. Such praise is accompanied by outbursts of joy.

Prayer and listening form one aspect of discipleship. Closely linked with this is the importance of 'doing', reaching out in compassion and unstinting service to those in need, and this as a permanent way of life, not just an occasional event. When it comes to the issue of discipleship, Jesus is demanding. He claims absolute loyalty; his urgent mission overrides family responsibilities and cultural traditions with disturbing radicality. Following him is not presented as a sinecure; the imagery of carrying one's cross is stark and forbidding. One area of Lukan concern that is striking highlights the area of riches and poverty. It is clear that he is ill at ease with growing affluence in his community and local churches. Aware of the dangers of wealth and complacency, which can stifle one's response to the Gospel, Luke includes words of Jesus that emphasise the need to share generously one's possessions with those in need. This is a message that is no less challenging for us today. Jesus well knows that disciples can fail; his initial group did so quite spectacularly. But he forgives, and his forgiveness is transformative and becomes integral to their proclamation to the nations.

It is my hope that, as we have walked through the Lukan narrative, exploring the evangelist's different themes, we have, like the Emmaus disciples, sensed Jesus' presence with us as our friend and saviour. Jesus continues to deepen our insight into God's love and purpose and our appreciation of God's providential care. Through our walking, perhaps our understanding of the meaning of discipleship has become clearer and its challenges sharper. I hope that there have been many occasions when we have felt "our hearts burning within us" and the urge to share the experience and message of Jesus with others.

Notes

1   Green, *Luke*, 22, maintains that the Holy Spirit is behind the realisation of the divine plan, putting into effect the will of God.

2   Powell, *The Gospels*, 104–107, stresses that for Luke, Jesus is saviour from the Infancy Narrative onwards and throughout his life; salvation is a present reality ("today"), not the result of Jesus' death or focused on the afterlife. Salvation is the result of a liberating encounter with Jesus.

3   Luke links the prophetic role of Jesus with both Moses and Elijah.

4   Women feature more frequently in Luke than in the other Synoptic Gospels. We have met Mary, Elizabeth and Anna in the Infancy Narrative. Mary Magdalene, Joanna and Susanna are named among the many who provided for Jesus and the disciples during the ministry; Mary Magdalene, Joanna and Mary the mother of James encounter the two angelic figures at the empty tomb. Mary and Martha welcome Jesus into their home. Jesus heals Simon's mother-in-law, raises the widow's son at Nain, is anointed by the woman in the house of Simon the Pharisee, raises Jairus' daughter to life, heals the woman afflicted with bleeding, heals a disabled woman in the synagogue, recognises the poor widow's generosity in the temple, addresses the "Daughters of Jerusalem" *en route* for Calvary, and includes women protagonists in parables. Some feminist scholars, however, consider Luke's portrait of women in the Gospel and Acts "ambiguous at best, and dangerous at worst." Rather than an advocate, he is considered as seeking to restrict and control. See, for example, Reid, *Parables*, 42–44.

Bibliography

On Luke

Byrne, Brendan. *The Hospitality of God: A Reading of Luke's Gospel.* Collegeville: Liturgical Press, 2000

Caird, G.B. *The Gospel of St. Luke.* Pelican Gospel Commentaries; Harmondsworth: Penguin, 1963

Carroll, John T. *Luke: A Commentary.* Louisville: Westminster John Knox Press, 2012

Catholic Bishops' Conference of England and Wales, and of Scotland, The. *The Gift of Scripture.* London: CTS, 2005

Chrupcala, L. Daniel. *Everyone Will See the Salvation of God: Studies in Lukan Theology.* Milan: Edizioni Terra Santa, 2015

Ellis, E. Earle. *The Gospel of Luke.* London: Oliphants, 1974

Evans, Christopher F. *Saint Luke.* London: SCM, 1990

Fallon, M. *Gospel According to St Luke: An Introductory Commentary.* Bangalore: Asian Trading Corporation, 1997

Fitzmyer, Joseph A. *The Gospel according to Luke*, 2 vols. New York: Doubleday, 1981, 1985

————. *Luke the Theologian: Aspects of his Teaching.* London: Geoffrey Chapman, 1989

Green, Joel B. *The Gospel of Luke*, NICNT. Cambridge: Eerdmans, 1997

Johnson, Luke T. *The Gospel of Luke*, Sacra Pagina 3. Collegeville MN: Liturgical Press, 1991

Karris, Robert J. *Luke: Artist and Theologian.* New York: Paulist, 1985

————. "God's Boundary-Breaking Mercy", *The Bible Today* 24, 1986

LaVerdiere, Eugene. *Luke.* Dublin: Veritas, 1980

Levine, Amy-Jill. "Luke: Introduction and Annotations" in *The Jewish Annotated New Testament*, eds. Amy-Jill Levine and Marc Zvi Brettler. New York: Oxford University Press, Inc., 2011

Marshall, I. Howard. *The Gospel of Luke: A Commentary on the Greek Text.* Exeter: Paternoster Press, 1978

372

McBride, Denis. *The Gospel of Luke: A Reflective Commentary.* Dublin: Dominican
Publications, 1991
Mosetto, F. *Lettura del Vangelo secondo Luca.* Rome: LAS, 2003
Powell, Mark A. *What is Narrative Criticism?* Minneapolis: Fortress, 1990
—————. *Fortress Introduction to The Gospels.* Minneapolis: Fortress, 1998
Reid, Barbara E. *A Retreat with Luke: Stepping Out on the Word of God.* Cincinnati:
St Anthony Messenger Press, 2000
Resseguie, James L. *Spiritual Landscape: Images of the Spiritual Life in the Gospel of
Luke.* Peabody MA: Hendrikson, 2004
—————. *Narrative Criticism of the New Testament. An Introduction.* Grand
Rapids: Baker Academic, 2005
Tannehill, Robert C. *Luke.* Nashville: Abingdon Press, 1996
Thompson, G.H.P. *The Gospel according to Luke.* Oxford: Clarendon Press, 1972
Tuckett, Christopher M. *Luke.* Sheffield: Sheffield Academic Press, 1996.
Wright, N. Tom. *Luke for Everyone.* London: SPCK, 2001

Further Reading

Bailey, Kenneth E. *Poet and* Peasant and *Through Peasant Eyes.* Grand Rapids:
Eerdmans, 1983
—————. *Jesus Through Middle Eastern Eyes.* London: SPCK, 2008
—————. *The Good Shepherd.* London: SPCK, 2015
Bauckham, Richard. *Jesus and the Eyewitnesses: The Gospels as Eyewitness Testimony.*
Grand Rapids: Eerdmans, 2006
Borg, Marcus J. *Jesus: The Life, Teachings, and Relevance of a Religious Revolutionary.*
New York: HarperOne, 2006
Borg, Marcus J. and Crossan, John Dominic. *The First Christmas: What the Gospels
Really Teach About Jesus's Birth.* New York: HarperOne, 2007
Boxall, Ian. "Luke's Nativity Story: A Narrative Reading", in *New Perspectives on
the Nativity,* ed. Jeremy Corley, London: T&T Clark, 2009
Boring, M. Eugene. *Mark: A Commentary.* London: Westminster John Knox
Press, 2006
Brown, Raymond E. *New Testament Essays.* New York: Paulist Press, 1965
—————. *The Gospel According to John,* Anchor Bible, 2 vols. New York:
Doubleday, 1966; London: Geoffrey Chapman, 1971
—————. *The Virginal Conception and Bodily Resurrection of Jesus.* London:
Geoffrey Chapman, 1974

—————. *An Adult Christ at Christmas*. Collegeville MN: The Liturgical Press, 1978

—————. *A Coming Christ in Advent*. Collegeville MN: The Liturgical Press, 1988

—————. *The Birth of the Messiah*. London: Geoffrey Chapman, 1993

—————. *The Death of the Messiah*, 2 vols. London, Geoffrey Chapman, 1994

—————. *An Introduction to the New Testament*. The Anchor Bible Reference Library. New York: Doubleday, 1997

Byrne, Brendan. *A Costly Freedom: A Theological Reading of Mark's Gospel*. Collegeville MN: The Liturgical Press, 2008

Coloe, Mary L. *God Dwells with Us: Temple Symbolism in the Fourth Gospel*. Collegeville, MN: The Liturgical Press, 2001

Corley, Jeremy, ed. *New Perspectives on the Nativity*. London: T&T Clark, 2009

Crossan, John Dominic. *In Parables: The Challenge of the Historical Jesus*. San Francisco: Harper & Row, 1973

Culpepper, R. Alan. *The Gospel and Letters of John*. Nashville: Abingdon Press, 1998

—————. *Mark*. Macon, GA: Smyth & Helwys Publishing, 2007

Dodd, Charles H. "The Appearances of the Risen Christ: An Essay in Form-Criticism of the Gospels," in *Studies in the Gospel: Essays in Memory of R.H. Lightfoot*, ed. Dennis E. Nineham. Oxford: Blackwell, 1957

—————. *The Parables of the Kingdom*. London: Collins, 1961

—————. *The Founder of Christianity*. London: Collins, 1971

Donahue, John R. *The Gospel in Parable*. Philadelphia: Fortress, 1988

Donahue, John R. and Harrington, Daniel J. *The Gospel of Mark*, Sacra Pagina 2. Collegeville MN: Liturgical Press, 2002

Dunn, James D.G. *Jesus Remembered: Christianity in the Making Vol 1*. Cambridge, Eerdmans, 2003

—————. *A New Perspective on Jesus: What the Quest for the Historical Jesus Missed*. London: SPCK, 2005

Fuller, Reginald H. *The Formation of the Resurrection Narratives*. London: SPCK, 1972

Harrington, Wilfrid. *Mark*. Dublin: Veritas, 1979

Hooker, Morna D. *The Gospel According to St Mark*. London: A&C Black, 1991

Jeremias, Joachim. *The Parables of Jesus*. Translated by S. H. Hooke. London: SCM, 1963

—————. *New Testament Theology*. Translated by John Bowden. London: SCM, 1971

Johnson, Elizabeth A. *Truly our Sister. A Theology of Mary in the Communion of Saints*. London: Continuum, 2002

Kasper, Walter. *Pope Francis' Revolution of Tenderness and Love*. Translated by
William Madges. New York: Paulist Press, 2015

Kauffman, Joel. *The Nazareth Jesus Knew*. Nazareth, USA: Nazareth Village, 2005

Keating, Thomas. *The Kingdom of God is like...* . Slough: St Paul's, 1993

King, Nicholas. "The Significance of the Inn for Luke's Infancy Narrative", in
New Perspectives on the Nativity, ed. Jeremy Corley, London: T&T Clark,
2009

Koester, Craig R. *The Word of Life: A Theology of John's Gospel*. Grand Rapids:
Eerdmans, 2008

Lambrecht, Jan. *Once More Astonished: The Parables of Jesus*. New York:
Crossroad, 1981

Lee, Dorothy. *Transfiguration: New Century Theology*. London: Continuum, 2004

Levine, Amy-Jill. *Short Stories by Jesus*. New York: HarperOne, 2014

Lincoln, Andrew T. *Born of a Virgin? Reconceiving Jesus in the Bible, Tradition, and
Theology*. London: SPCK, 2013

Lohfink, Gerhard. *Jesus of Nazareth. What He Wanted. Who He Was*. Translated
by Linda M Maloney. Collegeville, MN: The Liturgical Press, 2012

Luz, Ulrich. *Matthew*. 3 vols. Minneapolis, MN: Augsburg Fortress, 2001, 2005,
2007

Maluf, Leonard J. "Zechariah's 'Benedictus': A New Look at a Familiar Text",
in *New Perspectives on the Nativity*, ed. Jeremy Corley, London: T&T
Clark, 2009

Manson, Thomas W. *The Sayings of Jesus*. London: SCM Press, 1971

Martin, George. *The Gospel according to Mark: Meaning and Message*. Chicago:
Loyola Press, 2005

Martin, James. *Jesus: A Pilgrimage*. New York: HarperCollins, 2014

Matera, Frank J. *Passion Narratives and Gospel Theologies*. New York: Paulist Press,
1986

McBride, Denis. *The Gospel of Mark: A Reflective Commentary*. Dublin: Dominican
Publications, 1996

―――――. *The Parables of Jesus*. Chawton: Redemptorist Publications, 1999

McIver, Robert K. *Memory, Jesus and the Synoptic Gospels*. Resources for Biblical
Study 59. Atlanta: SBL, 2011

Meier, John P. *A Marginal Jew. Rethinking the Historical Jesus*. The Anchor Yale
Library, 5 vols. New York: Doubleday, 1991–2016

Moloney, Francis J. *This is the Gospel of the Lord: Reflections on the Gospel Readings
Year C*. Homebush: St Paul Publications, 1991

―――――. *The Gospel of John*, Sacra Pagina 4. Collegeville, MN: The Liturgical
Press, 1998

―――――. *The Gospel of Mark: A Commentary*. Peabody MA: Hendrickson, 2002

—————. *Love in the Gospel of John. An Exegetical, Theological and Literary Study.* Grand Rapids, MI: Baker Academic, 2013

—————. *The Resurrection of the Messiah: A Narrative Commentary on the Resurrection Accounts in the Four Gospels.* New York: Paulist Press, 2013

—————. *A Body Broken for a Broken People. Marriage, Divorce, and the Eucharist.* Mulgrave: Garratt, 2015

—————. *Reading the New Testament in the Church. A Primer for Pastors, Religious Educators, and Believers.* Grand Rapids, MI: Baker Academic, 2015

—————. *Reflections on Evangelical Consecration.* Bolton: Don Bosco Publications, 2015

Neyrey, Jerome. *The Passion according to Luke: A Redaction Study of Luke's Soteriology.* New York: Paulist Press, 1985

Nineham, Dennis E. *Saint Mark.* London: Penguin, 1963

O'Collins, Gerald. *The Easter Jesus.* London: Darton, Longman & Todd Ltd, 1973

—————. *Easter Faith: Believing in the Risen Jesus.* London: Darton, Longman, Todd, 2003

Pagola, José A. *Jesus, An Historical Approximation.* Miami: Convivium, 2011

Pixner, Bargil. *With Jesus through Galilee According to the Fifth Gospel.* Rosh Pina: Corazin Publishing, 1992

Powell, Mark A. *What is Narrative Criticism?* Minneapolis: Fortress, 1990

—————. *Fortress Introduction to The Gospels.* Minneapolis: Fortress, 1998

Ratzinger, Joseph, Pope Benedict XVI. *Jesus of Nazareth: Part 2: Holy Week— From the Entrance into Jerusalem to the Resurrection.* Translated by Philip J. Whitmore. San Francisco: Ignatius Press, 2011

Reid, Barbara E. *Parables for Preachers: Year C.* Collegeville MN: Liturgical Press, 2000

—————. "Prophetic Voices of Elizabeth, Mary and Anna in Luke 1-2", in *New Perspectives on the Nativity*, ed. Jeremy Corley, London: T&T Clark, 2009

Rhoads, David and Michie, Donald. *Mark as Story: An Introduction to the Narrative of a Gospel.* Philadelphia: Fortress, 1982

Thompson, G.H.P. *The Gospel according to Luke.* Oxford: Clarendon Press, 1972

Tournier, Paul. *Guilt and Grace.* London: Hodder & Stoughton, 1962

Voorwinde, Stephen. *Jesus' Emotions in the Gospels.* London: T&T Clark, 2011

Williams, Rowan. *Resurrection: Interpreting the Easter Gospel* (3rd edition). London: Darton, Longman, Todd, 2014

—————. *God with Us God with Us: The Meaning of The Cross and Resurrection— Then and Now.* London: SPCK, 2017

Winstanley, Michael T. *Come and See*. London: Darton, Longman and Todd, 1985

——. *Symbols and Spirituality*. Bolton: Don Bosco Publications, 2007

——. *Lenten Sundays*. Bolton: Don Bosco Publications, 2011

——. *Jesus and the Little People*. Bolton: Don Bosco Publications, 2012

——. *An Advent Journey*. Bolton: Don Bosco Publications, 2014

Wright, N. Tom. *Jesus and the Victory of God*. London: SPCK, 2000

——. *Mark for Everyone*. London: SPCK, 2001

——. *The Resurrection of the Son of God*. London: SPCK, 2003

——. *Surprised by Scripture: Engaging Contemporary Issues*. London: SPCK, 2014

Other Books by the Author

An Advent Journey. Bolton: Don Bosco Publications, 2014

Come and See. London: Darton, Longman and Todd, 1985

Don Bosco's Gospel Way. Bolton: Don Bosco Publications, 2002

Into Your Hands. Homebush, NSW: St Paul's Publications, 1994

Jesus and the Little People. Bolton: Don Bosco Publications, 2012

Lenten Sundays. Bolton: Don Bosco Publications, 2011

Scripture, Sacraments, Sprituality. Essex: McCrimmon Publishing Co. Ltd., 2002

Symbols and Spirituality. Bolton: Don Bosco Publications, 2007

About the Author

Michael T Winstanley is a Salesian of Don Bosco. He is a graduate of the Salesian Pontifical University, Rome, and London University. He lectured in biblical studies at Ushaw College, Durham, for seventeen years. Michael has spent many years in Formation Ministry, served twice as Provincial of the British Province, given retreats in many countries and been involved in a variety of adult education programmes. For twelve years, he worked with the Salesian volunteers at Savio Retreat House in Bollington. Currently, he is Vicar for Religious in the Salford Diocese. This is his ninth book.